Cancer in the Twentieth Century

Cancer in the Twentieth Century

Edited by *David Cantor*

THE JOHNS HOPKINS UNIVERSITY PRESS
Baltimore

© 2008 The Johns Hopkins University Press
All rights reserved. Published 2008
Printed in the United States of America on acid-free paper
9 8 7 6 5 4 3 2 1

The Johns Hopkins University Press
2715 North Charles Street
Baltimore, Maryland 21218-4363
www.press.jhu.edu

ISBN 10: 0-8018-8867-0
ISBN 13: 978-0-8018-8867-0

Library of Congress Control Number: 2007940407

A catalog record for this book is available from the British Library.

Book design by William Longhauser

Cover: American cancer education programs taught the public that early cancers were curable. This poster was the entry of Joseph Binder (1898–1972) in a 1940 poster competition organized by the American Society for the Control of Cancer (ASCC). Binder, a Viennese graphic designer, moved to the United States, where his innovative poster designs were hugely influential in the 1930s and 1940s. Informed by Cubist and DeStijl ideas, his illustrations employed geometric forms and color contrasts to enhance the psychological impact of the picture. The image reproduced here won fourth prize in the ASCC competition, for which Binder received $50.00. The original was in shades of beige and blue, with two geometrically arranged faces, "one turned up to the light of the cancer control sword, the other down to darkness" (quotation from "800 Enter Poster Competition," *Bull. Am. Soc. Control Cancer*, December 1940, *22* (12): 7–10, on p.7). Source of illustration: G. Terry Sharrer, Ph.D., National Museum of American History. Available at NCI Visuals Online, National Cancer Institute, U.S. National Institutes of Health (www.cancer.gov).

For more information about *Bulletin of the History of Medicine*, please see:
www.press.jhu.edu/journals/bulletin_of_the_history_of_medicine/

Special discounts are available for bulk purchases of this book. For more information, please contact Special Sales at 410-516-6936 or specialsales@press.jhu.edu.

Contents

Part III: Prevention and Risk

Preface

This book began life as a workshop entitled "Cancer in the Twentieth Century," held at the National Institutes of Health, Bethesda, Maryland, 15–17 November 2004. A selection of the papers presented at this meeting was published as a special issue of the *Bulletin of the History of Medicine* in Spring 2007. They are reprinted here with minor modifications.

Many people and institutions made the workshop, the special issue, and this book possible. The workshop was sponsored by the History of Medicine Division of the National Library of Medicine (NLM); the Wellcome Unit for the History of Medicine and the Centre for the History of Science, Technology, and Medicine at the University of Manchester; and the Society for the Social History of Medicine. Manchester's involvement in the workshop, the special issue, and this book was funded by a Wellcome Trust Programme Grant, Constructing Cancers, 1945–2000. The unit and I express our thanks to the trust for this support.

The special issue and book would not have happened without the help of many individuals, including Donald Lindberg, Elizabeth Fee, Paul Theerman, Ba Ba Chang, and Omar Echegoyén at the NLM; John Pickstone and Carsten Timmermann at the Wellcome Unit; and Randy Packard, Mary Fissell, and Susan Abrams at the *Bulletin*. My thanks to them all, but especially to Susan, who graciously guided this editor through the volume's first incarnation. Trevor Lipscombe at the Johns Hopkins University Press oversaw its rebirth as a book.

Finally, Matt Newson, then a graduate student at the University of Southern California, provided invaluable research assistance as a 2004 summer intern at the library.

Cancer in the Twentieth Century

Introduction: Cancer Control and Prevention in the Twentieth Century

DAVID CANTOR

At first sight the development of cancer control programs in Europe and in North America might seem to follow similar trajectories: on both continents they emerged in the late nineteenth and early twentieth centuries, and "early detection and treatment" were generally the cornerstone of policy.[1] From this perspective, control was most likely to succeed if

I thank Matt Newson for research assistance as a 2004 Summer Intern at the NLM. Also helpful in formulating my ideas for this introduction were the commentaries by Dorothy Porter, Patrice Pinell, Charles Rosenberg, Barbara Clow, John Parascandola, and Nikolai Krementsov at the "Cancer in the Twentieth Century" workshop held at the National Institutes of Health, Bethesda, Maryland, 15–17 November 2004. John Pickstone and Christine Holmberg read and made valuable comments on earlier versions of this paper, parts of which were presented at two "History of Cancer" conferences organized in France by the INCa Cancer Observatory and the Institute for the History of Medicine and Health of Geneva University: one at the National Cancer Institute, Boulogne Billancourt, Paris, 18–19 May 2006, and the other at Moulin XII, Ste Gemme Moronval, France, 18–20 October 2006.

1. On cancer control in the United States, see Lester Breslow, Daniel Wilner, Larry Agran, et al., *A History of Cancer Control in the United States, with Emphasis on the Period 1946–1971,* 4 vols., prepared by the History of Cancer Control Project, UCLA School of Public Health, pursuant to Contract no. N01-CN-55172 (Bethesda, Md.: Division of Cancer Control and Rehabilitation, National Cancer Institute, Bethesda; Dept. of Health, Education, and Welfare, Public Health Service, National Institutes of Health, National Cancer Institute, Division of Cancer Control and Rehabilitation, 1977); James T. Patterson, *The Dread Disease: Cancer and Modern American Culture* (Cambridge: Harvard University Press, 1987); Barron H. Lerner, *The Breast Cancer Wars: Fear, Hope and the Pursuit of a Cure in Twentieth-Century America* (New York: Oxford University Press, 2003); Kirsten E. Gardner, *Early Detection: Women, Cancer, and Awareness Campaigns in the Twentieth-Century United States* (Chapel Hill: University of North Carolina Press, 2006). On France, Germany, and Canada, see Patrice Pinell, *The Fight against Cancer: France 1890–1940* (London: Routledge, 2002); Robert N. Proctor, *The*

medical interventions began as early as possible in the development of the disease—or of a precursor to the disease—when, doctors[2] believed, the chance of successful treatment was greatest. Thus the key tasks of control programs were to identify the disease or the risk of the disease at the earliest possible stage; to get patients to their doctors as soon as the disease, or the possibility of disease, was identified; and to ensure their early treatment by experts using a recognized means of treatment—generally surgery, radiotherapy, chemotherapy, or some combination thereof.

The term "control" was carefully chosen. Until recently programs did not emphasize the elimination or eradication of the disease, nor of the suffering and death it caused, at least in the short term.[3] For most of the century, when mortality seemed to rise relentlessly, the assumption was that the disease and the risk of the disease would not go away, at least in the foreseeable future. Individual patients might be cured, but there was always the chance of recurrence. Mortality and incidence might eventually decline, but the disease or the risk of the disease would always be present in the population. It would always be in need of management or control. Thus, despite various "wars," "campaigns," and "crusades" to "conquer" the disease, the best that anticancer programs generally offered was the possibility of effective intervention if a cancer—or a precancerous condition—established itself in the body and was discovered early. To this end, they sought not only to control the disease therapeutically, but also to reform the behaviors, individuals, organizations, and social structures that encouraged delay.[4]

One of the standard stories goes that—with perhaps the exception of Nazi Germany[5]—"early detection and treatment" dominated control programs until the 1960s and 1970s, when they were challenged by a growing interest in cancer prevention.[6] In this account, attention broadened from

Nazi War on Cancer (Princeton: Princeton University Press, 1999); Charles Hayter, *Element of Hope: Radium and the Response to Cancer in Canada, 1900–1940* (Montreal: McGill-Queen's University Press, 2005).

2. The term "physician" has different meanings in Britain and the United States. In this essay I reserve the term for discussions of doctors in the United States. When discussing other countries or international events that include the United States, I use the terms "doctors," "medical practitioners," or "practitioners."

3. Andrew C. von Eschenbach, "NCI Sets Goal of Eliminating Suffering and Death Due to Cancer by 2015," *J. Nat. Med. Assoc.*, 2003, *95*: 637–39; "NCI Director Sets a Goal: Eliminate Suffering, Death from Cancer by 2015," *Cancer Lett.*, 2003, *29* (7): 1–7.

4. Robert A. Aronowitz, "Do Not Delay: Breast Cancer and Time, 1900–1970," *Milbank Quart.*, 2001, *79*: 355–86.

5. Proctor, *Nazi War on Cancer* (n. 1).

6. Breslow et al., *History of Cancer Control* (n. 1); Robert N. Proctor, *Cancer Wars: How Politics Shapes What We Know and Don't Know about Cancer* (New York: Basic Books, 1995).

the treatment of cancers at an early stage in their development to include the prevention of the disease before it started. The roots of this interest in cancer prevention are usually traced to Anglo-American work in the 1940s that identified smoking as a cause of cancer, which by the 1960s and 1970s widened to a range of other putative causes of cancer associated with occupation, environment, and lifestyle. The story traces the difficult birth of cancer prevention during this period, and of attempts by the state to identify and regulate carcinogenic substances.

The papers in this collection suggest that such a tale will have to be revised. Focusing primarily on Britain and the United States, the authors tell stories not of similar trajectories, but of a diversity of approaches to and meanings of *control*. In the first place, they suggest that the first phase—early detection and treatment—was characterized by many different approaches, including public education and the organization of cancer therapy. In Britain and America cancer agencies agreed that it was essential that people should seek medical attention as early as possible. They also agreed that expert surgery, radiotherapy, and chemotherapy were the only effective treatments. But they differed over how to get the public to go to the doctor, the role of public education, how cancer services should be delivered, who should provide them, and what forms of therapy were most appropriate to particular cancers.

In the second place, these papers also highlight a diversity of approaches to *prevention* in the twentieth century.[7] The standard account is a tale of the difficult birth of efforts to prevent cancer from the late 1960s and 1970s.[8] Papers in this collection lend support to this account; however, they also suggest that prevention meant much more than preventing environmental and lifestyle causes of cancer. They demonstrate that throughout the twentieth century "early detection and treatment" were themselves sometimes portrayed as a form of cancer prevention—preventing the further development of cancers already established in the body, or identifying and intervening against precancerous conditions before they turned cancerous. The difficult birth of the 1960s and 1970s was thus in part the result of struggles between therapeutic models of prevention and those based on targeting environmental and lifestyle causes of the disease. This struggle

---

7. I am particularly grateful to Ornella Moscucci for discussions about cancer prevention in the United Kingdom. She is working on a history of cancer prevention, and has independently come to a similar argument to the one presented here: Ornella Moscucci, "Preventing Cancer: Problems of Aetiology and Strategy in Early Twentieth Century United Kingdom" (Paper presented to the History of Cancer Conference held at Moulin XII, Ste Gemme Moronval, France, 18–20 October 2006).

8. Breslow et al., *History of Cancer Control* (n. 1); Proctor, *Cancer Wars* (n. 6).

was further complicated by tensions between those who focused prevention on efforts to reform individual behavior and those who focused on social-structural determinants of health and disease.

In what follows, I adopt a capacious definition of cancer control. Control has historically covered much more than scientific and medical efforts to control the disease as a biological entity, or to control cancer mortality and incidence: it has also involved efforts to control or manage human activities, structures, and emotions that affected these goals, including those that promoted delay or increased the risk of the disease. It has thus covered a very wide range of activities, undertaken by a very wide range of groups, that cover much of the field of cancer in the twentieth century. Contemporary commentators have attempted to narrow the definition of control: to demarcate it from prevention, biomedical research, and routine medical care; to separate it from the politics of cancer; and to divide the world of cancer into those who promote or impede the advance of control.[9] Such a narrowing may capture something of the drift of current Anglo-American approaches to control, but it does not capture the rich diversity of this subject in the twentieth century that this volume seeks to explore, nor does it capture how efforts to control the disease were embedded in a range of other related activities aimed at controlling social, economic, and cultural activities related to cancer.

Detection and Treatment, 1900–1970

American cancer-control programs provide a valuable starting point for an exploration of the first theme—the diversity of national approaches to "early detection and treatment." There is a substantial literature on the campaigns against cancer in the United States,[10] perhaps more than for

9. Breslow et al., *History of Cancer Control* (n. 1), esp. vol. 1, *Introductory Materials*, pp. 14–16; Proctor, *Cancer Wars* (n. 6); *A New Agenda for Cancer Control Research: Report of the Cancer Control Review Group*, National Cancer Institute, Cancer Control Program Review Group, 7 August 1997, NCI archives, Bethesda, Md., DC012878. An online version of the report is available at **http://deainfo.nci.nih.gov/ADVISORY/BSA/bsa_program/bsacacntrlmin.htm** (accessed 10 July 2006). The separation between prevention and control was implicit in the title of the National Cancer Institute's Division of Cancer Prevention and Control (DCPC), created in 1983. In 1997 the distinction widened when the NCI abolished the DCPC and created two new divisions: the Division of Cancer Control and Population Science under Barbara Rimer, and the Division of Cancer Prevention under Peter Greenwald: "DRCCA Will Become DCPC, Organize into Three Major Program Areas," *Cancer Lett.*, 1982, *8* (33): 4–6; "NCI Splits Prevention and Control Division; Rimer to Direct Division of Cancer Control," ibid., 1997, *23* (29): 1–5.

10. Breslow et al., *History of Cancer Control* (n. 1); Patterson, *Dread Disease* (n. 1); Lerner, *Breast Cancer Wars* (n. 1); Gardner, *Early Detection* (n. 1).

other countries. As the papers collected here show, the American story differs substantially from that of Britain and other countries.

The United States

Early detection and treatment dominated American approaches to cancer, and in particular the policies of the American Society for the Control of Cancer (ASCC). Founded in 1913 by a small group of surgeons who saw early surgical—and later radiotherapeutic—intervention as the key to cancer control, the ASCC came to dominate American approaches to cancer control in the first half of the century. The problem, the ASCC claimed, was that patients often arrived in the doctor's office long after the possibility of cure had gone.[11] Part of the reason was that the beginnings of the disease could be subtle, painless, and easily missed. There was often little to prompt the would-be patient to see his or her physician. All too often, the ASCC complained, the public was quite unaware of the nature of the warning signs of cancer, doubtful of the possibility of a cure, and overly fearful of the disease or its treatments, and so avoided the physician until pain and debility became too much—and by then it was often too late: the disease had progressed too far for successful treatment. Furthermore, "quacks" and ignorant orthodox physicians often compounded the issue by confusing the public, mistreating the disease, and encouraging further delay.

The ASCC's diagnosis of the cancer problem was shared by most other cancer organizations in the United States, including state health authorities (which became increasingly concerned about cancer from the late 1920s) and the federal government (which established a National Cancer Institute in 1937). To all these agencies, education was a key to transforming such attitudes. From the 1910s, vast public-education programs aggressively promoted early detection and treatment as creating the best opportunity for a cure; encouraged people to inspect themselves for the early warning signs of cancer[12] and to undergo regular medical check-ups; warned of the dangers of quackery and folk remedies;[13] and sought to undermine popular beliefs that might encourage delay. The message was that cancer was curable if caught early and treated by a recognized

11. Aronowitz, "Do Not Delay" (n. 4).

12. On efforts to promote breast self-examination in the 1950s, see, e.g., Lerner, *Breast Cancer Wars* (n. 1), pp. 54–60.

13. For a different approach to alternative medicine, see the account of Canadian responses to alternative medicine in Barbara Clow, *Negotiating Disease: Power and Cancer Care, 1900–1950* (Montreal: McGill-Queens University Press, 2001), esp. pp. 119–46.

physician, and the public was thus urged to turn to their physicians at the first suspicion of cancer—though cancer educators often sent different messages to men and women, some of which tended to undermine their own stated goals.[14] Public-education programs were complemented by medical-education programs that targeted ignorant physicians, who, the organizers of cancer campaigns feared, might undermine the control efforts. They also dovetailed with efforts to raise support for cancer organizations: public education often blurred seamlessly into fund-raising and political lobbying, thus laying the groundwork for the dramatic expansion of philanthropic and government support for cancer after World War II.

If cancer agencies sought to transform people's attitudes and behaviors toward the disease and its treatments, they also sought to reorganize cancer services.[15] In general, within each state they hoped to create a hierarchical network of care, beginning with the family physician (the port-of-first-call for many middle-class patients until the breakdown of family medicine in the 1960s), followed variously by local cancer clinics, regional cancer hospitals or centers, and, for some, a national cancer hospital. This hierarchy would be linked by a referral system that aimed to channel cancer patients into a few specialist centers, to tempt them away from domestic and alternative remedies, and to limit the role of family physicians in treating cancer. In the specialist centers they could be treated by teams of experts in the disease (supported by laboratory and technical services) who would also hone their skills on the large numbers of patients coming through, and would use such patients as a means of educating future generations of physicians.

In practice, the situation varied from state to state and from institution to institution. There were vast differences in provision according to geography and the economic class and race of patients. The market-driven nature of medical practice often resulted in a patchwork of provision, dependent on the ability of individual physicians to raise funds to purchase radium or other therapeutic technologies, on the perception of new therapeutic technologies as money-spinners for hospitals, or on the internecine struggles between practitioners of surgery and radiotherapy (and later, chemotherapy). It also created problems for efforts to rationalize cancer services. For many physicians, the creation of centralized

14. Leslie J. Reagan, "Engendering the Dread Disease: Women, Men, and Cancer," *Amer. J. Pub. Health*, 1997, *87*: 1779–87.

15. The model of cancer services described here is similar to Daniel M. Fox's model of hierarchical regionalism: see Fox, *Health Policies, Health Politics: The British and American Experience, 1911–1965* (Princeton: Princeton University Press, 1986).

referral systems and teamwork posed a challenge to individual private practice, especially where state or federal authorities were involved. And the problem was further complicated by disagreements among cancer experts on how control should be organized: some recommended the creation of cancer institutes, others wanted cancer clinics in existing hospitals, and others argued for combinations such as central units with satellite clinics.[16] Yet despite these differences and problems, the fantasy of a rational organization of cancer services persisted.

Reorganization extended not only to the provision of services, but also to the production of knowledge. In the mid-twentieth century, support for cancer research increased dramatically, both from the federal government and from voluntary agencies such as the ASCC.[17] Much of this research explored basic questions of the biological cause and mechanism of action of cancer, leading to fears of a divorce between research and control.[18] Programs of cancer control within the federally funded National Cancer Institute (NCI) became increasingly marginalized

16. See, e.g., the results of a Canadian survey of American opinion on cancer-control organization: Hayter, *Element of Hope* (n. 1), p. 117.

17. For earlier efforts at promoting research, see Victor A. Triolo and Ilse L. Riegel, "The American Association for Cancer Research, 1907–1940: Historical Review," *Cancer Res.*, 1961, *21*: 137–67; Hugh J. Creech, "Historical Review of the American Association of Cancer Research, Inc., 1941–1978," ibid., 1979, *39*: 1863–90; Karen A. Rader, *Making Mice: Standardizing Animals for American Biomedical Research, 1900–1955* (Princeton: Princeton University Press, 2004).

18. For example, American public-education programs informed the public that cancer was not a hereditary disease, at the same time that research organizations supported vast programs of experimental research into cancer genetics and heredity. See David Cantor, "The Frustrations of Families: Henry Lynch, Heredity and Cancer Control, 1962–1975," *Med. Hist.*, 2006, *50*: 279–302; on cancer genetic research see Ilana Löwy and Jean-Paul Gaudillière, "Disciplining Cancer: Mice and the Practice of Genetic Purity," in *The Invisible Industrialist: Manufactures and the Production of Scientific Knowledge*, ed. Jean-Paul Gaudillière and Ilana Löwy (Basingstoke: Macmillan, 1998), pp. 209–49; Jean-Paul Gaudillière, "Circulating Mice and Viruses: The Jackson Memorial Laboratory, the National Cancer Institute, and the Genetics of Breast Cancer, 1930–1965," in *The Practices of Human Genetics*, ed. Michael Fortun and Everett Mendelsohn (Dordrecht: Kluwer Academic, 1999), pp. 89–124; Gaudillière, "Mendelism and Medicine: Controlling Human Inheritance in Local Contexts, 1920–1960," *Comptes rendus de l'Académie des Sciences*, ser. 3, *Sciences de la vie*, 2000, *323*: 1117–26; Gaudillière, "Making Heredity in Mice and Men: The Production and Uses of Animal Models in Postwar Human Genetics," in *Heredity and Infection: The History of Disease Transmission*, ed. Gaudillière and Ilana Löwy (London: Routledge, 2001), pp. 181–202; Gaudillière, "Mapping as Technology: Genes, Mutant Mice, and Biomedical Research (1910–1965)," in *Classical Genetic Research and Its Legacy: The Mapping Cultures of Twentieth-Century Genetics*, ed. Hans-Jörg Rheinberger and Gaudillière (London: Routledge, 2004), pp. 173–203; Rader, *Making Mice* (n. 17).

institutionally in the 1940s.[19] The American Society for the Control of Cancer dropped the word "control" from its title in 1944 and became the American Cancer Society (ACS). Critics increasingly argued that the research had less to do with control than with the research agendas and careers of the scientists.[20] Nevertheless, research also identified trends in incidence, mortality, and survival, and aimed to develop new diagnostic and therapeutic interventions, including drug treatments for cancer such as chemotherapy and immunotherapy.[21] For example, from the 1940s vast programs of research aimed to identify new chemical compounds that might work against the disease, and to test the therapeutic value of these compounds.[22] Ideally, promising new compounds would be tested on animal models and through clinical trials on patients, especially the randomized double-blind clinical trial. The specialist hospitals and centers established to provide cancer care became centers of such research, since their large populations of patients and teams of experts made them ideal settings for therapeutic trials.

Thus, until the 1970s, American cancer-control programs had several objectives: they aimed to encourage the public to seek care at the earliest opportunity from competent orthodox physicians; to educate regular physicians to deal more effectively with the disease; to establish systems for channeling patients to appropriate specialist care; and, especially from the 1940s and 1950s, to improve knowledge and practice through research. These objectives were supported by legal restrictions on who could treat cancer, and on access to potentially harmful therapeutic technologies and substances, both orthodox and alternative. They were also supported by vast lobbying and marketing efforts promoted by the voluntary and federal cancer agencies, professional organizations, and, increasingly, corporations with interests in producing and distributing cancer products and services.

19. Breslow et al., *History of Cancer Control* (n. 1). On the importance of radium therapy to the NCI in the 1930s, see David Cantor, "Radium, Cancer Research, and the End of the New Deal" (paper presented at the "Biomedicine in the Twentieth Century: Practices, Policies, and Politics" conference held at the National Institutes of Health, Bethesda, Md., 5–6 December 2005).

20. Daniel S. Greenberg, *The Politics of Pure Science* (New York: New American Library, 1968).

21. Toine Pieters, *Interferon: The Science and Selling of a Miracle Drug* (London: Routledge, 2005); Sandra Panem, *The Interferon Crusade* (Washington, D.C.: Brookings Institution, 1984). See also Ilana Löwy, *Between Bench and Bedside: Science, Healing, and Interleukin-2 in a Cancer Ward* (Cambridge: Harvard University Press, 1996).

22. Jordan Goodman and Vivien Walsh, *The Story of Taxol: Nature and Politics in the Pursuit of an Anti-Cancer Drug* (Cambridge: Cambridge University Press, 2001).

Public Education

But what was characteristic of American cancer control was not necessarily characteristic of programs elsewhere. In the United States, vast programs of public education were instituted in the early twentieth century[23]—but elsewhere, others were more cautious about this approach. In the Netherlands, for example, public-education programs did not emerge until the 1950s, despite the beginnings of national efforts against cancer in the 1910s.[24] In this volume, Elizabeth Toon suggests that the British (who also began anticancer efforts in the early twentieth century) were similarly reluctant to promote public education until the 1950s and 1960s.[25]

Such differences reflected, in part, very different attitudes toward managing the public. Critics worried that American-style efforts to promote self-examination might encourage the public to self-diagnose the disease, and so ultimately to undermine programs of cancer control by challenging the authority of the doctor.[26] They also worried that such public-education efforts might blind the public to any educational message by inducing either a paralyzing fear of the disease, or an undue optimism about the possibility of a cure that would eventually be disappointed as the expected cure failed to materialize.[27] Such concerns led British and Dutch cancer agencies to adopt a much more cautious, paternalistic attitude toward public education, as did related fears that such programs might overwhelm general practitioners with trivial complaints from their patients, or undermine efforts to persuade the public to support cancer research or treatment. Educational efforts in these countries tended to focus less on the public than on the profession, and, where they did focus on the public, they tended to stress local (and often low-key) rather than

23. Similar programs were also instituted in France, Germany, and Canada, emphasizing early detection and treatment. See Pinell, *Fight against Cancer* (n. 1); Proctor, *Nazi War on Cancer* (n. 1); Hayter, *Element of Hope* (n. 1).

24. Stephen Snelders, Frans J. Meijman, and Toine Pieters, "Cancer Health Communication in the Netherlands 1910–1950: Paternalism or Popularization?" *Medizinhistorisches Journal*, 2006, *41*: 271–89.

25. See also Ornella Moscucci, "Fast Track to Treatment: Cancer Education in Britain, ca. 1900–1948" (paper presented at the "Patients and Pathways: Cancer Therapies in Historical and Sociological Perspective" conference held at the Centre for the History of Science, Technology and Medicine, University of Manchester, 6–8 October 2005).

26. Snelders, Meijman, and Pieters, "Cancer Health Communication" (n. 24); Moscucci, "Fast Track to Treatment" (n. 25).

27. On British medical attitudes toward public emotion, see David Cantor, "Representing 'The Public': Medicine, Charity and Emotion in Twentieth-Century Britain," in *Medicine, Health and the Public Sphere in Britain, 1600–2000*, ed. Steve Sturdy (London: Routledge, 2002), pp. 145–68.

national efforts. There was no equivalent to the ASCC in Britain; the two major cancer charities—the British Empire Cancer Campaign and the Imperial Cancer Research Fund—were more focused on research than was their American counterpart.[28]

None of this is to say that the Americans were not similarly concerned that educational programs might work against the objectives they were supposed to promote.[29] On the contrary, American cancer campaigns recognized that even the most careful public-education program might encourage people to delay. The point is illustrated by my paper in this volume on public-education movies, in which I argue that American cancer agencies tended to worry that these movies might undermine the very message they wished to get across by promoting undue fears or hopes in the public. But whereas such concerns prompted the British and Dutch to eschew public-education efforts, the Americans took a very different approach: they sought to embed the movies within a range of other educational efforts in order to counteract any tendency on the part of the public to misread the message. They also used the new technology to educate the public to manage their own fears of the disease, and they excluded from movies subjects (such as radical surgery) that they feared might deter would-be patients from seeking care from regular physicians. Gretchen Krueger's paper on public campaigns against childhood leukemia reinforces the last point: she shows that cancer agencies drew on older images of the child to promote their messages and agendas to the public, but that they also tended to underplay aspects of the disease and its treatment that they feared might work against their messages and agendas. The cancer organizations discussed in both of these papers saw the public as a fickle entity that needed to be managed both for its own benefit and for that of the organizations. It was such an approach to the public that helped to generate the vast expansion of political, philanthropic, and popular support for cancer after World War II. By embedding mass-media approaches to cancer education within broader communication systems that also emphasized the importance of personal communication between doctor and patient, the American cancer agencies were able to undertake aggressive, even sensationalist, public-education campaigns while, at the same time, counteracting any possibility that these campaigns might undermine the message of control.

28. Joan Austoker, *A History of the Imperial Cancer Research Fund, 1902–1986* (Oxford: Oxford University Press, 1988).

29. For a comparison of British and American responses to cancerphobia, see James T. Patterson, "Cancer, Cancerphobia, and Culture: Reflections on Attitudes in the United States and Great Britain," *Twent. Cent. Brit. Hist.*, 1991, 2: 137–49.

If the papers in this collection highlight the very different attitudes of the British and the Americans toward public education before the 1950s, they also show how, from the 1950s, the British sought to give up their earlier doubts about public education. Toon highlights the importance to this change of a survey conducted in the Northern English city of Manchester, which began to transform the image of the British general public. This survey suggested that some doctors no longer saw the British public as ignorant of the disease: in their view, it was in fact quite knowledgeable of the disease, albeit not in the way that doctors and scientists were. The public's knowledge came from local, everyday encounters with medicine and medical institutions. From this perspective, it was suggested that British control efforts should focus on changing people's experience of cancer. Put another way, the belief was that people would seek cancer care if cancer services improved—a problematic assumption, given the shortfalls in medical ability to tackle the disease, and political anxieties that the demand for health care risked creating an unmanageable tax burden. Perhaps for such reasons, the Manchester "experiment" had only a limited immediate impact: cancer education remained a low priority for the British until the 1960s. As Virginia Berridge notes in this volume, it was not until after the Royal College of Physicians 1962 report on the link between smoking and cancer that the British began to focus more attention on broader educational programs, and to use the media to get the message across.[30]

Therapy

The papers in this collection also illustrate how British approaches to cancer therapy differed from those in the United States. It has been noted that until the 1970s, orthodox practitioners in both countries tended to regard surgery, X rays, radium, and (from the 1940s) chemotherapy as the mainstays of therapy—but British and American practitioners differed over what forms of therapy were appropriate to particular cancers, how services should be organized, and who should provide them. John Pickstone highlights the point in his article in this volume. He sees the history of cancer therapy in the twentieth century as a successive addition of modalities: surgery, radiotherapy, and chemotherapy layered on one another, so that by the end of the century cancers would often be treated with combinations of these modalities that varied depending on

---

30. See also Virginia Berridge and Kelly Loughlin, "Smoking and the New Health Education in Britain, 1950s–1970s," *Amer. J. Pub. Health*, 2005, *95*: 956–64.

the type of cancer, its location, its stage of development, and the effectiveness of other interventions. He argues that historians have yet to engage with this kind of "contested cumulation" of therapies, but he also stresses that these additions were negotiated in different ways in Britain and the United States, with different long-term consequences for the development of services and specialization. In each country negotiations were framed by the specific political, economic, social, and health-care structures in which they developed. In Britain, health-care organization tended to be centralized and tax-funded; in America, it tended to be individualized and market-funded.

Radium provides a good illustration of such differences before World War II. As Pickstone and Ornella Moscucci note, radium emerged as an alternative and supplement to surgery after World War I.[31] But it was often hard to obtain, and as medical demand grew in the late 1920s, attention in Britain focused on a national shortfall in supplies. In 1929 the government, in association with voluntary organizations, established the Radium Trust and Radium Commission: the former to purchase radium with government and voluntary monies, the latter to distribute the radium to hospitals across the country.[32] During the 1930s the Radium Trust was perhaps the world's largest purchaser of radium, able to negotiate price reductions in the world's most expensive substance due to its purchasing power, and through imperial agreements after 1932 when Canadian sources of radium challenged an older Belgian dominance of supply.[33] The Commission

31. For the significance of radium to French and Canadian cancer services see, respectively, Pinell, *Fight against Cancer* (n. 1), and Hayter, *Element of Hope* (n. 1).

32. The exception was that radium in London was purchased and distributed through the King Edward's Hospital Fund. On radium therapy in Britain, see Caroline Murphy, "A History of Radiotherapy to 1950: Cancer and Radiotherapy in Britain 1850–1950" (Ph.D. diss., University of Manchester, 1986); Murphy, "From Friedenheim to Hospice: A Century of Cancer Hospitals," in *The Hospital in History*, ed. Lindsay Granshaw and Roy Porter (New York: Routledge, 1989), pp. 221–41; David Cantor, "The Definition of Radiobiology: The Medical Research Council's Support for Research into the Biological Effects of Radiation in Britain, 1919–1939" (Ph.D. diss., Lancaster University, 1987); Cantor, "The MRC's Support for Experimental Radiology during the Inter-war Years," in *Historical Perspectives on the Role of the MRC: Essays in the History of the Medical Research Council of the United Kingdom and Its Predecessor, the Medical Research Committee, 1913–1953*, ed. Joan Austoker and Linda Bryder (Oxford: Oxford University Press, 1989), pp. 181–204. For an older account of the Commission, see F. G. Spear and K. Griffiths, *The Radium Commission: A Short History of Its Origin and Work, 1929–1948* (London: His Majesty's Stationery Office, 1951). On the King's Fund, see F. K. Prochaska, *Philanthropy and the Hospitals of London: The King's Fund, 1897–1990* (Oxford: Clarendon Press, 2002), pp. 115–17, 141–42.

33. For an account of radium production and supply, see Edward R. Landa, "The First Nuclear Industry," *Sci. Amer.*, 1982, *247* (5): 180–93.

used the vast supplies provided by the Trust to reshape cancer services in the country: Hospitals that wanted Commission radium were encouraged to adopt certain standards of therapeutic practice. The Commission also enforced a closer coordination between X-ray and radium therapy, the appointment of physicists or radium officers to measure dosage and ensure radiation protection, and the creation of teams of physicists/ radium officers, pathologists, surgeons, and radiotherapists to manage care. It encouraged the separation of radiotherapy from the diagnostic uses of X rays. And it was instrumental in transforming the approach of Medical Officers of Health (MOsH) toward cancer: their early interest in social, preventive, and holistic approaches had by the 1930s given way to individualized, reductive, and therapeutic approaches; they had become administrators of clinical and laboratory approaches to cancer.[34]

These efforts to reform cancer services did not go unchallenged. Local radium committees contested the Commission's authority; surgeons and radiologists were sometimes reluctant to adopt its standards; doctors worried that treatment might be determined by the accidents of referral; and (as in America) there were continual mutterings of medical discontent about the increased role of the state in medicine, and the subordination of the individual practitioner to the team. But the Commission—together with a related radium-research scheme organized by the Medical Research Council (MRC)[35]—provided an institutional framework for the development of cancer therapy in the 1930s. MRC and Commission radium was used to promote a variety of profession and political agendas, including those of radiotherapists, hospital physics, and, as Moscucci shows in this volume, feminist doctors. It was a means to improve access to beds, shape the development of therapeutic practice, and improve women's health and women's access to medical education.

The story of radium is very different in the United States. Despite similar concerns about a national shortfall of radium for cancer services, American physicians were reluctant to create a centralized purchasing and distribution system—though some states, including Missouri, came close to such a system. Some American physicians argued for the creation of a federal organization equivalent to the British Radium Trust and Commission as a solution to the shortage, but efforts in this direction were stymied by fears of growing involvement of government in cancer and

34. Rosa M. Medina-Domenech and Claudia A. Castañada, "Redefining Cancer during the Inter-War Period: British Medical Officers of Health, State Policy, Managerialism, and Public Health," *Amer. J. Pub. Health,* in press.
35. Cantor, "MRC's Support for Experimental Radiology" (n. 32).

radium. After a brief flirtation with federal purchase and distribution of medical radium, in the late 1930s physicians persuaded the government to shift its focus to improving medical training and encouraging research.[36] Thereafter the vast bulk of American medical radium was purchased by a diverse range of organizations and individuals, with the result that practice developed very differently in different parts of the country and in different institutions, and it tended to remain under the control of surgeons. There was no central agency to standardize practice, to enforce either a union between X-ray and radium therapy or their separation from the diagnostic uses of radiation (which remained closely linked to therapeutics in the United States at least until the 1960s).

Such differences are striking, given that the Americans and the British had very similar radium problems. Interwar American physicians complained that the development of radium therapy in their country was hampered by inadequate supplies of the element. In their view, therapeutics was at the mercy of the international trade in radium, much of it under the control of European imperial powers, and certain key technical developments in radium therapy (notably radium beam therapy) were difficult to develop in the United States because they required huge quantities of radium. In America most medical radium (generally, in the form of one of its salts) was used in milligram quantities contained in tubes, needles, or plaques that were implanted into or placed upon the surface of the body. Alternatively, it was used to produce radon gas, which was held in containers called "seeds" and implanted in the body in similar ways to the salt. By contrast, radium beam therapy involved the use of large quantities of radium—perhaps half a gram or more—to generate a beam of radiation at some distance from the body that was used therapeutically in a manner akin to X rays. It was becoming almost a routine treatment in Europe in the late 1930s, but it remained an experimental technique in the United States—partly because of the radium shortage, partly because many American physicians were not convinced by the European experience of beam therapy, and partly because they began to look to alternative technologies such as supervoltage X-ray machines or the cyclotron.

If Europeans dominated the new therapies of the 1920s and 1930s, the situation was very different after World War II. Against a backdrop of economic growth in the United States, American spending on cancer soared, rapidly overtaking anything in war-devastated Europe, which was struggling to recover economically. A new "biomedical complex" emerged around cancer, characterized by new relationships between the biological

36. Cantor, "Radium, Cancer Research" (n. 19).

sciences, clinical medicine, the pharmaceutical industry, and the federal government as a major supporter of research, as well as by a vast increase in the scale of investment, the numbers of research institutions, and the size of the scientific and medical communities, and all increasingly entangled in emergent Cold War politics. In other words, the postwar years saw the development of a new system of cancer research that involved new relations between medical innovation and biology.[37] This development affected Britain as well, but in different ways and to varying degrees.

For the British, the scale of American cancer research was so vast that it raised important questions about how to fit into this research world. In new areas such as chemotherapy it seemed to make little sense to compete directly with the Americans, and they therefore shifted focus to develop programs that built on British research strengths within the larger American program.[38] At the same time, they remained much less enthusiastic about chemotherapy than their American counterparts, and a clinical specialty of oncology based on chemotherapy did not emerge in the United Kingdom before the 1970s. As Pickstone and Carsten Timmermann suggest, the British continued to focus much more effort on radiotherapeutics. Yet even here Americans often dominated: major new developments in radiotherapeutic technology often came from the United States, and British and European innovations were often more effectively developed in the United States. The British repeatedly found themselves struggling to keep up with American research on a range of new therapeutic devices, including the cobalt bomb, the cyclotron, the betatron, the linear accelerator, and the nuclear pile, a source of radioisotopes.[39]

37. Jean-Paul Gaudillière, *Inventer la biomédicine: La France, l'Amérique et la production des savoirs du vivant (1945–1965)* (Paris: La Découverte, 2002). For a valuable account of cancer research and Cold War politics in the USSR, see Nikolai Krementsov, *The Cure: A Story of Cancer and Politics from the Annals of the Cold War* (Chicago: University of Chicago Press, 2002).

38. For a history of cancer research in Britain, see Austoker, *History of the Imperial Cancer Research Fund* (n. 28).

39. Angela N. H. Creager, "Tracing the Politics of Changing Postwar Research Practices: The Export of 'American' Radioisotopes to European Biologists," *Stud. Hist. & Philos. Sci.*, part C: *Biol. & Biomed. Sci.*, 2002, *33*: 367–88; Creager, "The Industrialization of Radioisotopes by the U.S. Atomic Energy Commission," in *The Science-Industry Nexus: History, Policy, Implications: Nobel Symposium 123*, ed. Karl Grandin, Nina Wormbs, and Sven Widmalm (Sagamore Beach, Mass.: Science History Publications/USA, 2004), pp. 143–67. On links between postwar nuclear physics and cancer, see Stuart M. Feffer, "Atoms, Cancer, and Politics: Supporting Atomic Science at the University of Chicago, 1944–1950," *Hist. Stud. Phys. & Biol. Sci.*, 1992, *22*: 233–61. On British medical isotopes, see Alison Kraft, "Between Medicine and Industry: Medical Physics and the Rise of the Radioisotope, 1945–65," *Contemp. Brit. Hist.*, 2006, *20*: 1–35.

The scale and nature of postwar American efforts is well illustrated by chemotherapy, which emerged in the 1940s and 1950s especially against childhood leukemia. As budgets for cancer grew, American governmental and private agencies developed vast programs on an industrial scale to identify chemicals of possible value in treatment.[40] Such programs involved the study of tens of thousands of different compounds for possible anticancer properties;[41] if any showed these properties, they would be tested on animals, and eventually on humans. Peter Keating and Alberto Cambrosio argue in this volume that a new "style of practice"—the clinical trial—emerged at this time that brought together oncologists, patients, and institutions to explore the value of these substances for the treatment of cancer, to shape research agendas, and to formalize guidelines for research and eventually routine treatment.[42] But the process was painstaking, often taking years, and only a few compounds ever made it to clinical practice. Nothing on this scale existed in Britain, or indeed anywhere else in the world. Keating and Cambrosio suggest that European clinical-trial programs in the 1960s developed in ways that were often quite different from those in the United States.[43]

None of this is to say that the British therapeutics was shaped entirely by developments in America. It has already been noted that the British were much less enthusiastic about chemotherapy than the Americans; similarly, they were much less enamored of radical surgical techniques, such as the radical mastectomy. Pickstone shows how such differences can be attributed, at least in part, to the institutional strength of radiotherapy within the newly created National Health Service (created 1948),

40. R. F. Bud, "Strategy in American Cancer Research after World War II: A Case Study," *Soc. Stud. Sci.*, 1978, *8*: 425–59; C. Gordon Zubrod, "Origins and Development of Chemotherapy Research at the National Cancer Institute," *Cancer Treat. Rep.*, 1984, *68*: 9–19.

41. Goodman and Walsh, *Story of Taxol* (n. 22).

42. Keating and Cambrosio's account is part of a broader effort to trace the contours of the cancer clinical trial. See also Peter Keating and Alberto Cambrosio, "Real Compared to What? Diagnosing Leukemias and Lymphomas," in *Living and Working with the New Medical Technologies: Intersections of Inquiry*, ed. Margaret Lock, Allan Young, and Alberto Cambrosio (Cambridge: Cambridge University Press, 2000), pp. 103–34; Keating and Cambrosio, "The New Genetics and Cancer: The Contributions of Clinical Medicine in the Era of Biomedicine," *J. Hist. Med. & Allied Sci.*, 2001, *56*: 321–52; Keating and Cambrosio, "From Screening to Clinical Research: The Cure of Leukemia and the Early Development of the Cooperative Oncology Groups, 1955–1966," *Bull. Hist. Med.*, 2002, *76*: 299–334; Keating and Cambrosio, "Beyond 'Bad News': The Diagnosis, Prognosis and Classification of Lymphomas and Lymphoma Patients in the Era of Biomedicine (1945–1995)," *Med. Hist.*, 2003, *47*: 291–312.

43. For a general history of the clinical trial in the United States, see Harry M. Marks, *The Progress of Experiment: Science and Therapeutic Reform in the United States, 1900–1990* (Cambridge: Cambridge University Press, 1997).

a legacy of the efforts by the National Radium Commission to reshape radiotherapy in the 1930s. Such institutional strength allowed radiotherapists to challenge surgeons in areas they regarded as their own. Indeed, as Barron Lerner has noted elsewhere, U.S. surgeons who doubted the value of the radical mastectomy turned for evidence to their British and European colleagues.[44] In this volume Lerner shows how American critics of chemotherapy also looked to Europe and Canada. Thus a comparative focus on British and American cancer therapy allows us to explore what was specifically British or American about that therapy, and how the two traditions shaped each other.

Prevention

The second major focus of this collection is on the diversity of approaches to and meanings of prevention in the twentieth century. A standard story is of the marginalization of prevention within programs of cancer control in the first fifty to sixty years of the century, followed by its difficult birth in the 1960s and 1970s. But the papers in this collection tell a different story. In the first place, they problematize the account of marginalization by suggesting that "prevention" was a very malleable term. Indeed, for much of the twentieth century "prevention" tended to be a part of "early detection and treatment" and so, ironically, to be at the heart of cancer control. What were marginal—in both British and American control programs—were prevention efforts focused on environmental and lifestyle causes of the disease, which until the 1960s and 1970s tended to be subordinated to "early detection and treatment." In the second place, these papers also suggest that these different approaches to prevention came into conflict in the 1960s and 1970s, as political concerns about environmental and lifestyle causes of cancer emerged.

Reinventing Prevention

It should first be noted, however, that the 1960s and 1970s did not witness so much a difficult *birth* of approaches to prevention that focused on environmental and lifestyle causes of cancer, as a difficult *reinvention* of an older tradition of interest in these possible causes. This tradition can be traced back to antiquity, but it gained particular prominence in the early modern period with medical reports that said mortality from the disease was increasing, and that associated cancer with overindulgence,

44. Lerner, *Breast Cancer Wars* (n. 1), pp. 93–106.

for example in meat.[45] Medical and domestic health texts advised people to avoid activities that might excite the onset of cancer, such as a sharp knock, the wearing of corsets by women, or an excessive or wrong diet; to take sufficient exercise; and to maintain an easy and cheery disposition.[46] It was commonly recognized that not everyone who wore corsets, or ate too much or the wrong sorts of food, or was affected by depression, succumbed to cancer. Nor did everyone with a constitutional or hereditary predisposition get the disease. Rather, cancer was the outcome of a combination of exciting and predisposing causes, neither of which was sufficient in itself. It was not possible to identify everyone who might fall victim to the disease, but it was sometimes possible to modify the habits and conditions that might encourage it.

From the 1840s, statistical evidence reinforced earlier reports that cancer mortality rates were increasing in "civilized" nations (though it remained unsettled until the early twentieth century as to whether this increase was real, or the product of better diagnosis or greater awareness of the disease). A growing literature argued that so-called primitive or uncivilized peoples had a lower incidence of cancer than those in urban industrial nations, and that cancer mortality was lower among rural than urban populations.[47] Commentators claimed that it was caused by the

45. William Nisbet, *An Inquiry into the History, Nature, Causes, and Different Modes of Treatment Hitherto Pursued in the Cure of Scrophula and Cancer* (Edinburgh: Chapman, 1795), pp. 182–84; Nisbet, *An Inquiry into the History, Nature, Causes, and Different Modes of Treatment Hitherto Pursued in the Cure of Scrophula, Pulmonary Consumption, and Cancer to which is Appended an Appendix Containing a Letter to a Celebrated Professor of Edinburgh*, 2nd ed. (London: Scott, 1800), pp. 182–84; John O'Connor, *"An Inaugural Essay on Carcinoma or Cancer," submitted to the examination of Charles Alexander Warfield and the Medical Faculty of the College of Maryland on 1st May 1812 for the degree of Doctor of Physic* (Baltimore: Edes, 1812), p. 20.

46. For example, see William Hayle Walshe, *The Nature and Treatment of Cancer* (London: Taylor and Walton, 1846), pp. 191–92; William Buchan and William Nisbet, *The New Domestic Medicine, or, a Treatise on the Prevention and Cure of Diseases, by Regimen and Simple Medicines. With an Appendix, Containing A Dispensatory for the Use of Private Practitioners. To which is now added, Memoirs of the Life of Dr. Buchan: And Important Extracts from Other Works, Particularly His Advice to Mothers, On the Subject of Their Own Health, and the Means of Promoting the Health, Strength, and Beauty of Their Offspring, etc.* (London: Kelly, 1809), pp. 421–26, esp. p. 426. On Buchan and *Domestic Medicine*, see C. J. Lawrence, "William Buchan: Medicine Laid Open," *Med. Hist.*, 1975, *19*: 20–35; Charles E. Rosenberg, "Medical Text and Social Context: Explaining William Buchan's *Domestic Medicine*," *Bull. Hist. Med.*, 1983, *57*: 22–42; Richard B. Sher, "William Buchan's *Domestic Medicine*: Laying Book History Open," in *The Human Face of the Book Trade: Print Culture and Its Creators*, ed. Peter Isaac and Barry McKay (Winchester, U.K.: St. Paul's Bibliographies; New Castle, Del.: Oak Knoll Press, 1999), pp. 45–64.

47. For a discussion of cancer as a disease of civilization, see Proctor, *Cancer Wars* (n. 6), pp. 16–34.

stress of urban living; by the quality of the food and water supplies in the cities; and, especially from the late nineteenth and early twentieth centuries, by occupational hazards, including radiation, asbestos, dyes, and other chemicals.[48] Such concerns caused renewed attention to efforts to change people's habits to prevent cancer—but they also highlighted the need for broader social and political responses to the problem.

Thus by the early twentieth century cancer was often seen as a disease of urban-industrial populations, one that could be prevented through individual or social action to reduce exposure to risk. The point can be made by looking at arguments that attributed the rise of incidence or mortality to the changing diet of the urban population. Commentators variously argued that cancer was a result of the increase in meat consumption, the poor quality of urban food, modern methods of food preservation, the sheer quantity of food available, or the availability of new and exotic foodstuffs made possible by the growth of international trade and transportation. Such interest in diet and nutrition was supported by evidence that diet was crucial to the successful uptake of transplantable tumors in mice; by reports that cancer mortality fell with declines in meat consumption in Denmark and the United Kingdom during World War I; and by statistical correlations between the rise in cancer mortality and nineteenth-century changes in diet.[49] Vegetarians and temperance reformers seized upon

48. On radiation, see Claudia Clark, *Radium Girls: Women and Industrial Health Reform, 1910–1935* (Chapel Hill: University of North Carolina Press, 1997); Daniel Paul Serwer, *The Rise of Radiation Protection: Science, Medicine and Technology in Society, 1896–1935,* Informal Report BNL 22279, Brookhaven National Laboratory, 1976. For research on chemicals and cancer and its relationship to irritation theories of cancer causation, see Austoker, *History of the Imperial Cancer Research Fund* (n. 28), pp. 118–25. More generally on early-to-mid-century environmentalist approaches to environmental and occupational causes of cancer, see Proctor, *Cancer Wars* (n. 6), pp. 35–53. On asbestos, see Geoffrey Tweedale, with additional research by Philip Hansen, *Magic Mineral to Killer Dust: Turner and Newall and the Asbestos Hazard* (Oxford: Oxford University Press, 2000). On mule spinners' cancer, see T. Wyke, "Mule Spinners' Cancer," in *The Barefoot Aristocrats: A History of the Amalgamated Association of Operative Cotton Spinners,* ed. A. Fowler and T. Wyke (Littleborough: Kelsall, 1987), pp. 184–96.

49. On transplantation studies see, e.g., C. Moreschi, "Beziehungen zwischen Ernährung und Tumorwachstum," *Zeitschrift für Immunitätsforschung. Originale,* 1909, *2:* 651–75; Peyton Rous, "The Rate of Tumor Growth in Underfed Hosts," *Proc. Soc. Exp. Biol. & Med.,* 1910–11, *8:* 128–30; Rous, "The Influence of Diet on Transplanted and Spontaneous Mouse Tumors," *J. Exp. Med.,* 1914, *20:* 433–51; Eleanor Van Ness Van Alstyne and S. P. Beebe, "Diet Studies in Transplantable Tumors I," *J. Med. Res.,* 1913–14, *29:* 217–32; J. E. Sweet, Ellen P. Corson-White, and G. J. Saxon, "The Relation of Diets and of Castration to the Transmissible Tumors of Rats and Mice," *J. Biol. Chem.,* 1913, *15:* 181–91; Sweet, Corson-White, and Saxon, "On the Influence of Certain Diets upon the Growth of Experimental Tumors," *Proc. Soc. Exp. Biol. &*

the evidence of associations between meat and alcohol consumption and cancer to argue that dietary and alcohol reform would help prevent cancer.[50] For many other commentators, it was clear that moderation in food consumption, especially meat, was a key to prevention.

However, such concerns had little impact on American cancer-control programs that emerged in the early twentieth century. Led by the physician-dominated ASCC, these programs paid little attention to the causal role of environment or habit in cancer. Instead, they tended to focus on "early detection and treatment," which some came to define as "prevention"[51]—preventing the further growth of cancers established in the body, or preventing the onset of cancer by the removal of precancerous conditions. The ASCC was not persuaded by claims that certain habits such as diet caused cancer. Indeed, it often associated suggestions that diet caused or cured cancer with quackery and food faddism; its educational pamphlets stated that diet was not a cause of cancer, and that changes in diet would do little or nothing to prevent or treat the disease. The evidence for some environmental causes—notably radiation and some environmental chemicals[52]—was probably more widely accepted among cancer experts, some of whom were exposed to such dangers themselves. Nevertheless, at

---

Med., 1912–13, *10*: 175–76. On declines in meat consumption, see S. Monckton Copeman and Major Greenwood, *Reports on Public Health and Medical Subjects*, no. 36, *Diet and Cancer with Special Reference to the Incidence of Cancer upon Members of Certain Religious Orders* (London: HMSO, 1926). For discussions of evidence of low cancer rates in "primitive" peoples, and statistical correlations between rising mortality in the West and changes in diet, see Frederick L. Hoffman, *Cancer and Diet, with Facts and Observations on Related Subjects* (Baltimore: Williams & Wilkins, 1937).

50. W. Roger Williams, *The Natural History of Cancer with Special Reference to Its Causation and Prevention* (London: Heinemann, 1908); Francis Albert Rollo Russell, *Preventable Cancer: A Statistical Research* (New York: Longmans, Green, 1912); J. Ellis Barker, *Cancer: How It Is Caused, How It Can Be Prevented* (New York: Dutton, 1924). On how alcohol might cause cancer, see the wonderful illustrations used by John Harvey Kellogg during his lectures: *Dr. Kellogg's Temperance Charts: Showing in a Series of Ten Plates the Physical Effects of Alcohol and Tobacco* (Battle Creek, Mich.: Health Publishing, 1882); copies available in the National Library of Medicine, NLM Unique ID: 101136438.

51. See, e.g., American Medical Association, Council on Health and Public Instruction, American Society for the Control of Cancer, *Prevention of Cancer Series*, Pamphlets 1–10 (1915–24). Even Germany with its focus on environmental and social causes of cancer also gave considerable emphasis to early detection and treatment: Proctor, *Nazi War on Cancer* (n. 1). For an extended review of this book, see David Cantor, "Cancer and the Nazis," *Sci. Cult.*, 2001, *10*: 121–33.

52. Clark, *Radium Girls* (n. 48); Serwer, *Rise of Radiation Protection* (n. 48); Austoker, *History of the Imperial Cancer Research Fund* (n. 28), pp. 118–25; Proctor, *Cancer Wars* (n. 6), pp. 35–53.

a time when doctors were besieged by cancer patients for whom they could do little, the priority shifted to patient care, and prevention was redefined in therapeutic and individualized terms that made the surgeons—and later the radiotherapists—who dominated control organizations central to the definition. Such a shift also meant that practitioners generally did not have to address the tricky political problem of intervention against the producers of environmental cancers.

The British seem to have abandoned environmental and hereditarian explanations of cancer less quickly than did their American counterparts, perhaps because the leaders of the British Empire Cancer Campaign were also prominent supporters of holistic and Hippocratic approaches to medicine.[53] Nevertheless, in Britain, as in the United States, therapeutic prevention came to displace—but not entirely replace—prevention aimed at reforming individual habits.[54] Thus, while individuals might be advised to reduce their exposure to irritants or infections by changing their clothing, diet, or dental habits, such recommendations seem to have given ground to advice to have surgeons or dentists remove sources of irritation or infection such as warts, moles, or bad teeth.[55] Few practitioners stopped giving hygienic advice about cancer prevention to their patients, but therapeutic prevention measures came to dominate the message of British cancer-control organizations in the early twentieth century.

In this volume two papers explore the therapeutic approaches to cancer prevention in the United States. Ilana Löwy's paper on differential diagnosis in breast cancer nicely traces the elision between cancer therapy and cancer prevention. She shows how, on the one hand, pre–World War I American physicians saw in differential diagnosis the hope of reducing the number of unnecessary surgical operations for breast cancer by identifying precancerous conditions before they turned cancerous. On the other

---

53. On the BECC, see Austoker, *History of the Imperial Cancer Research Fund* (n. 28). On holism and Hippocratism, see Christopher Lawrence and George Weisz, eds., *Greater than the Parts: Holism in Biomedicine, 1920–1950* (New York: Oxford University Press, 1998); David Cantor, ed., *Reinventing Hippocrates* (Aldershot: Ashgate, 2002).

54. Such definitions of prevention can be traced back to at least the mid-nineteenth century and to growing interest in prophylactic surgery. See, e.g., recommendations for circumcision as a preventive for cancer of the penis for individuals belonging to cancerous families: Walshe, *Nature and Treatment of Cancer* (n. 46), pp. 192–93.

55. For example, the British surgeon W. Sampson Handley, who claimed that a common factor in all cancers was chronic lymph stasis (essentially a general sluggishness of the lymph system), argued that cancer was often caused by dental infection—and secondary infections of the mouth, stomach, and bowel—and urged greater attention to dental hygiene: "Cancer of a dentally clean mouth is a rarity," he claimed (W. Sampson Handley, *The Genesis of Cancer* [London: Paul, Trench, Trubner, 1931], p. 222).

hand, she also shows how it promoted prophylactic surgery by identifying conditions that might lead to cancer. Women with such precancerous conditions were often told that the best hope of preventing cancer was the removal of their breasts. Raul Necochea shows how from the 1960s the American physician Henry Lynch turned to family pedigrees and then to molecular genetics to identify hereditary cancers—or precancerous conditions—at an earlier stage than they could otherwise be identified, and so to prevent the disease from establishing itself or, once established, from progressing further. Lynch, an advocate of prophylatic surgery, was also a strong proponent of a national registry system of cancer families to identify patients at risk of the disease, and to help in the estimation of risk for particular target organs. These papers build on a growing historical literature that highlights the importance to control/prevention of innovations in diagnostic technology, and of efforts to determine the forms and stages of cancer most amenable to intervention.[56]

"Early detection and treatment" dominated American and British approaches to cancer prevention until the 1970s, and they remain important today[57]—but in the 1960s and 1970s they were joined by a revived interest in environmental and lifestyle causes of cancer. Early twentieth-century doctors and scientists had focused some attention on such causes, but they tended to be subordinated to efforts to improve early detection and treatment. In both the United States and the United Kingdom this began to change in the late 1940s, with epidemiologic research undertaken in both countries that identified cigarette smoking as a cause of lung cancer.[58] Reports by the Royal College of Physicians (1962) and the

56. On staging, see Marie Ménoret, "The Genesis of the Notion of Stages in Oncology: The French Permanent Cancer Survey (1943–1952)," *Soc. Hist. Med.*, 2002, *15*: 291–302. On new technologies such as the Pap smear, see Monica J. Casper and Adele E. Clarke, "Making the Pap Smear into the 'Right Tool' for the Job: Cervical Cancer Screening in the USA, circa 1940–95," *Soc. Stud. Sci.*, 1998, *28*: 255–90; A. E. Clarke and M. J. Casper, "From Simple Technology to Complex Arena: Classification of Pap Smears, 1917–90," *Med. Anthrop. Quart.*, 1996, *10*: 601–23. For work on family histories, see Cantor, "Frustrations of Families" (n. 18); Paolo Palladino, "Between Knowledge and Practice: On Medical Professionals, Patients, and the Making of the Genetics of Cancer," *Soc. Stud. Sci.*, 2002, *22*: 137–65.

57. Breslow et al., *History of Cancer Control* (n. 1).

58. Allan M. Brandt, "Cigarette Risk and American Culture," *Daedalus*, 1990, *119*: 155–76. On the vast historical literature on smoking and cancer, see John C. Burnham, "American Physicians and Tobacco Use: Two Surgeons General, 1929 and 1964," *Bull. Hist. Med.*, 1989, *63*: 1–31; John Parascandola, "The Surgeons General and Smoking," *Pub. Health Rep.*, 1997, *112*: 440–42; Mark Parascandola, "Cigarettes and the US Public Health Service in the 1950s," *Amer. J. Pub. Health*, 2001, *91*: 196–205; Colin Talley, Howard I. Kushner, and Claire E. Sterk, "Lung Cancer, Chronic Disease Epidemiology, and Medicine, 1948–1964," *J. Hist. Med. & Allied Sci.*, 2004, *59*: 329–74; Richard Kluger, *Ashes to Ashes: America's Hundred-Year Cigarette*

U.S. Surgeon General (1964) marked a shift in official attitudes toward the acceptance of epidemiologic proof that smoking "caused" cancer; the triumph of multicausal explanations of the onset of disease, a key moment in the emergence of the "risk factor" concept of disease; and the disciplinary formation of chronic-disease epidemiology.[59]

In some ways these changes were not entirely new. As I have mentioned, nineteenth- and early twentieth-century physicians had seen cancer as the outcome of many different causes. It was dependent on both constitutional and environmental factors, neither of which was sufficient to promote cancer. Diet, nervous stress, environment, heredity, and individual susceptibility might all contribute to the onset of the disease, but it was rarely the case that any one factor was sufficient in itself. Rather, cancer was the outcome of an often unknowable combination of factors. What was different about the new interest in the 1960s and 1970s in multifactorial causation was that it was built upon statistical calculations of risk and a new acceptance that statistical association could be deemed a cause under certain conditions. For such reasons, I refer to this new interest in lifestyle and environmental cancers not as a revival but as a *reinvention* of these concepts and their relation to cancer.

War, the Public Health, and the Unabashed Triumph of Philip Morris (New York: Knopf, 1996); John C. Burnham, *Bad Habits: Drinking, Smoking, Taking Drugs, Gambling, Sexual Misbehavior and Swearing in American History* (London: New York University Press, 1993); Amy Fairchild and James Cosgrove, "Out of the Ashes: The Life, Death, and Rebirth of the 'Safer' Cigarette in the United States," *Amer. J. Pub. Health*, 2004, *94*: 192–204; Matthew Hilton, *Smoking in British Popular Culture, 1800–2000: Perfect Pleasures* (Manchester: Manchester University Press, 2000); Stephen Lock, Lois Reynolds, and E. M. Tansey, eds., *Ashes to Ashes: The History of Smoking and Health* (Amsterdam: Rodopi, 1998); Jon M. Harkness, "The U.S. Public Health Service and Smoking in the 1950s: The Tale of Two More Statements," *J. Hist. Med. & Allied Sci.*, Advance Access published 15 September 2006, **doi:10.1093/jhmas/jrl015**. For additional citations, see nn. 59 and 60.

59. Mervyn Susser, "Epidemiology in the United States after World War II: The Evolution of Technique," *Epidemiol. Rev.*, 1985, *7*: 147–77, on pp. 150–51; Brandt, "Cigarette Risk" (n. 58), pp. 160–64; William G. Rothstein, *Public Health and the Risk Factor: A History of an Uneven Medical Revolution* (Rochester, N.Y.: University of Rochester Press, 2003), pp. 238–50; Mark Parascandola, "Skepticism, Statistical Methods, and the Cigarette: A Historical Analysis of a Methodological Debate," *Perspect. Biol. & Med.*, 2004, *47*: 244–61; Luc Berlivet, "'Association or Causation?' The Debate on the Scientific Status of Risk Factor Epidemiology, 1947–c. 1965," in *Making Health Policy: Networks in Research and Policy after 1945*, ed. Virginia Berridge (Amsterdam: Rodopi, 2005), pp. 39–74; Mark Parascandola, "Epidemiology in Transition: Tobacco and Lung Cancer in the 1950s," in *Body Counts: Medical Quantification in Historical and Sociological Perspectives*, ed. Gérard Jorland, Annick Opinel, and George Weisz (Montreal: McGill-Queen's University Press, 2005), pp. 226–48; Harkness, "U.S. Public Health Service and Smoking" (n. 58).

In a series of recent articles, Virginia Berridge has traced the particular trajectory of this transition in Britain.[60] In this volume she highlights the importance of the smoking/lung cancer debate to certain other transformations. It will be recalled that British cancer agencies had been remarkably reluctant to direct cancer-education programs toward the public. Berridge suggests that the 1962 RCP report was the harbinger of a major change in policy: after 1962, medical and public health agencies gave up their earlier anxieties about public education and embraced media health campaigns aimed at the public. Coming at a time of increasing cultural emphasis on "permissiveness" regarding lifestyle, such campaigns, Berridge argues, marked the beginnings of attempts by the state to regulate or control the new emphasis on tolerance and open-mindedness. She sees the embrace of the media as part of a broader emergence of what she calls a "coercive permissiveness" that emphasized both individual responsibility and governmental intervention in individual behavior.

The Politics of Prevention

The new interest in lifestyle causes of cancer posed a major threat to the centrality of therapeutics to control and prevention. From the 1960s, critics argued that despite an enormous investment in therapeutics, the survival rates for most cancers—except for some cancers in children—had not increased substantially in thirty years.[61] Indeed, as Carsten Timmermann demonstrates in this volume, research into the treatment of lung cancer had been particularly disappointing. Increasingly, these critics claimed that therapeutics should give way to other approaches. Efforts

---

60. Virginia Berridge, "Science and Policy: The Case of Postwar British Smoking Policy," in Lock, Reynolds, and Tansey, Ashes to Ashes (n. 58), pp. 143–63; Berridge, "Passive Smoking and Its Pre-History in Britain: Policy Speaks to Science?" Soc. Sci. & Med., 1999, 49: 1183–95; Berridge, "Post-war Smoking Policy in the UK and the Redefinition of Public Health," Twent. Cent. Brit. Hist., 2003, 14: 61–82; Virginia Berridge and Penny Starns, "The 'Invisible Industrialist' and Public Health: The Rise and Fall of 'Safer Smoking' in the 1970s," in Medicine, the Market and the Mass Media: Producing Health in the Twentieth Century, ed. Virginia Berridge and Kelly Loughlin (London: Routledge, 2005), pp. 172–91. See also Berridge and Loughlin, "Smoking and the New Health Education" (n. 30).

61. "The War on Cancer—Are We Winning It?" first published in Newsday, January 1977; reprinted in Senate Committee on Agriculture, Nutrition, and Forestry, Subcommittee on Nutrition, Nutrition and Cancer Research: Hearings before the Subcommittee on Nutrition of the Committee on Agriculture, Nutrition, and Forestry, United States Senate, Ninety-fifth Congress, Second Session, on Overview of Nutrition Research at the National Institutes of Health with Particular Emphasis on the National Cancer Institute, June 12 and 13, 1978 (Washington, D.C.: U.S. Government Printing Office, 1978), pp. 100–137.

targeted at smoking and other lifestyle causes of cancer seemed to have much better prospects of reducing cancer mortality and incidence, as did efforts that targeted environmental and occupational causes of this group of diseases. I conclude this section with a brief account of how these challenges to therapeutics played out in the second half of the twentieth century, and their impact on the meanings of prevention in this period. My argument here focuses primarily on the United States, where the secondary literature is strongest.

To advocates of therapeutic approaches to cancer control and prevention, the new emphasis on lifestyle was particularly worrying, since it seemed to find increasing popular and political support. From the late 1960s, Congress and advocacy groups began to pressure cancer agencies to shift attention to tobacco and (from the 1970s) also to diet, which critics argued was the second preventable cause of cancer after smoking.[62] At the same time, there was growing interest in environmental and occupational causes of cancer associated with industrial chemicals, pesticides, food additives, radiation, asbestos, and new drugs.[63] The ACS, the NCI,

---

62. Stephen Hilgartner, *Science on Stage: Expert Advice as Public Drama* (Stanford, Calif.: Stanford University Press, 2000); David Cantor, "Between Prevention and Therapy: Gio Batta Gori and the National Cancer Institute's Diet, Nutrition and Cancer Program, 1974–1978," unpublished ms.

63. On asbestos, see Tweedale and Hansen, *Magic Mineral* (n. 48); Jock McCulloch, *Asbestos Blues: Labour, Capital, Physicians and the State in South Africa* (Oxford: James Currey; Bloomington: Indiana University Press, 2002); Ronald Johnston and Arthur McIvor, *Lethal Work: A History of the Asbestos Tragedy in Scotland* (East Linton, Scotland: Tuckwell, 2000). For alternative perspectives on industry responses to the health effects of asbestos, see Peter Bartrip, *The Way from Dusty Death: Turner and Newall and the Regulation of Occupational Health in the British Asbestos Industry, 1890s–1970* (London: Athlone, 2001); Rachel Maines, *Asbestos and Fire: Technological Trade-Offs and the Body at Risk* (New Brunswick, N.J.: Rutgers University Press, 2005). On radiation, see J. Samuel Walker, *Permissible Dose: A History of Radiation Protection in the Twentieth Century* (Berkeley and Los Angeles: University of California Press, 2000); Sarah Dry, "The Population as Patient: Alice Stewart and the Controversy over Low-Level Radiation in the 1950s," in *The Risks of Medical Innovation: Risk Perception and Assessment in Historical Context*, ed. Thomas Schlich and Ulrich Tröhler (London: Routledge, 2006), pp. 116–32. On drugs, see the complex debates on the relation of the Pill and cancer in Lara V. Marks, *Sexual Chemistry: A History of the Contraceptive Pill* (New Haven: Yale University Press, 2001), chap. 7; Elizabeth Siegel Watkins, *On the Pill: A Social History of Oral Contraceptives, 1950–1970* (Baltimore: Johns Hopkins University Press, 1998), esp. chap. 4; Jean-Paul Gaudillière, "Hormones at Risk: Cancer and the Medical Uses of Industrially-Produced Sex Steroids in Germany, 1930–1960," in Schlich and Tröhler, *Risks of Medical Innovation* (n. 63), pp. 148–69. On food hormones such as DES, see Alan I. Marcus, *Cancer from Beef: DES, Federal Food Regulation, and Consumer Confidence* (Baltimore: Johns Hopkins University Press, 1994). On chemicals, see Gerald Markowitz and David Rosner, *Deceit and Denial: The Deadly Politics of Industrial Pollution* (Berkeley and Los Angeles: University of California Press; New

and other cancer agencies found themselves under growing pressure to divert resources from therapy-related activities to work that focused on lifestyle or environmental causes of the disease.

Against such a backdrop, therapists adopted two political strategies. First, they increasingly sought common cause with lay advocacy groups to persuade Congress and the public to put more resources into finding a cure for cancer. In their view, the new preventive strategies offered little immediate prospect of reducing cancer mortality or incidence, with perhaps the exception of lung cancer and some occupational cancers; more importantly, they offered little for the many thousands of people who faced cancer in the 1960s and 1970s, for whom the urgent need was for better treatment. Therapeutic approaches to cancer might not have resulted in a decline in cancer mortality, they claimed, but that was no argument for abandoning those who fell victim to the disease; rather, it made a strong case for more effort in this direction. Whatever their sympathy for prevention efforts focused on lifestyle, environment, or occupation, physicians remained focused on their sick patients, and were anxious that resources might disappear into a seemingly bottomless hole of preventive policies that offered little prospect of reducing cancer incidence or mortality for many years, if ever.

Second, therapists also began to revive the older notion of "early detection and treatment" as prevention, and so to piggyback therapeutics onto the new interest in prevention. It was a timely move, given new technical developments—such as the Pap smear (1940s), the use of mammography in screening (from 1960s), and later genetic testing (1980s–1990s)[64]—that

York: Milbank Memorial Fund, 2002). On hormone replacement therapy and cancer, see the survey by Nancy Krieger, Ilana Löwy, Robert Aronowitz, et al., "Hormone Replacement Therapy, Cancer, Controversies, and Women's Health: Historical, Epidemiological, Biological, Clinical, and Advocacy Perspectives," *J. Epidemiol. & Commun. Health*, 2005, *59*: 740–48. On the growth of EPA interest in cancer prevention, see Edmund P. Russell III, "Lost among the Parts per Billion: Ecological Protection at the United States Environmental Protection Agency, 1970–1993," *Envir. Hist.*, 1997, *2*: 29–51.

64. On the Pap smear, see Casper and Clarke, "Making the Pap Smear" (n. 56); Clarke and Casper, "From Simple Technology" (n. 56). On mammography, see Barron H. Lerner, "'To See Today with the Eyes of Tomorrow': A History of Screening Mammography" (Background paper for the Institute of Medicine report, *Mammography and Beyond: Developing Technologies for the Early Detection of Breast Cancer*, March 2001); Barron H. Lerner, "'To See Today with the Eyes of Tomorrow': A History of Screening Mammography," *Can. Bull. Med. Hist.*, 2003, *20*: 299–321; Lerner, *Breast Cancer Wars* (n. 1), pp. 196–222, 242–50; Gardner, *Early Detection* (n. 1), pp. 179–86. On cancer genetics, see Shobita Parthasarathy, "Architectures of Genetic Medicine: Comparing Genetic Testing for Breast Cancer in the USA and the UK," *Soc. Stud. Sci.*, 2005, *35*: 5–40; Pascale Bourret, "BRCA Patients and Clinical

allowed the identification of cancers and of risks of cancer at earlier stages than had hitherto been possible. Such innovations generated considerable medical, scientific, and commercial interest in promoting "early detection and treatment" as a form of prevention, and revived older interests in prophylactic surgery, for example against breast cancer. Radiological, imaging, pharmaceutical, and genomics companies thus joined with physicians to promote new medicalized and individualized notions of prevention—a move that divided the growing number of lay advocacy groups, some of which (perhaps the most visible) came to press for greater resources for cancer therapy, while others rejected preventive efforts that did not focus on environmental or lifestyle causes of cancer.[65]

Such a revival of older notions of prevention attracted support from biomedical scientists who found advocates of environmentalist and lifestyle approaches to cancer to be critical of the investment in basic research, for example in viruses after the 1971 Cancer Act.[66] It also found support from industries that were threatened by the environmentalist lobby and its supporters in Congress. Many companies sought to deny or obscure evidence that their products or processes caused cancer, to muffle the

---

Collectives: New Configurations of Action in Cancer Genetics Practices," ibid., pp. 41–68; Jean-Paul Gaudillière and Ilana Löwy, "Science, Markets and Public Health: Contemporary Testing for Breast Cancer Predispostion," in Berridge and Loughlin, *Medicine, the Market and the Mass Media* (n. 60), pp. 266–88.

65. On women's advocacy in particular, see Lerner, *Breast Cancer Wars* (n. 1); Gardner, *Early Detection* (n. 1); Ellen Leopold, *A Darker Ribbon: Breast Cancer, Women, and Their Doctors in the Twentieth Century* (Boston: Beacon Press, 1999); James S. Olson, *Bathsheba's Breast: Women, Cancer, and History* (Baltimore: Johns Hopkins University Press, 2002); Amy Sue Bix, "Diseases Chasing Money and Power: Breast Cancer and AIDS Activism Challenging Authority," in *Health Care Policy in Contemporary America*, ed. Alan I. Marcus and Hamilton Cravens (University Park: Penn State University Press, 1997), pp. 5–32; Maren Klawiter, "Chemicals, Cancer and Prevention: The Synergy of Synthetic Social Movements" in *Synthetic Planet: Chemical Politics and the Hazards of Modern Life*, ed. Monica J. Casper (New York: Routledge, 2003), pp. 155–75; Klawiter, "Risk, Prevention and the Breast Cancer Continuum: The NCI, the FDA, Health Activism and the Pharmaceutical Industry," *Hist. & Technol.*, 2002, *18*: 309–53; Klawiter, "From Private Stigma to Global Assembly: Transforming the Terrain of Breast Cancer," in *Global Ethnography: Forces, Connections, and Imaginations in a Postmodern World*, ed. Michael Burawoy, Joseph A. Blum, Sheba George, et al. (Berkeley and Los Angeles: University of California Press, 2000), pp. 299–334. On the role of advocacy groups in testing for breast cancer predisposition see Gaudillière and Löwy, "Science, Markets and Public Health" (n. 64).

66. For an example of such an attack on virus research, see Cantor, "Between Prevention and Therapy" (n. 62). On virus research, see Angela N. H. Creager and Jean-Paul Gaudillière, "Experimental Platforms and Technologies of Visualisation: Cancer as Viral Epidemic," in Gaudillière and Löwy, *Heredity and Infection* (n. 18), pp. 203–41.

public pronouncements of those of their own scientists who suggested that such dangers were real, and to garner political support against the public health lobby. Such responses formed a constant problem for those seeking to promote concern about lifestyle and environmental causes of cancer: too often, they complained, the industries concerned attempted to thwart their efforts to identify such risks, to shift responsibility from themselves to individuals affected by the disease by suggesting that their behaviors were the problem and not the actions of the industries concerned, and to promote forms of intervention that did not compromise their commercial interests.[67]

The consequence was particularly hard for those interested in occupational and environmental causes of cancer.[68] Following a growth of interest in these causes during the 1960s and 1970s, policy began to drift elsewhere with growing scientific criticism that their contribution to the overall cancer burden had been overestimated, and, in the early 1980s, with the election of President Ronald Reagan. The Reagan administration and its ideologues found medicalized notions of prevention that emphasized individual responsibility much less threatening than environmentalist lobbies that promoted greater regulation. Thus policies aimed at prevention based on lifestyle (smoking and diet) and "early detection and treatment" grew at the expense of prevention strategies aimed at challenging occupational and environmental cancers through governmental intervention. Critics responded that the NCI and the ACS downplayed the evidence for increasing cancer rates and their relation to avoidable exposure to industrial and environmental carcinogens. Instead, such critics claimed, these organizations, together with the chemical, radiation, and other industries, focused attention on dietary fat (ignoring industrial contaminants such as pesticides) and smoking (ignoring increasing lung-cancer rates in nonsmokers, and the important role of occupational exposure and urban air pollution) as the predominant causes of cancer mortality and incidence. They were obsessed with diagnosis, treatment, and basic research, and indifferent to cancer cause and prevention.[69]

Such criticisms highlight a further fracture in the debates over cancer prevention in the last third of the twentieth century. As occupational and environmental causes of cancer were increasingly ignored, critics came to worry that an emphasis on lifestyle factors distracted attention from

67. See the citations in n. 63.
68. Proctor, *Cancer Wars* (n. 6), pp. 75–100.
69. Samuel S. Epstein, "Losing the 'War against Cancer': A Need for Public Policy Reforms," *Internat. J. Health Sci.*, 1992, *22*: 455–69.

broader structural factors that promoted cancer.[70] In their view, lifestyle approaches to cancer were often characterized by an outlook on disease that emphasized the role of individual behavior rather than environmental and social factors in disease causation, and so focused attention more on efforts to change individual conduct than on social institutions, industrial production, or governmental regulation. Others argued that such individualist approaches also carried moralistic values that held individuals responsible for their cancers despite evidence that social-structural factors played an important role in determining disease in populations. Put another way, critics suggested, the new emphasis on lifestyle focused mainly on *apparent* choices, conceiving of individuals as consumers who could be educated to make more informed decisions regarding their health—but this was to ignore that personal choices were shaped largely by social structures.

The result of such debates has often been a confusion of preventions. Despite efforts since the 1950s to rationalize the different approaches to cancer prevention by creating categories of primary, secondary, and tertiary prevention (see Glossary for recent guidelines),[71] there remains disagreement on where the boundaries between therapy and prevention lie, on whether tertiary prevention is an attempt by therapists to sponge off of the new enthusiasm for prevention, and on what constitutes each of the three approaches.[72] The labels have been used in quite contradictory ways, and some interventions seem to fit into more than one category. Others reject the label "prevention" being attached to anything that

70. Christopher Sellers, "Discovering Environmental Cancer: Wilhelm Hueper, Post–World War II Epidemiology, and the Vanishing Clinician's Eye," *Amer. J. Pub. Health,* 1997, *87*: 1824–35. See also Proctor, *Cancer Wars* (n. 6), esp. chaps. 3–4. For an example of the debates in the 1980s, see the debate between Richard Peto and Samuel Epstein in Richard Peto, "Distorting the Epidemiology of Cancer: The Need for a More Balanced Overview," *Nature,* 1980, *284*: 297–300; Samuel S. Epstein and Joel B. Swartz, "Fallacies of Lifestyle Cancer Theories," *Nature,* 1981, *289*: 127–30.

71. In 1957 the U.S. Commission on Chronic Illness classified prevention into primary, secondary, and tertiary prevention: primary prevention aimed at the reduction of the incidence of a specific illness; secondary prevention, the reduction of the prevalence of an illness; and tertiary prevention, the reduction of the amount of disability resulting from a specific illness. See U.S. Commission on Chronic Illness, *Chronic Illness in the United States,* vol. 1: *Prevention of Chronic Illness* (Cambridge: Harvard University Press, 1957), pp. 126–43; H. R. Leavell and E. G. Clark, *Preventive Medicine for the Doctor in His Community: An Epidemiologic Approach* (New York: McGraw-Hill, 1965).

72. For example, chemoprevention is sometimes labeled as tertiary prevention, sometimes as having the goal of primary prevention (preventing the occurrence of the disease), sometimes as secondary prevention (early detection and reversion of tumors at a premalignant stage), and sometimes as some combination of the three.

does not focus on environmental or occupational causes.[73] In part, these divisions are derived from technical debates within cancer control—but they also reflect the harsh politics of the latter part of the century, the struggle for resources, ideological divisions over public policy, and efforts of powerful vested interests to shape cancer policy to their own interests. Prevention, like control, involved a multiplicity of (sometimes contradictory) meanings and approaches—a confusion of meanings shaped as much by politics as by science.

The Essays

The essays that follow are divided into three parts. The papers in Part I—Between Education and Marketing—explore the ways in which cancer-control organizations have sought to persuade people to change their behaviors regarding cancer, set this in the context of broader media representations of cancer, and discuss the different approaches to cancer education in Britain and the United States. Three of the essays—those by Gretchen Krueger, Elizabeth Toon, and me—have already been summarized in the context of the discussion of different British and American approaches to cancer education. Here I wish to make a further point, that these essays can also be read as accounts of different approaches to the marketing of cancer, especially when read alongside Susan Lederer's essay on Hollywood portrayals of cancer.

The intertwining of marketing and education is well illustrated by the situation of American cancer control in the first half of the twentieth century. Physician leaders of cancer-control organizations such as the ASCC/ACS saw themselves as competing for patients and public support with alternative practitioners, purveyors of patent medicines, folk healers, and physicians whom they regarded as ignorant of the disease and

---

73. Silvio De Flora, Alberto Izzottia, Francesco D'Agostinia, Roumen M. Balanskyb, Douglas Noonanc, and Adriana Albinic, "Multiple Points of Intervention in the Prevention of Cancer and Other Mutation-Related Diseases," *Mutat. Res./Fund. & Molec. Mech. Mutagen.*, 2001, *480–81*: 9–22; "A Comprehensive Approach to Cancer Prevention and Control: A Vision for the Future," in *Prevention Strategies That Work* (Steps to a Healthier U.S. Initiative, U.S. Department of Health and Human Services, 2003), esp. p. 25; Gail L. Shaw, "Editorial: Cancer Prevention—Perspectives and Implications," *Cancer Control J.*, March/April 1997, *4* (2): https://www.moffitt.usf.edu/pubs/ccj/ (accessed 18 September 2006). On chemoprevention, see Jennifer Fosket, "Constructing 'High-Risk Women': The Development and Standardization of a Breast Cancer Risk Assessment Tool," *Sci. Technol. & Hum. Val.*, 2004, *29*: 291–313; Fosket, "Breast Cancer Risk and the Politics of Prevention: Analysis of a Clinical Trial" (Ph.D. diss., University of California, San Francisco, 2002).

its treatments. Their efforts to educate the public about early detection and treatment thus were not only about appropriate care, but were also attempts to control a highly competitive market in cancer care by dissuading patients from going elsewhere for treatment. For such reasons, these leaders were doubly anxious to ensure that their educational efforts did not scare off the public: anxious that they did not undermine public compliance with the message of early detection and treatment, and anxious that they did not undermine the opportunities that such compliance created for controlling the market in cancer care.

Thus my essay account of how the educational technology of the movie threatened to undermine cancer-control programs can also be read as an account of how it threatened to undermine ASCC/ACS efforts to manage a volatile market in cancer care. To the extent that the technology promoted awareness of the value of early diagnosis, it was good for expanding therapeutic business opportunities (at least for those not defined as "quacks," purveyors of patent medicines, or ignorant physicians). To the extent that it promoted excessive fear of the disease or its treatment, it could ultimately undermine such opportunities by dissuading people from seeking help and driving them into the arms of the competition. Therefore, the control organizations needed to develop strategies that did not defeat the original purposes of the campaigns. Cancer control was as much about controlling markets and personal behaviors as it was about controlling disease.

Gretchen Krueger's essay also highlights the intertwining of education and marketing, with reference to leukemia. She argues that in media campaigns for this disease the image of the child was central to efforts to promote programs of early detection and treatment. But such images were not only about promoting the health of the child, they were also about efforts to build a business of leukemia around chemotherapeutic approaches to the disease, and to encourage donations for further research in the field. Once again, efforts to control markets and publics went hand in hand with efforts to control diseases—a point that is stressed in both of our papers when we highlight how the 1944 takeover of the ACS by advertisers and business people transformed cancer education and marketing. Where I show how moviemaking expanded, diversified, and became better integrated with Hollywood and the entertainment industry, Krueger shows that the takeover was important to promoting the new field of chemotherapy, and the flexible responsiveness of cancer marketing to changing client expectations and the effectiveness of therapeutics.

Susan Lederer's essay broadens the focus to set these developments in public education and marketing in the context of Hollywood's portrayal of cancer. Lederer argues that Hollywood took a much greater interest in cancer than has previously been realized, and that this interest began to be more focused in the late 1930s, at about the same time that cancer agencies revived interest in using movies as a tool of public education. But whereas the development of the public health movie was driven by the imperatives of cancer control and the medical market in cancer diagnosis and therapy, Hollywood was driven by the imperatives of the business of entertainment. Thus, for example, Lederer shows that while the ASCC/ACS and Hollywood sought to exclude certain issues from their films, Hollywood's concerns were very different from those of the public-education cancer movie. Where the ASCC/ACS worried that movie portrayals of the operating room and recovery process might undermine programs of cancer control, Hollywood was often happy to follow patients into the operating theater, and to show surgeons failing to cure. For Hollywood, it was issues of mercy killing and aesthetics that structured what was shown: the industry tended to exclude the possibility of euthanasia from its movies, and to focus on nondisfiguring cancers such as brain tumors. Given the cultural prominence of Hollywood's portrayal of cancer, these were imperatives with which the public-education efforts discussed by Krueger and by me had to engage.

How different things were in Britain. In the first place, British cancer agencies seem to have been less concerned than their American counterparts by the competition of quacks, patent-medicine purveyors, folk healers, and others—in part because such competition was less of a threat within highly centralized organizations such as the NRC and later the NHS. In the second place, while the transformation of cancer marketing and education in America after 1944 occurred in the context of vast economic growth, an unprecedented consumer boom, the expansion of state and private support for research, and the impetus of a market-driven health-care system, the situation in postwar Britain was very different. The country was more or else bankrupted by war, the economy was in the doldrums, rationing continued until the early 1950s, and the country was moving toward a taxation-driven health-care system. Marketing cancer—or simply educating people about it—was quite problematic in such a context, as Elizabeth Toon's essay demonstrates. Her account of the unwillingness of the British to educate the public (as opposed to the profession) can be read as an account of how the British also sought to control the spending of tax revenue on health care. The relative failure of the Manchester experiment illustrates the point. One of the implications of the Manchester experiment was that people's attitudes toward cancer control would change if cancer services improved—yet such improvements would have required vast inputs of Treasury monies, and would also have needed substantial innovations in therapy and care, neither of which could easily be promised. No small wonder, then, that the British were unwilling to go down the American route of vast, aggressive cancer-education programs: while such campaigns were welcomed as stimulating demand in a market-driven health system, they were less welcome for the same reason in a taxation-driven health-care system where the imperative was to limit costs. Cancer control, in Toon's account, was as much about controlling costs as it was about controlling disease.

❖

While Part I focuses on how cancer agencies sought to attract public support for their programs of control, Part II—Therapeutics—focuses on the therapeutic modalities at the heart of control. The authors trace the different meanings of and approaches to therapy—especially radiotherapy and chemotherapy—in Britain and the United States, the ways in which different professional groups and individuals sought to create opportunities for themselves through these modalities, how state and market medicine shaped cancer services, and how patients responded to this.

Ornella Moscucci's paper explores why British feminist doctors turned to radium therapy in the first three decades of the twentieth century. Focusing on cervical cancer, Moscucci argues that radium was of particular interest to feminists because of their long history of opposition to gynecological surgery. Radium provided both an opportunity to improve cure rates, and an alternative to the severe mutilation associated with surgical interventions against cervical cancer. Cancer control, in Moscucci's account, was as much about controlling the activities of male surgeons as it was about controlling the disease. But feminists also had another interest in radium: Moscucci argues that it provided a means of improving women's access to medical education at a time when they were often excluded from training posts and honorary appointments at voluntary hospitals. She thus highlights the way in which the introduction of radiotherapy was tied up with feminist efforts to reform medicine, as both a practice and a profession. She also highlights the importance of the state to such feminist politics, for it provided the radium that feminist surgeons used to promote their agendas.

John Pickstone expands on the role of the state in his essay on the three major therapeutic modalities that developed in the first sixty to seventy years of the twentieth century: surgery, radiotherapy, and chemotherapy. In his account, interwar British radium therapy exemplified a model of centralized—and partly state-supported—health care. As we have shown earlier, the modality was shaped by the National Radium Commission and later the National Health Service, which institutionalized radiotherapy in British medicine, and encouraged the development of teamwork in therapy at a time when most clinicians espoused a more individualist approach to medical work. But Pickstone also makes a further point: he argues that this organization of radiotherapy was associated with a particular form of knowledge, an analytic "way of knowing." Radiotherapeutic organizations broke complex things and events into their elements, promoted specialization in these elements, and then, to coordinate and rationalize their work, organized the specialists into teams, standardized the techniques, and systematically collected statistics to assess the impact of interventions.

The contrast with chemotherapy is striking. If radiotherapy under the NRC/NHS exemplified an analytic/rationalist model, Pickstone argues that post–World War II American chemotherapy exemplified a more inventive and experimentalist mode, which, through the practice of trials, shaped the new subprofession of medical oncology. Paradoxically, this experimentalist mode began with a huge investment by the state, notably through the federally funded National Cancer Institute. But while the Americans focused state involvement on trials research, they severely limited its involvement in routine cancer care: there was no centralized organization in the United States equivalent to the National Radium Commission or the National Health Service in Britain. Thus while initially developed with federal monies, Pickstone argues, American chemotherapy's prominence and professional form were shaped by the imperatives of the medical market.

Peter Keating and Alberto Cambrosio look more closely at the chemotherapeutic trial in post–World War II North America and Europe, exploring how various groups came together to shape its development. Their discussion of the protocol and its normalized version, the clinical practice guideline, makes the point. The authors show that the development of the protocol in the postwar period lies at the heart of modern cancer treatment research and practice. Protocols came to be linked in complex ways to all the key components of modern cancer treatment research: government agencies, pharmaceutical companies, nonprofit organizations, patients, and physicians were all involved in different ways with the protocol, both in its creation and in its application. Keating and Cambrosio's account thus employs the protocol—and the trial more generally—as a window onto the interrelations between all these groups and institutions as they contributed to the creation, evolution, and implementation of the clinical trial, and the development of treatment modalities, research methodologies, disease concepts, and biological models. Put another way, protocols provide an opportunity to explore the dynamics of biomedical research at many different levels and across many different component parts of the cancer treatment/research enterprise. Pickstone argues that chemotherapy trials embodied modes of experimentalism and invention. Keating and Cambrosio show how trials also sought to rationalize the organization of chemotherapeutic research and practice.

Finally, Barron Lerner returns to the relations of cancer to feminism raised earlier by Moscucci, but from the perspective of one exceptional American patient in the 1970s. He examines how Rose Kushner built on her earlier campaigns against radical mastectomies as the treatment of choice for breast cancer in the United States to raise questions about the use of adjuvant chemotherapy for breast cancer. As Lerner notes, Kushner's activism emerged from a combination of feminist politics, journalistic experience, and her personal unwillingness to accept the public health message put out by the cancer agencies. Her relative success in challenging the public health message laid the groundwork for some of the breast cancer activists of the 1980s. It also raises questions about the boundaries between lay and expert knowledge that were becoming politicized during this period, and about the politicization of control. If the physicians who ran cancer-control programs routinely sought to control the behaviors of patients as much as the disease itself, Kushner shows how patients could mirror these meanings of control: they sought to control not only the disease, but also the behaviors of the physicians who treated them.

It should be clear by now that cancer control meant many different things. For most of the twentieth century it was focused on the control of the disease as a biological entity through early detection and treatment—attempts to control its development in the body, and, by extension, to control mortality from the disease, and perhaps its incidence. But such efforts were generally embedded in a range of other activities—attempts to control health behaviors, markets, health-care costs, and the activities of quacks, folk healers, the media, and "ignorant" medical practitioners—all of which had an effect on attempts to control the biological disease. Part III of this collection—Prevention and Risk—problematizes the distinction between cancer control and prevention. The authors explore the ways in which prevention/control was shaped by the development of new innovations in diagnostic and screening technology, molecular genetics, and the statistical calculation of risk; and how the emergence of interest in lifestyle causes of cancer in Britain was embedded in broader shifts in approaches to controlling human health behaviors.

The complex interrelations of therapeutics, control, and prevention are explored in the first essay in this section. Ilana Löwy argues that, from before World War I, American physicians saw improvements in the differential diagnosis of breast lesions as a means of reducing the number of unnecessary radical surgeries, encouraging women to see a physician as soon as possible, and preventing malignant pathologies by removing lesions before they turned cancerous. In her account, the development of new pathological techniques—such as the frozen section—facilitated the identification of precancerous lesions so that they might be surgically removed. Surgery thus became a form of prevention. For example, women who were diagnosed with "chronic mastitis" or "cystic disease of the breast" were commonly advised to have a mastectomy, in the belief that this reduced their risk of cancer. Yet difficulties in stabilizing the prognostic meaning of so-called precancerous lesions problematized this approach: it remained unclear whether they were really precancerous, and, if precancerous, what the chances were of their developing into cancer. Löwy argues that from the 1950s these conditions were replaced by "carcinoma in situ," and that recent developments of tests for hereditary predisposition to breast cancer are a continuation of attempts to detect what she calls an "embodied risk" of cancer, and to eliminate this risk by cutting it out.

Raul Necochea's paper on the American physician Henry Lynch develops Löwy's point, about the continuity between early detection and treatment and contemporary interest in hereditary predispositions to cancer, from a different perspective. Beginning in the 1960s, Lynch used family studies to identify a statistical *risk* of cancer among individuals with relatives who had cancer, a risk that could be identified long before the onset of the disease or of precancerous signs or symptoms. Lynch hoped that by identifying a hereditary risk of cancer among relatives of patients with cancer he might be able to improve programs of early detection and treatment. But the evidence from family studies was unpersuasive to most scientists and doctors, prompting Lynch to begin a long search for more convincing means of identifying risk. Focusing on hereditary nonpolyposis colorectal cancer (HNPCC), Necochea argues that it was only in the 1990s that the identification of genes associated with the disease transformed it from one that a few physicians believed ran in families to one with precise genetic components that researchers generally accepted, and that could be detected through genetic tests. The irony of such wide acceptance, however, was, as Necochea notes, that the "cancer family" construct was crucial in the search for the HNPCC genes, and that the diagnosis of HNPCC continued to require that the mutated genes be found within a kin group that is generally accepted as a "cancer family."

Löwy's and Necochea's papers both problematize the distinction between cancer control and cancer prevention. Both approaches were cast as preventive, but both were also located within the dominant early twentieth-century framework of control by means of early detection and treatment. Paradoxically, the paper by Virginia Berridge on lung cancer and smoking also problematizes the distinction between control and prevention, but in a different way. In the first place, hers is an account of the rebirth or reinvention of interest in lifestyle causes of cancer in 1960s and 1970s Britain. She argues that the 1962 Royal College of Physicians (RCP) report marked the creation of what she calls a "policy community" around public health that linked government civil servants to medical experts outside, shifted the focus of public health toward individual behavior legitimated through population-based epidemiology, stimulated new attitudes on the part of the government in relation to the public on health issues, and encouraged a heightened role for research-based surveillance. It was thus a very different approach to prevention from that described by Löwy and Necochea.

In the second place, however, Berridge's account also reveals the interwoven nature of control and prevention. She shows how efforts to control rising cancer mortality were embedded in new efforts to control or shape human behavior. The RCP report, she argues, marked a new willingness on the part of medicine to speak to the public and to use the media to do so. Put another way, Berridge argues that efforts to prevent/control cancer were crucially tied up with new "mediatized" attempts to shape or control human behaviors. In her view, the report and the media efforts that followed it were heralds of a "coercive permissiveness" that embodied contradictions in approaches to public health in the 1960s. Health became a matter of individual responsibility, but the British conceived of individual responsibility within a new framework of governmental intervention in individual behavior. Members of the public could modify their own habits and lifestyles to attain better health, but that modification was increasingly state ordained and supported.

Finally, Carsten Timmermann returns us to the complex relations between therapeutics and prevention/control after World War II. It is often claimed that the identification of smoking as a cause of lung cancer has resulted in the neglect of therapy. Timmermann aims to debunk this claim, at least for Britain before the 1970s. In the first place, he suggests, research on lung-cancer therapy was not undermined by the stigma associated with an allegedly self-inflicted illness, for the simple reason that smoking and lung cancer were not stigmatized before the 1970s. In the second place, Timmermann argues that from the 1950s the MRC in fact undertook a vigorous program of research to develop new therapeutic procedures against lung cancers. He claims that the failure to develop a successful treatment had more to do with the technical and ethical difficulties associated with the disease than with any stigma. More broadly, this failure also helped to ease the emergence, from the 1960s and 1970s, of policies aimed at preventing/controlling smoking. If Löwy and Necochea show how prevention could also *be* therapy and control, Timmermann shows how therapeutic failures could open the door to other approaches to prevention and control.

Glossary

Recent definition of primary, secondary, and tertiary prevention, Centers for Disease Control, National Center for Chronic Disease Prevention and Health Promotion

Primary prevention refers to the complete prevention of disease, often through methods that inhibit exposure to risk factors (e.g., preventing exposure to tobacco smoke).

Secondary prevention is meant to inhibit or reverse the effects of disease in its early stages, mainly through early detection (e.g., using the Pap test to discover and treat cervical neoplasia).

Tertiary prevention identifies the disease process and attempts to prevent further disability and restore a higher level of functioning (e.g., pain management or use of prostheses where indicated).

Source: Guidance for Comprehensive Cancer Control Planning, vol. 1: *Guidelines*, Division of Cancer Prevention and Control, Centers for Disease Control and Prevention, 4770 Buford Highway, NE, Atlanta, GA 30341, 25 March 2002, p. 122. Online version: **http://www.cdc.gov/cancer/ncccp/cccpdf/Guidance-Guidelines .pdf** (accessed 18 September 2006).

Part I / Between Education and Marketing

Uncertain Enthusiasm:
The American Cancer Society,
Public Education, and the
Problems of the Movie, 1921–1960

DAVID CANTOR

SUMMARY: Historians have highlighted a growing medical enthusiasm for public health education movies in the early twentieth century. This essay suggests that there is another historiographic tale to tell, of concerns that films might *undermine* the public health messages they were designed to promote—concerns that threatened continued interest in movies during the Depression of the 1930s. First, focusing on cancer-education movies aimed at the general public released by the American Society for the Control of Cancer (ASCC, founded 1913), the paper argues that the organization's initial enthusiasm for movies was tempered from the late 1920s by a combination of high production costs, uncertainty as to the effectiveness of movies as public-education tools, and the hard economic situation. It was only after 1944 that motion pictures became a stable part of the propaganda efforts of the renamed American Cancer Society. This transformation followed the takeover of the Society by advertisers and businesspeople, led by Mary Lasker, who introduced business models of fund-raising and education, and made expensive communication technologies, such as movies, central to cancer control. Second, the article also traces the persistence of anxieties that movies might undermine cancer control by encouraging emotional responses

This article would have been impossible but for the help of archivists and curators of movie collections at the National Library of Medicine, the National Archives, the National Film Board of Canada, the American Cancer Society, and the Library of Congress. I am particularly grateful to Bill Stine and Peter Carlin who provided me with access to the American Cancer Society's unrivaled collection of historical cancer-education movies, and to Ken Weissman and his colleagues at the Motion Picture Conservation Center, Library of Congress, who allowed me to view what was then the only copy of *Reward of Courage*, now fortunately preserved and duplicated. The Rockefeller Archive Center kindly allowed me to view their records on the making of this movie. Mike Sappol commented on an earlier draft of this paper, as did participants in meetings of the National Institutes of Health's Biomedical Research History Interest Group, 15 June 2004; of the workshop, "Mediating Biomedicine: Engaging, Resisting, Negotiating," held at the University of Manchester, 10–11 September 2004; and of the "Cancer in the Twentieth Century Workshop," held at the NIH, 15–17 November 2004.

that led audiences to ignore the lessons the movies were intended to encourage. But whereas such anxieties dampened ASCC enthusiasm for cancer-education movies during the hard economic times of the 1930s, they had no such effect after 1944, and attention shifted to developing techniques of controlling unwanted audience responses.

KEYWORDS: public-education movies; cancer education; American Society for the Control of Cancer; American Cancer Society; cancerphobia

When in 1921 the American Society for the Control of Cancer (ASCC) released its first public-education movie, the hope was that this would open a new era in cancer education. Crusaders against tuberculosis and venereal diseases had used movies for similar purposes long before the Society took an interest in the medium, as had commentators on a range of controversial issues such as birth control, euthanasia, and eugenics. There seemed every reason to believe that the fight against cancer would benefit from the success of the new medium as a tool of public education. Historians have documented the enthusiasm with which early twentieth-century public health officials turned to movies for such public-education purposes.[1] The ASCC shared the excitement.

But, in the case of cancer, the initial enthusiasm was short-lived. The 1929 economic crash ended most movie production for seven or eight years as concerns about high production costs, poor distribution, and the effectiveness of movies as a public-education tool made the cancer organization—still young, and financially vulnerable—wary of committing monies to the medium. The projectors began to roll again in 1937 with the beginnings of federal involvement in cancer research, but ASCC doubts about the cost-effectiveness of public-education movies did not immediately dissipate. It was only after 1944 that the Society's enthusiasm for the movie as a means of educating the public about cancer came into its own.

1. Martin S. Pernick, "Thomas Edison's Tuberculosis Films: Mass Media and Health Propaganda," *Hastings Cent. Rep.*, June 1978, pp. 21–27; Pernick, *The Black Stork: Eugenics and the Death of "Defective" Babies in American Medicine and Motion Pictures since 1915* (New York: Oxford University Press, 1996). See also Susan E. Lederer and Naomi Rogers, "Media," in *Medicine in the Twentieth Century*, ed. Roger Cooter and John Pickstone (Amsterdam: Harwood Academic Publishers, 2000), pp. 487–502; Lisa Cartwright, *Screening the Body: Tracing Medicine's Visual Culture* (Minneapolis: University of Minnesota Press, 1995); Adolf Nichtenhauser, "A History of Motion Pictures in Medicine" (unpublished book MS, ca. 1950), Adolf Nichtenhauser History of Motion Pictures in Medicine Collection, MS C 380, Archives and Modern Manuscripts Program, History of Medicine Division, National Library of Medicine, Bethesda, Md.

This paper is thus about why the ASCC saw the movie as a very uncertain tool for raising the public visibility of cancer until the mid-1940s, and why this changed after 1944. For all their enthusiasm about the new medium, the leaders of the ASCC—physicians, scientists, and a few lay supporters—often found other means of public education to be cheaper and more effective. Newspapers, magazines, and radio reached much broader audiences than did public-education movies, and there were also cheaper means of presenting a cancer-control message in the sorts of venues in which the movie was generally shown—mothers' meetings, women's clubs, factories, churches, schools, movie theaters, and so on. Then, in 1944, the old ASCC leadership was ousted by a small group of influential business people and advertisers, who took over the organization and renamed it the American Cancer Society (ACS).[2] Much more willing than their forebears to spend money in order to raise money, the new leaders had little patience for what they saw as the penny-pinching of the old guard and introduced business models of fund-raising and education to the organization that involved substantial outlays of resources. Income dramatically increased, and expensive communication technologies such as the movie became more feasible: indeed, they became a key to the new ways of education and raising money.

If this paper is about the ASCC's anxieties about the cost of movies, it is also about its concerns about the potential of the movie to undermine its own educational message. Two issues in particular worried the pre-1944 ASCC. The first was that movies had the power to generate fears of the disease or its treatment that could overwhelm any rational response on the part of the public to the message of early detection and treatment, and so could weaken the very programs of cancer control that they were designed to promote. The second, which gained attention in the early 1940s, was the anxiety that an emphasis on the need for cancer *research* might promote a view among the public that physicians did not know as much about cancer as they claimed, and so might undercut cancer *control* by raising questions about the limitations of medical knowledge. Such issues worried the physician leaders of the ASCC; helped to dampen their enthusiasm for movies as public-education tools, especially when financial times tightened; and persisted after 1944. Nevertheless, whereas these issues prompted the physician leaders of the ASCC to limit the role of the movie in public education,

---

2. James T. Patterson, *The Dread Disease: Cancer and Modern American Culture* (Cambridge: Harvard University Press, 1987), pp. 172–79; Kirsten E. Gardner, *Early Detection: Women, Cancer, and Awareness Campaigns in the Twentieth-Century United States* (Chapel Hill: University of North Carolina Press, 2006), pp. 95–104.

they had no such effect on the post-1944 leadership; on the contrary, the new leaders saw the movie as an indispensable part of an integrated range of mutually supportive methods of public education and cancer control. Part of the historiographic aim of this paper is to explain why.

1921–1937

In the Beginning . . .

The early enthusiasm for movies as a public-education tool came at an opportune time for the ASCC. From its beginnings in 1913, the Society argued that for cancer control to succeed, millions of men and women had to be persuaded to abandon the habits of generations and to seek qualified medical assistance at the first sign of what might be cancer. In the view of its founding physicians, control depended on identifying the disease as early in its development as possible while the tumor was still a local condition, before it spread to other parts of the body and constitutional complications set in. Yet, the early signs of cancer could be subtle and easily missed, and there was often no pain or debility to prompt patients to see their physicians before the disease had spread and become incurable. Thus, the ASCC began a program of public education with the aim of teaching people to identify the early signs of the disease, to go for a regular health check-up, and to seek early treatment if cancer was diagnosed. Initial educational efforts focused on newspapers, magazines, lantern slides, and innumerable talks by physicians, but the Society was also keen to find new ways of getting its message across. After a delay in organizing the campaign caused by World War I, in 1921 the ASCC launched its first cancer week—an intense effort at fund-raising and education—and it was there that it saw a role for the motion picture. Its first movie, *Reward of Courage*, was to be a centerpiece of this effort.[3]

For the young organization, making a movie was expensive. It secured a grant of $8,500 from the Rockefeller Foundation, and hired a small

---

3. "Consolidated Report of the President and Executive Committee," *Campaign Notes of the American Society for the Control of Cancer* (hereafter *Camp. Notes ASCC*), 1922, *4* (3): [3–4, at p. 3] (early issues of some of these journals are unpaginated; bracketed numbers are my own pagination); "'The Reward of Courage,'" ibid., *4* (2): [1]. For other reports of the showing of this movie, see "Colorado," ibid., 1921, *3* (12): [2]; "West Virginia," ibid., 1922, *4* (1): [4]. For its showing in Canada, see Shannon Macdonald, "The History of Cancer Treatment in Nova Scotia," *Dalhousie Med. J.*, Spring 2003, **http://medjournal.medicine.dal .ca/DMJONLIN/spring03/history%20ccns.htm** (accessed 19 May 2004). For a history of the lantern slide, see Maren Stange, "Jacob Riis and Urban Visual Culture: The Lanternslide Exhibition as Entertainment and Ideology," *J. Urb. Hist.*, 1989, *15*: 274–303.

commercial film company, the Eastern Film Corporation (220 West 42nd St., New York), to make the movie. Founded in 1908, and with studios in Rhode Island, the Eastern Film Corporation was a vigorous promoter of movies as a tool of salesmanship.[4] It assured the ASCC that it had produced most of the movies made for the U.S. Red Cross during the First World War.[5] The $8,500 allowed Eastern to make a movie of higher quality than many public health movies. The film included some animated diagrams demonstrating the growth and extension of cancer. It was also tinted: happy parts were tinted pink; sad parts were tinted blue; and the rest was standard amber. In 1921, Frank J. Osborne (Executive Secretary, ASCC) wrote that Eastern had agreed to alter a scenario that he had written, "by introducing more action and human appeal material in the way of a love story."[6]

The movie tells the tale of Eugene (Gene) Barnes and his fiancée Dorothy Flint, the daughter of Marshall Flint, the owner of the Pleasantville Accessories Supply Company where Gene is superintendent. The movie opens with Gene reporting to Marshall that a newly installed company clinic has paid for itself by preventing time lost on account of sickness, and has saved the workers money as well. Flint is impressed and he and Gene visit the clinic. When Dr. Dale—the clinic physician—shows them some cases of cancer he has identified among the workers and their families, Flint asks how they *caught* the disease. This provides Dale with an opportunity to explain (the ASCC position) that cancer is not contagious (it cannot be caught), that "quack" treatments are dangerous, that early treatment can lead to cure, and that any lump in the breast is dangerous. Flint reports the last warning to his wife, Anna, who, unknown to him, has spotted such a lump in her own breast. The lump is diagnosed as cancer by the family surgeon, Dr. Clinton.

Anna's diagnosis prompts Dorothy (the movie now tinted blue) to break off her engagement to Gene, fearful that the disease is hereditary. It also prompts Mrs. Flint to turn for help to Gene's rival as suitor to Dorothy, Mr. Morris Maxwell, whom Anna prefers as a potential son-in-law. Maxwell claims to be associated with a philanthropic group of scientists, including

4. Frank A. Tichenor (president of the Eastern Film Corporation), "Motion Pictures as Trade Getters," *Ann. Amer. Acad. Polit. & Soc. Sci.*, 1926, *128*: 84–93; Tichenor was a coeditor of this special issue on motion pictures, which included Joseph Franklin Montague, "What Motion Pictures Can Do for Medical Education," on pp. 139–42.

5. Frank J. Osborne to Mrs. Mead, 2 March 1921, Laura Spelman Rockefeller Memorial Archives, series III, box 5, folder "American Society for the Control of Cancer, 1921–23," Rockefeller Archive Center, Sleepy Hollow, N.Y. (hereafter LSR, "ASCC").

6. Ibid.

some of the best cancer specialists. In fact, he is the "quack" owner of the "Scientific Cancer Cure Institute," which offers a cancer treatment called Radiumized Paste ("NO KNIFE, NO PAIN, No Failure Recorded"), and his interest in Anna is mercenary: he wants her to encourage her husband to support his Institute, and persuades her to write a check for $200 for her own treatment. But just as she hands over the money her husband bursts into the room accompanied by Dale, and they confront the quack. They are joined by Gene and a Post Office inspector, who arrests Maxwell. Gene and Dorothy marry after Dr. Clinton informs them that cancer is not hereditary. The movie ends with a happy family scene (the film now tinted pink), comprising Dorothy, Gene, their new baby, and Mr. and Mrs. Flint (who has been cured by surgery). The movie thus urged viewers to seek help from authoritative medical sources at the first suspicion of cancer; aimed to correct the "false" impressions that cancer was contagious or hereditary; and exposed the dangers of unscientific, mercenary, "quack" treatments.

The movie is remarkable for including perhaps the first cinematographic depiction of a breast examination, albeit discreetly shot. It also contains some shots of the industrial clinic, the animated drawings mentioned above, and some scenes in which Dr. Dale examines a patient—but there are no scenes showing cancer therapy. Frank J. Osborne later wrote that all operative, technique, and hospital scenes had been eliminated:

> I believe [he concluded] the public will respond much more readily to the suggestion of immediate attention to anything suggesting cancer, if the arrangements for radical treatment are kept in the background and left to the physician after the patient has applied for advice.[7]

As such comments suggest, the ASCC may have seen movies as a means of educating the public about cancer. But it was also concerned that disturbing scenes—such as hints of radical treatment—had the potential to undermine their efforts by frightening people away from their physicians. Such scenes, the ASCC believed, had no place in the public forum of the movie screen; they were best dealt with elsewhere where the fears could be more easily managed. Perhaps for these reasons, the movie was described as both a "dramatic presentation, [and] entirely unobjectionable."[8] By 1923, thirty-six copies of the two-reel movie were in circulation.[9] It was still available in 1926.[10]

7. Frank J. Osborne to W. S. Richardson, 29 July 1921, ibid.

8. "Cooperation of Health Departments in the Control of Cancer," *Camp. Notes ASCC*, August 1926, *8* (8): [1–3, at p. 2].

9. Osborne to Richardson, 25 January 1923, LSR, "ASCC."

10. "Cooperation of Health Departments" (n. 8), [pp. 2–3].

Conversions

We know little about audience reactions to *Reward of Courage*, but the ASCC was clearly converted to the possibility of the movie as a public-education tool. On 10 February 1925 it released a second movie, *A Fortunate Accident*—a melodrama, first shown before the St. Louis Medical Society.[11] There followed, in 1928, a British movie, *The Cultivation of Living Tissue*—the first time-lapse photography of cells grown in culture, filmed by the British pathologist R. G. Canti.[12] Then in 1929 the Society released two other movies: *By the Way*, about which no details appear to have survived,[13] and another melodrama, *This Great Peril*, the first reel of which survives in the ACS archives.[14]

The ASCC was not only converted to the movie, it was particularly converted to the melodrama as a means of education. Scientific movies like the Canti film apparently generated little public interest. Thus while the ASCC initially viewed the Canti film as having both public and professional appeal, in time it appears to have shown the movie mainly to medical audiences, and to have viewed it as a technical rather than a public-education movie.[15] Instead of dry science, the ASCC wrapped its control message in

11. "'A Fortunate Accident' the New Cancer Film," *Camp. Notes ASCC*, 1925, *7* (2): [p. 4]. The film was shown at a meeting in which George A. Soper, Ph.D. (managing director of the ASCC), and Gideon Wells, M.D., spoke before the St. Louis Medical Society, 10 February 1925: George A. Soper, "Methods and Results of Efforts to Control Cancer by Education," *Weekly Bull. St. Louis Med. Soc.*, 1925, *19* (27): 9–13; Gideon Wells, "Statistical Studies in Cancer," ibid., pp. 13–14. For the use of the movie in a "Country Entertainment," see "Cancer as a Subject for Popular Entertainment," *Camp. Notes ASCC*, 1925, *7* (6): [1–3, at p. 2].

12. "The New Cancer Film," *Camp. Notes ASCC*, 1928, *10* (11): [4]. On Canti and the Strangeways Laboratory, see David Cantor, "The Definition of Radiobiology: The Medical Research Council's Support for Research into the Biological Effects of Radiation in Britain, 1919–1939" (Ph.D. diss., Lancaster University, 1987); Duncan Wilson, "The Early History of Tissue Culture in Britain: The Interwar Years," *Soc. Hist. Med.*, 2005, *18*: 225–43. See also Nichtenhauser, "History of Motion Pictures in Medicine" (n. 1), pp. III-268–IV Supplement SF 36–7.

13. "Society Holds Semi-Annual Meeting," *Camp. Notes ASCC*, 1929, *11* (11): 3.

14. Kirsten Gardner seems to have seen another version of the movie (also from the ACS archives) that included a list of credits; the copy I viewed did not include the credits. Gardner wrongly notes that the movie was released in 1920: Gardner, *Early Detection* (n. 2), p. 228 n. 77, p. 257.

15. "New Cancer Film" (n. 12), [p. 4]; "Interest Shown in the Canti Film," *Camp. Notes ASCC*, 1928, *10* (12): [4]; "Society Received Many Requests for the Booking Film," ibid., 1929, *11* (2): [4]; "Dental Society Cancer Program," ibid., 1929, *11* (5): [4]; "Association Sees Film," ibid., 1929, *11* (8): 6. By 1930 it seems to have been regarded as a technical film rather than a movie for the public, as was another movie of cells by Warren H. Lewis: see "The Lewis Cancer Film," *Bulletin of the American Society for the Control of Cancer* (hereafter *Bull. ASCC*), 1928, *12* (10): 8.

a dramatic narrative: the suggestion that movies should include human interest and action had been taken to heart.

An example of a human-interest and action story is provided by *A Fortunate Accident*. I have found no copy of this movie; however, the ASCC provides a synopsis in its newsletter, *Campaign Notes*.[16] According to the synopsis, the accident in question happens to a Mrs. Brown-Jones, a woman of wealth and social position in an unnamed small town. She is involved in an automobile collision with a coal truck outside the offices of Dr. Strong, a young, well-trained physician who has recently arrived in town with his mother hoping to establish himself in practice, only to find that establishing a practice is not an easy thing to do. Strong examines Brown-Jones, and finds that she is not seriously injured—but while she is briefly unconscious, he discovers what he thinks may be an early breast cancer. Mrs. Brown-Jones is indignant, believing that this implies a hereditary taint; she dismisses Strong, and seeks a second opinion of the lump in her breast from an eminent surgeon. He confirms Strong's diagnosis, recommends an immediate operation, and refers Brown-Jones to what he calls a capable physician in her hometown; this physician turns out to be Dr. Strong. Mrs. Brown-Jones accepts the referral and reengages Strong, who arranges for the operation that saves her life. The automobile accident is thus fortunate for Mrs. Brown-Jones, whose cancer is detected early enough to be treated successfully; for Dr. Strong, who is now able to establish himself in practice; and for the crusade against cancer, which gains an influential supporter in the person of Mrs. Brown-Jones. The synopsis concludes:

> Mrs. Brown-Jones is thus converted to the modern doctrine of cancer control, and becomes a center of intelligent and useful information in regard to cancer within her large sphere of social and philanthropic influence.[17]

The key word here is "converted." As the term suggests, this movie was a conversion narrative, telling the tale of how (what the synopsis portrays as) an ignorant woman is persuaded to seek early treatment and eventually to become a missionary for the cancer crusade. It is a story of a transition from darkness to light, from ignorance to knowledge, from tradition to modernity, and from impending death to life, and of how medical authority trumps class (in the guise of a society lady)—all through the intervention of circumstance and a knowledgeable physician.

Conversion narratives were a common plot-device in movies aimed at the general public. In general they dramatized the processes by which

16. "'A Fortunate Accident' the New Cancer Film," *Camp. Notes ASCC*, 1925, 7 (2): [4].
17. Ibid.

individuals were persuaded to accept medical advice regarding cancer, and the penalties for those who failed to convert. Sometimes the language of these narratives echoed that of religious conversion, with individuals being "saved," "choosing to live," and coming to accept the "doctrine" of cancer control. But these were not religious conversion stories. The orthodoxy that they sought to promote was early detection and treatment. The devils that they sought to exorcise were those of quackery, ignorance, fear, and a lack of deference to medical authority—and the gods they sought to install were those of the doctor's office, the hospital, and later the laboratory. Thus, these stories may have drawn on the language and structure of the religious conversion narrative, but they turned them into something else: a medical or biomedical conversion account.

The first cancer movie to use this structure was *Reward of Courage* in 1921 (though it was by no means the first public health movie to do so), and like many other movies it asserted not only medical but also male authority over women's beliefs about cancer. In this film it is Marshall Flint—husband, father, and employer—who is converted to the medical approach to cancer, and it is he who saves his wife (and, in a different way, his daughter) from falling into Maurice Maxwell's hands. In *A Fortunate Accident* it is the unnamed eminent male surgeon who converts Mrs. Brown-Jones to the modern doctrine of cancer control. And the theme of medical/male authority is reiterated in a third movie, *This Great Peril* (1929), where a young physician persuades his former fiancée to save her mother. The figure of the mother in this movie, as in *Reward of Courage*, represents gullibility, ignorance, tradition, and outmoded belief. In both films, it is the mother who stands in the way of progress, who endangers herself through her credulity and lack of knowledge, and who seeks to interfere with her daughter's marriage prospects.[18]

Produced by Visualgraphic Pictures of New York for the ASCC, *This Great Peril* tells the story of a young physician, Gordon Crane, who leaves home to train with a world-famous New York cancer specialist, George Gwyn. Crane asks his fiancée, Margaret, to wait two more years to marry; instead, she breaks off the engagement, swayed in part by her mother who thinks that Gordon is impractical and selfish. However, Margaret's mother has cancer, turns to a "quack," and ends up in a "sanitarium." In desperation, Margaret abandons her earlier doubts about Gordon and appeals for help to her former fiancé, now himself a successful cancer specialist.

18. For another example of maternal culpability in public health movies, see Lisa Cartwright's discussion of the antituberculosis movie *Let My People Live* (1938) in her *Screening the Body* (n. 1), pp. 149–50.

He insists on the dismissal of the charlatan and then, heroically, operates on the mother despite the late stage of the cancer. The operation is a success, and in more ways than one: not only is the mother cured, she also changes her attitude toward Gordon, and encourages reconciliation with Margaret. Thus the hero gets the girl, the mother gets her life, quackery is vanquished, and orthodox medicine triumphs—and all because Gordon was willing to sacrifice his future happiness for his healing vocation.[19]

Demise

By 1933 the ASCC's involvement in motion pictures had faded. The failure of the Canti film to attract public interest has been noted (though several versions of it remained in circulation as a technical movie until at least the 1940s).[20] The melodramas fared little better: by 1933 *Reward of Courage* and *A Fortunate Accident* had long since disappeared from the screens, and *This Great Peril* was soon to go. An ASCC report that year noted that *This Great Peril*—a silent movie made after the advent of sound in 1927—"no longer holds anything of interest or value and is rarely called for."[21] The report recommended the making of a new film "suitable for presentation to intelligent groups who are interested in having some technical material presented in simplified form."[22] Yet no new cancer motion picture was made until 1937.

The roots of the decline went back to the 1929 economic crash. Making a movie was not cheap, and the crash led the ASCC, still searching for funds, to be wary of such expenditure, when cheaper and perhaps more effective measures were available to promote the cancer-control message—pamphlets, radio talks, magazine articles, and especially newspaper articles were less expensive to produce, and perhaps better at reaching a mass audience.[23] For example, a 1931 report noted that movies came

19. "'This Great Peril'—Society's New Film for Laymen—Ready for Release," *Camp. Notes ASCC*, 1929, *11* (6): 4–6.

20. "Report of Activities of the American Society for the Control of Cancer: 1929–1933," *Bull. ASCC*, 1933, *15* (10): 1–15, at p. 4; *Catalog of Educational Material* (New York [?]: American Society for the Control of Cancer, n.d.) (copy available in the National Library of Medicine at call number QZ200 qA518c 1941).

21. "Report of Activities of the American Society for the Control of Cancer: 1929–1933," *Bull. ASCC*, 1933, *15* (10): 1–15, at p. 4.

22. Ibid. In contrast to the Canti film, *This Great Peril* was no longer listed as available in the 1940s *Catalog of Educational Material* (n. 20). For an example of a call for movies for the medical profession, see "Fifteenth Annual Meeting of the Members of the Society. March 3, 1928," *Camp. Notes ASCC*, 1928, *10* (2): [1–4, at p. 4].

23. On the importance of newspaper publicity and its comparison to movies, see Harry C. Saltzstein, "Newspaper Publicity in the Control of Cancer," in American Society for the Con-

very far down the list of the reasons people gave for turning to an ASCC information bureau; magazines, posters, car cards, newspapers, radio talks, pamphlets, and exhibits were all cited more often than movies.[24] As *This Great Peril* neared the end of its run, there was little incentive to invest new money in such an expensive technology.

It could be argued that movies were never intended for the sorts of mass audiences that could be reached by newspapers, radio, and magazines. They tended to be shown in smaller venues—women's clubs, factories, movie theaters, and so on—often as an accompaniment to a lecture by a physician. But even here, there were reasons to avoid the expense of movie production: many places did not have the projection equipment to show movies; movie-theater owners could be reluctant to allow their equipment to be used; and the ASCC was poorly organized in parts of the country, making it difficult to put on film events. Moreover, cheaper technologies could substitute for the motion picture in these settings. Thus, during the 1930s, the ASCC's interest in film was limited to an updated version of the lantern slide: the filmstrip, a series of still pictures that could be shown with a standard hand-operated film slide projector.[25] For all such reasons, even before the passing of *This Great Peril*, movies were rarely shown at educational events. The projectors went dark.

1937–1944

Revival

The darkness ended in 1937 with the beginnings of federal support for cancer. In January 1937, Time Inc. released *Conquering Cancer* as part of its *March of Time* series to coincide with the creation of the National Cancer Institute (also 1937).[26] Movie screens came to life with cancer, and

---

trol of Cancer, *Cancer Control: Report of an International Symposium Held under the Auspices of the American Society for the Control of Cancer, Lake Mohonk, New York, U.S.A., September 20–24, 1926* (Chicago: Surgical Publishing Co. of Chicago, 1927), pp. 299–307, esp. p. 299.

24. Ella Hoffman Rigney, "A Practical Program in Cancer Publicity," *Bull. ASCC,* 1931, *13* (11): 5–6, at p. 6.

25. "New Medical Filmstrips Issued," *Bull. ASCC,* 1940, *22* (1): 10. The history of the celluloid filmstrip as a technology is told in Reece V. Jenkins, *Images and Enterprise: Technology and the American Photographic Industry, 1839–1925* (Baltimore: Johns Hopkins University Press, 1975), chap. 6. For a popular history of the educational uses of the filmstrip, see Danny Gregory, *Change Your Underwear Twice a Week: Lessons from the Golden Age of the Classroom Filmstrip* (New York: Artisan, 2004).

26. The movie was released in the *March of Time* series as part of a broader campaign by the publishers to promote cancer. The campaign also included influential articles in a

for the first time the auditoriums were filled with sound. As far as can be determined, all the movies of the 1920s had been silent. *Conquering Cancer* took belated advantage of the development of talkies, the wiring of (movie) theaters for sound, and the development of equipment that allowed them to be heard in other venues.

Conquering Cancer was of a very different genre from the movies of the 1920s, which were predominantly melodramas: it was a newsreel.[27] It also gave much more prominence to cancer research, and portrayed it as a very different enterprise. In the reel that survives of *This Great Peril,* knowledge is produced not in the laboratory, but in the doctor's office, and technology tends to be in the background.[28] In *Conquering Cancer,* the focus of research was the hospital and laboratory, which included dedicated buildings full of teams of researchers, technicians, animal houses, and sophisticated equipment. At a time when cancer researchers repeatedly complained about the poor status of their field and the lack of opportunities for research and career advancement, *Conquering Cancer* hinted at the promise that research offered Americans for understanding and curing the disease.[29]

Conquering Cancer aimed to provide "the technical information in simplified form" that the ASCC had called for in 1933, but it did so without the financial help of the ASCC. The Society argued that its newly appointed publicity director, Clifton R. Read, had played a key role in encouraging Time Inc. to launch its movie, and that it encouraged a spurt in private donations—but it also noted that the film was produced "entirely without

---

number of Time Inc. publications: "Cancer: The Great Darkness," *Fortune,* March 1937, *15*: 112; "U.S. Science Wars Against an Unknown Enemy: Cancer," *Life,* 1 March 1937, pp. 11–17. See "Publicity," *Bull. ASCC,* 1937, *19* (1): 11–12, at p. 12; "With the Women's Field Army," ibid., *19* (3): 10–12, at p. 10; "With the Women's Field Army," ibid., *19* (4): 10–12, at p. 11; "Revised Cancer Film Prepared for England," ibid., *19* (7): 9–10; "Report of Activities of the American Society for the Control of Cancer: 1935–36; 1936–37," ibid., *19* (10): 1–16, esp. pp. 2, 13; "An Extraordinary Year in the History of Cancer," ibid., *19* (12): 10–11, esp. p. 10; "The Cancer Front—1937," ibid., 1938, *20* (3): 8–9, esp. p. 9; "Movie Wins Medal of Cancer Group Here; March of Time Honored for War on Disease," *New York Times,* 28 October 1937, p. 30.

27. On the history of the newsreel, see Raymond Fielding, *The American Newsreel, 1911–1967* (Norman: University of Oklahoma Press, 1972); Fielding, *The March of Time, 1935–1951* (New York: Oxford University Press, 1978).

28. In an early scene, Gordon Crane finishes a scientific paper in the office he shares with his physician father; in another, George Gwyn and Gordon examine an X-ray film in their office, while a brightly lit room—possibly the surgery or consulting room—is partially revealed through a door behind them.

29. "Cancer: The Great Darkness" (n. 26).

cost to the Society."[30] Despite periodic calls for the ASCC to release new films,[31] movies remained costly to produce, and the organization did not immediately put monies into the medium.[32]

The situation changed in the early 1940s when the ASCC joined with the U.S. Public Health Service (PHS) to coproduce two new movies, *Choose to Live* (1940) and *Enemy X* (1942). Yet the ASCC's return to movie production was faltering at best. As I shall discuss in a moment, the movies were severely criticized as both confusing to the public and misleading about the nature of cancer treatment. As in the 1920s, the ASCC worried that any depiction of radical surgery might dissuade people from seeking help, and both it and the PHS were happy to call for cuts of the sort that Frank J. Osborne had advocated in 1921. Yet, to some critics, such cuts came at the cost of informing the public about the true nature of the disease and its treatments. They also raised a new concern: that the growing emphasis on research in cancer-education movies might work against efforts to persuade people to seek early detection and treatment, by suggesting that doctors did not know as much as they claimed about cancer, and raising questions about their current ability to treat the disease.

Choose to Live *(1940)*

These criticisms are well illustrated by *Choose to Live*. Combining the melodramatic genre of the 1920s with elements of a documentary or newsreel genre, *Choose to Live* tells the story of Mary Brown, who has detected what may be cancer in her breast. Mary's story begins with her being caught between her fear of cancer and her obligations to her family. Then she attends a meeting of her women's club where an eminent physician talks about the disease, prompting her to consult her family physician. The lump is diagnosed as cancer, and Mary's decision to seek help is vindicated by her joyful return home after a successful operation. The movie ends with a grateful Mary joining the ASCC's Women's Field Army, a nationwide fund-raising, educational, and volunteer body founded in

30. "Report of Activities . . . 1935–36; 1936–37" (n. 26), p. 2.

31. Marjorie B. Illig, "With the Women's Field Army," *Bull. ASCC*, 1938, *20* (10): 10–12, at p. 10.

32. The one exception was the release in 1938 of a 42-second trailer—possibly for the *March of Time* film—for use in motion picture houses: "April: Cancer Control Month," *Bull. ASCC*, 1938, *20* (4): 9. It may also be that the ASCC rereleased *Conquering Cancer* under a new title: *Cancer—Its Cure and Prevention* (1937). A copy of the movie with this last title is in the ACS archives in Atlanta, Ga.; a copy of *Conquering Cancer* is in the National Archives, College Park, Md.

1936 that Henry R. Luce, president of Time Inc., described as "the largest evangelistic movement ever launched against a disease."[33] By the end of 1940 more than two hundred prints of the original 16 mm (18-minute) version had been made, and a shortened 11-minute version was available at a lower cost.[34]

As the above account suggests, the movie has a similar structure to *A Fortunate Accident*. It is a conversion account in which an ignorant and fearful Mary is persuaded to seek early treatment from a recognized physician, and, like the fictional Mrs. Brown-Jones before her, eventually to become a missionary (evangelist?) for the ASCC.[35] In particular, the movie stresses the importance of conversion as an emotional event. The opening scenes focus on the anxieties that Mary feels about the possibility that she might have cancer; on how such anxieties prompt her to delay; and on how they conflict with her sense of responsibility toward her husband and children. Her eventual decision to seek help involves a transition not only from ignorance to knowledge, but also from fear to relief. Even before she knows the diagnosis of her condition, she finds that her decision to see her physician has lifted an immense emotional burden: "It's been such a relief to tell someone what I was afraid of," she tells her family physician.

Choose to Live thus marks the return of the conversion narrative to cancer control. It also seems to be the first such narrative to put the pathological laboratory at the heart of the story. As far as can be determined, the medical heroes of the 1920s movies had been practicing physicians such as Drs. Dale, Strong, and Crane. *Choose to Live*, however, subordinates the physician to the laboratory: the laboratory alone can determine whether a growth is a cancer. When Mary asks her family physician if she has cancer he tells her that he cannot say, and refers her to the hospital. The film shows how a section removed from Mary is processed and examined in the pathological laboratory, while she remains in the operating theater surrounded by surgeons, all awaiting the word of the pathologist. In Mary's case the lump is diagnosed as cancer, and the surgeons operate immediately without waking their patient. The next scene shows Mary reunited with her family and returning happily home. Her conversion has not only

33. "Extraordinary Year in the History of Cancer" (n. 26), p. 11. On women and the ASCC, see Gardner, *Early Detection* (n. 2).

34. "A New Film," *Bull. ASCC*, 1940, *22* (4): 9; "'Choose to Live,'" ibid., *22* (7): 7–8; Clifton R. Reed, "Service of Supply," ibid., *22* (9): 6–9, at p. 6; "'Choose to Live,'" ibid., *22* (11): 10.

35. Note, however, that Mary does not have the wealth or social position of the hyphenated Brown-Jones.

saved her and her family, it has also affirmed the diagnostic authority of the laboratory over her, her family physician, and her surgeons.

Choose to Live thus dramatized both the psychological consequences of Mary's conversion, and the processes by which the lump she had detected was transformed into the medical diagnosis of cancer. But it said much less about the surgical operation or its outcomes, and so drew criticism that it was less than truthful about the consequences of conversion. A review probably written by the movie expert Adolf Nichtenhauser, then pressing for a greater role of movies in public health education, argued that the film never expressly stated that Mary Brown had cancer;[36] that the nature of the operation was not mentioned; and that there was no clear indication of a convalescent period after treatment—Mary apparently leaves the hospital immediately after the operation.[37] But there were potential costs to such cuts and evasions: when cancer organizations failed to address issues that were already the subject of public concern, it could appear that they had something to hide, which could undermine their ability to persuade people to seek early detection and treatment. Nichtenhauser was not alone in criticizing the overly optimistic message of the ASCC.[38]

Nichtenhauser also raised another concern. The central part of *Choose to Live* is a lecture by a fictional eminent physician that includes a long discussion of cancer research, almost a documentary or newsreel illustrated by shots of laboratories, laboratory animals, and laboratory equipment. This lecture-cum-documentary is the stimulus to Mary Brown's decision to see her physician, but Nichtenhauser worried that it did not do the work it was intended to do.[39] In his view, the story of Mary Brown was not organically built into the lecture. The lecture itself he described as "a crowded affair. A great many things are mentioned, but no clear understanding is achieved."[40] The visual material, he suggested, was disjointed and consisted largely of shots of laboratories and apparatus, incomprehensible to lay audiences.

36. Review of *Choose to Live* contained in Adolf Nichtenhauser Papers, MS C 277, box 4, folder "Cancer 1948," Archives and Modern Manuscripts Program, History of Medicine Division, National Library of Medicine (hereafter Nichtenhauser Papers). The reviewer is actually wrong on this point: the narrator notes that the pathologist diagnoses cancer.

37. Adolf Nichtenhauser to Louis J. Neff (Executive Secretary, ASCC), 22 March 1944, Nichtenhauser Papers, MS C 277, box 4, folder "Cancer 1948."

38. Robert A. Aronowitz, "Do Not Delay: Breast Cancer and Time, 1900–1970," *Milbank Quart.*, 2001, *79*: 355–86; Gardner, *Early Detection* (n. 2), pp. 85–91.

39. The tension between research and control was not entirely new. In *This Great Peril*, Margaret's mother (who fears she may have cancer) comments that she does not trust young doctors (such as the research-oriented Gordon Crane) with pet theories.

40. Review of *Choose to Live* (n. 36).

And, perhaps most importantly, he concluded that people who had seen the film had been led to the belief that doctors did not know much about cancer because so much research was going on in laboratories.[41] In Nichtenhauser's view, the film failed to reconcile the tension between educating the public about research and educating it about practical measures of control. It could not be recommended, he wrote the ASCC.[42]

Enemy X *(1942)*

The second movie, *Enemy X*, was equally problematic to Nichtenhauser. It concerns an unknown killer who is murdering four hundred people a day in New York City, and marking them with an *X* on the forehead. "No mention of cancer until audience interest has been clinched [an ASCC catalog enthused]. Then the subject of cancer is delivered with a surprise punch that retains the interest and gets the message across vividly and forcefully."[43] The surprise punch comes when a voice cries "cut," and the camera pulls back to reveal (surprise!) a film set.

The actors in this murder mystery take a break from production, and go over to talk to one of New York's most eminent surgeons, the fictional Dr. Crandall. Among other things, Dr. Crandall becomes the vehicle for promoting yearly physical examinations as a means of preventing cancer. *Enemy X* was not the first movie to advocate regular physical examinations; for example, in a brief scene in *This Great Peril* Gordon Crane urges an audience to have a health examination once a year, and in *Reward of Courage* it is the routine examination of patients in the industrial clinic that allows Dr. Dale to catch early cancers among Flint's workers. But *Enemy X* articulates the case for a yearly physical much more extensively than do these early movies. For Crandall, the point is not to wait for symptoms to appear, for most people do not recognize early signs of the disease. Only a qualified physician could identify the subtle beginnings of the disease, especially among those patients who feel quite healthy. The actors are persuaded of the point, and the movie closes with their being called back to work. The ASCC catalog described *Enemy X* as "the best 'short' film on cancer so far produced."[44] Adolf Nichtenhauser had a brutally different

41. Ibid.; Nichtenhauser to Neff, 22 March 1944 (n. 37).

42. Nichtenhauser to Neff, 22 March 1944 (n. 37).

43. *Catalog of Educational Material* (n. 20). For other reports on *Enemy X*, see "A New Cancer Film," *Bull. ASCC*, 1941, *23* (12): 3.

44. *Catalog of Educational Material* (n. 20). For a different opinion, see "Motion Picture Films," 15 May 1943, Nichtenhauser Papers, MS C 277, box 1, folder "Amer. Cancer Society."

assessment: without elaborating, he wrote the ASCC that *Enemy X* was "a great mistake in every respect."[45]

Problems

With both of the ASCC's forays into moviemaking under question, older questions about the high cost of the technology came to the fore again. As one ASCC representative put it in 1943, "the expense of [motion picture] production is great and the needed money accumulates slowly."[46] Movies were not only expensive to produce, they remained difficult to distribute. The ASCC had expanded substantially since the 1920s, and the Women's Field Army provided new opportunities to get the cancer-control message across, yet movies tended to remain marginal to its efforts. In 1943 the Iowa Department of Health released a cancer-education movie called *Cancer,* but the ASCC rarely mentioned movies in articles on cancer education.[47] Nor were they often a feature of reports on the educational and fund-raising activities of the organization. As in the 1930s, the filmstrip remained a popular, cheaper alternative to the movie, as did the short two-minute "trailer." As the above-mentioned ASCC representative noted in 1943: "The less expensive similar things such as film strips and trailers can be produced in greater number."[48]

To add to these difficulties, the ASCC became concerned that movie theaters (in the 1920s a common venue for cancer shows) were increasingly closing their doors to the organization. Between 75 percent and 90 percent of the population went to the movies weekly, an ASCC booklet on how to generate publicity noted in 1942—but, it argued, this group was "one of the most difficult to crash."[49] It warned local organizers that

45. Nichtenhauser to Neff, 22 March 1944 (n. 37).

46. Herman C. Pitts, "Educational Program of American Society for the Control of Cancer," *Bull. ASCC,* 1943, *25* (11): 122–26, at p. 124.

47. For an exception, see Frank E. Adair, "The Teaching of Cancer," *Bull. ASCC,* 1937, *19* (7): 1–6, esp. p. 3. On the movie produced by the Iowa State Department of Health in 1943, see Edmund G. Zimmerer, "War-time Cancer Education," ibid., 1944, *26* (2): 14–16, esp. pp. 15–16; State of Iowa, *Report of the State Department of Heath for the Biennial Period Ending June 30, 1944* (Des Moines: State of Iowa, 1944), p. 45. It should also be noted that *Public Health in New York State* (1937), produced by the Division of Public Health Education, New York State Department of Health, included an account of the Department's efforts at cancer control as part of a survey of its activities.

48. Pitts, "Educational Program" (n. 46), pp. 124–25.

49. *Cancer Publicity: What It Is and How to Get It* (New York: ASCC, c. 1942), p. 13 (distributed free to officers of the WFA, *not* for general distribution), in *Catalog of Educational Material* (n. 20).

the Hays Office, the official board of censors of the movie industry, had
decreed that the great function of the entertainment screen is to entertain (and by implication, not to educate?); that the public went to be
amused and resented paying to see commercial or propaganda movies;
and that theater managers were constantly bombarded with requests to
show such films for various causes and often made a blanket rule never
to show any.[50] The best that could be hoped for was that theater owners
might show "shorts" (up to 15 minutes) or "trailers" (up to two minutes).
Such problems led the authors of the booklet to recommend that organizers should approach movie-theater owners only once a year, during the
annual April campaign.

1944–1960

Growth

All this changed in 1944, when the ASCC was taken over by a group of lay
businesspeople led by Mary Lasker, the wife of advertising tycoon Albert
Lasker, and was renamed the American Cancer Society (ACS).[51] This
takeover revolutionized the organization. The old leadership—dominated
by physicians and scientists—was sidelined. The new leaders reorganized
fund-raising and publicity along business models, lavishing resources on
education, and making movies central to their efforts. Suddenly monies were available as never before, and concerns about the high cost of
motion pictures lost their bite. The National Cancer Institute's budget for
movies also increased at the same time, but the ACS far outstripped the
government agency in the number and range of public-education films it
produced (see Tables 1 and 2). In 1946 it had five movies in circulation;[52]
another was released in 1947, and four more in 1948.[53] This growth was
accompanied by a broadening of the range of genres (cartoons, from

50. On the Hays Code, see Grey D. Black, *Hollywood Censored: Morality Codes, Catholics and the Movies* (Cambridge: Cambridge University Press, 1994).

51. Patterson, *Dread Disease* (n. 2), pp. 172–79; Gardner, *Early Detection* (n. 2), pp. 95–104.

52. ACS, *Annual Report for the Year Ending August 31st 1947* (New York[?]: American Can-cer Society), p. 32. It notes that the ACS also released two slide films produced by Zurich Insurance Co. of Chicago: *Search Everyone* and *An Enemy in Our Midst.*

53. See Table 1. For movies released by 1950, see American Cancer Society, *Annual Report 1950* (New York[?]: American Cancer Society), pp. 14–16.

Table 1. Cancer-education movies produced or released by ASCC/ACS and USPHS/NCI, 1921–1960 (excluding trailers and spots)

Year	Title	Released/ produced by
1921	*Reward of Courage*	ASCC
1925	*A Fortunate Accident*	ASCC
1928	*The Cultivation of Living Tissue* (The Canti movie, also called *Living Cells*)	ASCC
1929	*By the Way*	ASCC
	This Great Peril	ASCC
1937	*Cancer—Its Cure and Prevention* (orig. released by Time Inc. as *Conquering Cancer*)	ASCC
1940	*Choose to Live*	USPHS/ASCC
1942	*Enemy X*	USPHS/ASCC
1946	*The Traitor Within*	ACS
	Time Is Life	ACS
	On Guard	ACS
	Miracle Money (originally released by MGM in 1938)	ACS
	You Are the Switchman	ACS
1947	*The Battle Against Cancer*	ACS
1948	*You, Time, and Cancer*	ACS
	Life Saving Fingers	ACS, Idaho Div.
	The Doctor Speaks His Mind	ACS
1949	*We Speak Again*	ACS
	To Save These Lives	ACS
1950	*From One Cell*	ACS
	Challenge: Science Against Cancer (32 min.)	NCI & Canadian Department of Health and Welfare

Four other versions of this movie were released:
   Alerte: Science contre cancer (French version of *Challenge*) (32 min.)
   The Fight: Science Against Cancer (21 min.)
   The Outlaw Within, 1951[?] (11 min.)
   Cancer, 1951[?] (French version of *The Outlaw Within*) (11 min.)

	Breast Self-Examination	ACS/NCI
	To Save These Lives	ACS
1952	*Man Alive*	ACS
	Crusade	ACS
1953	*The Warning Shadow*	ACS
	Living Insurance	ACS, Idaho Div.

(*Continued on p. 58*)

Table 1 *(continued)*. Cancer-education movies produced or released by
ASCC/ACS and USPHS/NCI, 1921–1960 (excluding trailers and spots)

Year	Title	Released/ produced by
1955	*The House-to-House Campaign*	ACS, Iowa Div.
1956	*Sappy Homiens*	ACS
1957	*Much Ado About Something*	ACS
	The Man on the Other Side of the Desk	ACS
	Eight Out of Ten	ACS
	The Other City	ACS
	Time and Two Women	ACS
1958	*Never Alone*	ACS
	After Mastectomy	ACS, Oregon Div.
1960	*Inside Magoo*	ACS

Sources: Compiled from ASCC/ACS Bulletins, Newsletters, and Annual Reports (1913–60); and the collections of the Library of Congress, Film Division* (Washington, D.C.); National Archives* (College Park, Md.); National Library of Medicine* (Bethesda, Md.); ACS film collection* (Atlanta, Ga.); and NCI archives* (Bethesda). Copies of some of these movies are available at locations marked *.

1946;[54] "how-to" instructional movies, from 1948[55]). It was also accompanied by a growing tendency to target movies at particular audiences—television audiences, from 1947/48; schoolchildren, from 1950;[56] ACS volunteers and organizers, from 1955; and especially from the late 1940s, people suffering from or at risk for a variety of different cancers.

54. *The Traitor Within* (1946), an informational movie that outlines the nature of cancer and its treatment, the early warning signs of the disease, and the dangers of folk knowledge and patent medicines; *Man Alive* (1952), the story of Ed Parmlee who fears he may have cancer and is persuaded to see a physician; *Sappy Homiens* (1956), a cartoon/live-action movie in which a cartoonist at the UPA Studios translates the human race into the cartoon character Sappy Homiens, who advocates regular physical check-ups and contributions to the American Cancer Society; *Inside Magoo* (1960), the story of how short-sighted Mr. Magoo is persuaded to "see" a physician for a check-up.

55. American Cancer Society, *Annual Report 1949* (New York[?]: American Cancer Society), p. 43. Instructional movies on breast self-examination included *Life Saving Fingers* (1948) and *Breast Self-Examination* (1950). *We Speak Again* (1949) taught patients with operations for cancer of the larynx to "belch talk." *After Mastectomy* (1958) explored the problems of women living with the results of mastectomy. For reports on *Breast Self-Examination*, see "Film Has Long Way to Go," *ACS Bull.*, 1951, *1* (4): 4; "Store Employees Review BSE Film," ibid., 1952, *1* (18): 3.

56. *From One Cell* (1950): American Cancer Society, *Annual Report 1950* (n. 53), p. 16.

Table 2. Other cancer-education movies (excluding trailers and spots)

Year	Title	Released/produced by
1943	*Cancer*	Iowa State Health Department
1953	*Cancer*	Encyclopedia Britannica Films, Inc.
1954[?]	*One in 20,000*	International Temperance Society
1956	*The Charlatan*	CBS
1957	*Wide Wide World: The Creative Spirit*	NBC Kinescope

Sources: Compiled from ASCC/ACS Bulletins, Newsletters, and Annual Reports (1913–60); and the collections of the Library of Congress, Film Division* (Washington, D.C.); National Archives* (College Park, Md.); National Library of Medicine* (Bethesda, Md.); ACS film collection* (Atlanta, Ga.); and NCI archives* (Bethesda). Copies of some of these movies are available at locations marked *.

The new enthusiasm for movies was facilitated by a new willingness on the part of the ACS leadership to spend money in order to raise money. The leadership believed that the technology offered immense possibilities for fund-raising, especially as the postwar economy boomed. It also believed that movies had great potential for public education. During the war, governmental and medical enthusiasm for (noncancer) public health films aimed at mass audiences of military personnel and civilians had grown substantially as part of a broader effort to mobilize the population for war.[57] The wartime boom had been facilitated in part by a willingness on the part of Hollywood to promote public health issues of importance to the war effort, and the new leadership of the ACS was quick to learn the lesson. It had good connections with Hollywood studios, and increasingly used their stars (and also leading figures from sports, television, and elsewhere) to promote the fight against cancer, following the precedent set by the polio campaigns of the 1930s.[58] The move was timely, given

57. Nichtenhauser, "History of Motion Pictures in Medicine" (n. 1), pp III-281–III-356; Mary Losey, *A Report on the Outlook for the Profitable Production of Documentary Films for the Non-Theatrical Market* (Sugar Research Foundation; Film Program Services, 1948).

58. For the polio campaigns, see David M. Oshinsky, *Polio: An American Story* (New York: Oxford University Press, 2005); Tony Gould, *A Summer Plague: Polio and Its Survivors* (New Haven: Yale University Press, 1995), pp. 54–84; Jane S. Smith, *Patenting the Sun: Polio and the Salk Vaccine* (New York: Morrow, 1990), pp. 72–76; Hugh Gregory Gallagher, *F.D.R.'s Splendid Deception* (New York: Dodd, Mead, 1985), pp. 145–52. For the earlier history of polio, see Naomi Rogers, *Dirt and Disease: Polio Before FDR* (New Brunswick, N.J.: Rutgers University Press, 1992).

the widely publicized deaths from cancer of (among others) Humphrey Bogart and Babe Ruth. Many Hollywood and sports stars appeared in ACS trailers,[59] and the proceeds from opening nights of Hollywood movies were sometimes given over to cancer.[60]

Hollywood also became involved in the production of ACS movies. One of the ACS's first educational movies—*Miracle Money* (1946)—was a rerelease of a prewar Metro-Goldwyn-Mayer dramatic short (originally released in 1938): an antiquackery film, to which the ACS added some information of its own.[61] More commonly the ACS commissioned new movies, especially cartoons, from some of the Hollywood studios: John Sutherland Productions produced *The Traitor Within* (1946), and UPA produced *Man Alive* (1952), *Sappy Homiens* (1956), and *Inside Magoo* (1960).[62] These entertaining and visually imaginative movies allowed the ACS to begin to reopen the doors of cinemas, which the ASCC had felt had closed in the early 1940s. They also gained some recognition from the film industry: *Man Alive* was nominated for an Oscar in 1952.

If Hollywood offered fresh opportunities to get the ACS's message across, so too did the new medium of television.[63] In its advice to local organizers, the ACS stressed the difficulty of forcing an entry into the television market, especially given the competition for airtime from other charities. But from about 1947/48 the ACS produced a profusion of television trailers and "spots" (the latter were one-to-two-minute public service announcements designed to fit into television programming); new ones were usually released in time for the annual cancer week.[64] Some televi-

59. For trailers for movies, see "Bing Crosby's Campaign Motion Picture Trailer Previewed," *ACS Camp. Bull.*, 1948, no. *38*: 1, 4; "Celeste Holm and Five Friends Film 1952 Campaign Trailer," *ACS Bull.*, 1952, *1* (10): 1.

60. "Boston Film Premiere Nets $6,000 for ACS Campaign in Massachusetts," *ACS Camp. Bull.*, 1948, no. *49*: 4.

61. ACS, "Films List," 18 September 1946, Nichtenhauser Papers, MS C 277, box 1, folder "Amer. Cancer Society." For further information on *Miracle Money*, see **http://www.imdb.com/title/tt0030454/** (accessed 24 August 2006).

62. For a review of *The Traitor Within*, see Nichtenhauser Papers, MS C 277, box 19, folder "Reviews C–D." For a content description of the movie, see ibid., box 20, folder "Reviews (Misc.) (3)."

63. For a history of medicine in television, see Joseph Turow, *Playing Doctor: Television, Storytelling, and Medical Power* (New York: Oxford University Press, 1989).

64. "2 ACS Films Set for Television," *ACS Camp. Bull.*, 1948, no. *48*: 3; "Dr. Cameron Featured in New ACS Trailer," *ACS Bull.*, 1952, *1* (9): 2. On the growing importance of television to the ACS, see *Annual Report 1950* (n. 53), p. 15; "Key Men Advise About Radio, TV," *ACS Bull.*, 1952, *1* (11): 1–2; "Volunteer Chairmen Hold Key to Radio, TV Drive," ibid., p. 4; "Radio, TV Policy May Set Pattern," ibid., 1952, *1* (14): 1; "Radio, TV Stations

sion companies broadcast longer ACS propaganda movies,[65] and there is other evidence that television took a growing interest in cancer during this period: cancer became a staple of news reports, current affairs programs, documentaries, educational programs, telethons, and made-for-television movies.[66] In April 1949 the comedian Milton Berle ran a sixteen-hour television "marathon" to raise money for cancer research.[67] In 1956, CBS released *The Charlatan*, a melodrama about a "quack," played by George Sanders, who gets cancer and turns to an orthodox physician for help after his own treatments fail to cure him.[68]

Television and Hollywood may have been crucial to the ACS's efforts to expand education and fund-raising, but so too was a strategy of segmenting the audience to which it sought to appeal. Such segmentation had begun before 1944, with a number of movies specially targeted to women and breast cancer—this even before the creation in 1936 of the Women's Field Army.[69] But the targeting of movies expanded substantially after 1944 as the ACS released films to promote a number of discrete campaigns against breast cancer (from 1948),[70] cancer of the larynx (ca. 1949),[71] lung cancer (1953),[72] and uterine cancer (1957).[73] This targeting

---

Extend ACS Appeal," ibid., *1* (17): 1. Copies of TV spots are available in the ACS audiovisual archive in Atlanta.

65. Such as *You, Time, and Cancer* (1948): "New Cancer Film Prepared for Campaign Use," *Cancer News*, 1948, *2* (4): 16; "New Film Ready for Use in Drive," *ACS Camp. Bull.*, 1948, no. *42*: 2; "Murphy Seeks Check on Film," ibid., no. *44*: 2.

66. The first ACS report of a documentary show was in 1947: "Philadelphia Cancer Television Program," *Cancer News*, 1947, *1* (5): 12; "Television 'Eyes' a Cancer Clinic," *ACS Camp. Bull.*, 1948, no. *31*: 2. Examples of news reports are available in the film collections of the National Archives in College Park and the Library of Congress.

67. Patterson, *Dread Disease* (n. 2), p. 177.

68. According to IMDB the movie was released as part of CBS's *General Electric Theater* series (1953–62), hosted by Ronald Reagan; *The Charlatan* was episode #5.8, 11 November 1956: http://www.imdb.com/title/tt0586283/ (accessed 18 July 2006). IMDB also notes that it was part of the *Studio 57* series in 1956 in open syndication, released 7 November 1956: http://www.imdb.com/title/tt0712106/ (accessed 18 July 2006).

69. Notably *A Fortunate Accident, This Great Peril,* and *Choose to Live.*

70. Gardner, *Early Detection* (n. 2), pp. 110–20.

71. *We Speak Again* was part of a broader program against cancer of the larynx.

72. *The Warning Shadow* (1953) taught about the value of early diagnosis and treatment for lung cancer as part of a broader campaign against this disease: American Cancer Society, *Annual Report 1953* (New York[?]: American Cancer Society), p. 14.

73. *Time and Two Women* (1957) shifted the focus to the dangers of uterine cancer and the value of the Pap smear. In 1958 *Time and Two Women* was seen by 220,000 women; in 1959, by nearly 900,000: American Cancer Society, *Annual Report 1959* (New York[?]: American Cancer Society, 1960), p. 12; Gardner, *Early Detection* (n. 2), pp. 120–26.

provided new opportunities to appeal to groups and individuals about those cancers with which they were particularly concerned. It allowed the ACS both to offer specific information on particular cancers, and to slant, in ways that might appeal to the target group, its general control message: that early detection and treatment were the key to cancer control; that people should learn the early signs of the disease and see a physician the moment they noticed any of these signs; and that they should undergo regular physical examinations.[74] Earlier movies had urged people to examine themselves for the early signs of the disease, and to go for routine *medical* examinations even in the absence of signs or symptoms of the disease. The movies of the 1950s expanded and emphasized these tendencies. They also promoted new techniques of *self*-surveillance of asymptomatic individuals, such as breast self-examination.[75]

The ACS not only targeted movies to particular disease campaigns, it also increasingly targeted them to cancer research, then expanding as never before. It has already been noted that movies had begun to give greater attention to cancer research in the 1930s, but that this new interest in research raised concerns that it might undermine cancer control. Such concerns were largely abandoned after 1944, as the ACS sought to portray research and control as complementary activities. Moreover, with growing concern that the recruitment of scientists into cancer research was low, which might undermine the future expansion of the field, the ACS also began to produce a new type of movie: one aimed more at recruitment than control. Thus in 1950 *From One Cell* was released to educate secondary biology classes about cancer, and so to act as a means of encouraging students into research.[76] Reviews collected by Nichtenhauser were particularly critical of this movie, which, in their view, was ill-focused: "An excellent example of a bad instructional film," one noted.[77] The reviews

74. E.g., *Inside Magoo* (1960) promotes regular check-ups. *The Doctor Speaks His Mind* (1948) recommends check-ups every six months.

75. Gardner, *Early Detection* (n. 2), pp. 110–20. On *Breast Self-Examination*, see American Cancer Society, *Annual Report 1950* (n. 53), pp. 15, 16; *Annual Report 1951* (New York: American Cancer Society), pp. 20–22; "Film Has Long Way to Go; Illinois Makes Plan," *ACS Bull.*, 1951, *1* (4): 4; American Cancer Society, *Annual Report 1952* (New York: American Cancer Society), pp. 15–16, 24; "Self-examination of the Breasts," *Good Housekeeping*, November 1955, p. 32; "A Frank Film Helps Detect Breast Cancer," *Look*, 19 December 1950, p. 87. For a review of *Breast Self Examination* prepared by John L Meyer II in May 1951, see Nichtenhauser Papers, MS C 277, box 19, folder "Reviews N."

76. American Cancer Society, *Annual Report 1950* (n. 53), p. 16.

77. Quoted in memo from Erik Cripps and Marie L. Coleman to Medical Audio-Visual Institute: Drs Ruhe and Nichtenhauser, "Cancer Film Recommendations to State Dept.,"

preferred *Challenge: Science Against Cancer* (1950), released by the National Cancer Institute at the same time for a similar purpose.[78]

Finally, the ACS also began to target the lay volunteers and officials who ran the expanded organization. Lay volunteers had been included in early-detection-and-treatment movies such as *A Fortunate Accident* (1925), *Choose to Live* (1940), and *Time Is Life* (1946), all of which showed women volunteering in the campaign against cancer. But in the late 1940s, the ACS began to produce a new type of educational movie, one focused on the management of a local campaign, rather than on the management of the disease. *To Save These Lives* (1949) aimed to aid the recruitment of volunteers for ACS public-education programs;[79] *The House-to-House Campaign* (1955) taught ACS volunteers and officials how to organize successful door-to-door campaigns; *The Man on the Other Side of the Desk* (1957) showed them how to persuade local radio and TV producers to publicize the ACS; and *Eight Out of Ten* (1957) demonstrated how to organize a state cancer program. Other movies were less pragmatic and more self-congratulatory, such as *Much Ado About Something* (1957), which was an "All Star" round-up that showed how more than a dozen celebrities helped the Society.[80] Finally, the ACS produced *Never Alone* (1958), a celebratory story of the ACS and its work.[81]

---

4 February 1952, Nichtenhauser Papers, MS C 277, box 19, folder "Reviews C–D." See also Medical Audio-Visual Institute of the Association of American Medical Colleges, "Selection of Medical Motion Picture for Use by the Department of State Order No.: NY-14547-(14)-52," "Title of Film: From One Cell," 23 February 1952, ibid.

78. There are two reports on *Challenge: Science Against Cancer* in the Nichtenhauser Papers, one recommending its distribution by the State department, the other not recommending it (the negative recommendation was "no" on the grounds that the movie did not meet the Department of State's specification of a general-audience film in the field of cancer education); the more positive recommendation seems to be in accord with Nichtenhauser's views: Medical Audio-Visual Institute of the Association of American Medical Colleges, "Selection of Medical Motion Picture for Use by the Department of State," "Title of Film: Challenge: Science Against Cancer," [probably March 1952]; Medical Audio-Visual Institute of the Association of American Medical Colleges, "Selection of Medical Motion Picture for Use by the Department of State Order No.: NY-14547-(14)-52," "Title of Film: Challenge: Science Against Cancer," 17 March 1952; both in Nichtenhauser Papers, MS C 277, box 20, folder "Reviews R–S."

79. American Cancer Society, *Annual Report 1950* (n. 53), p. 16. Richard Braddock, "Films for Teaching Mass Communication," *Engl. J.*, 1955, *44* (3): 156–58, 167, at p. 167.

80. American Cancer Society, *Annual Report 1957* (New York [?]: American Cancer Society, 1958), p. 32.

81. American Cancer Society, *ACS Annual Report, 1958* (New York [?]: American Cancer Society), p. 32.

None of this is to say that the ACS abandoned older, pre-1944 uses of the movie.[82] It continued to produce movies to be shown at small, local meetings in town halls, movie theaters, churches, schools, women's clubs, and so on.[83] The standard format for these meetings would have been very familiar to audiences from the 1920s to the early 1940s: educational material such as pamphlets was distributed, and there were lectures and question-and-answer sessions. Like their forebears, many of the new movies were melodramas and conversion narratives that promoted regular examinations and early diagnosis and treatment, and argued that cancer was neither contagious nor hereditary; they also continued to assert medical/male authority over women's beliefs about cancer, but they increasingly sought to supplement this with efforts to convert men to medically approved approaches to cancer.[84] Some post-1944 movies, such as *The Doctor Speaks His Mind* (1948), were "human interest film[s] designed to help the medical speaker by putting his audience in a sympathetic and receptive frame of mind before he has to take the floor."[85] Others such as the tentatively titled *Ask to Live* (1948) were designed for programs where no professional speaker was present.[86] Many movies came with associated educational literature,[87] and were accompanied by newspaper, radio, and television publicity to attract audiences. The huge audiences that attended

82. See, e.g., *The Man on the Other Side of the Desk* and *One in Eight*.

83. For example, the ACS recommended that *You, Time, and Cancer* (1948) be shown to organized groups such as management, labor, fraternal, service, veterans', governmental, agricultural, and women's organizations: "New Cancer Film Prepared for Campaign Use" (n. 65), p. 16; "New Film Ready for Use in Drive" (n. 65), p. 2; "Murphy Seeks Check on Film" (n. 65), p. 2. On women's clubs and post-1944 movies, see Gardner, *Early Detection* (n. 2).

84. For melodramas, see *The Doctor Speaks His Mind* (1948), *Time Is Life* (1946), and *Time and Two Women* (1957). On male/medical authority over women, see *Choose to Live* (1940), *Breast Self-Examination* (1950), *Time Is Life* (1946), and *Time and Two Women* (1957). For movies aimed at men, see esp. *The Traitor Within* (1946), *Man Alive* (1952), and *Inside Magoo* (1960), all cartoons.

85. *The Doctor Speaks His Mind* (1948) follows the response of a physician to the fact that he has had to give the bad news to an old friend who left it too late to go to the doctor—which prompts him to reflect on the various patients he has seen, some of whom delayed and died, others of whom went for a regular check-up and survived. See "New Tools for Lay Education Programs," *Cancer News*, 1948, *2* (10–11): 8–11, at p. 10. For a negative review, see Nichtenhauser Papers, MS C 277, box 19, folder "Reviews C–D."

86. "New Tools for Lay Education Programs" (n. 85), p. 10. The movie was either never produced or retitled, and hence it does not appear in Table 1.

87. The ACS recommended that *The Traitor Within* (1946) be supplemented at each showing with a talk, and the distribution of an ACS folder stressed important points covered in the film: "New Material Developed by Education Department," *Cancer News*, 1947, *1* (5): 8–10, at p. 9; "'The Traitor Within' Seen by 960 Montanans," *ACS Camp. Bull.*, 1948, no. *36*: 2.

Breast Self-Examination (1950) and *Time and Two Women* (1957) were evidence, the ACS felt, of the educational value of the medium. The movie had become an integral part of cancer education.

Managing Responses to the Movies

The movie might have become integral to cancer control, but this did not mean that medical anxieties about its potential to undermine the ACS's educational message had disappeared. To many physicians, movies remained a double-edged sword: they had the power to persuade people to seek early detection and treatment, but they also had the power to dissuade them from this course. They provided a valuable tool for creating a healthy fear of the disease, one that prompted people to see their physicians, especially in the early stages of the disease when the symptoms were least alarming. Yet, movies could also do quite the opposite, promoting delay by creating an unhealthy, debilitating fear—a particular concern at a time when some physicians argued that cancerphobia could result from even the most benign forms of cancer education. The ACS thus had the delicate task of attempting to pick a path between such healthy and unhealthy fears. Yet all too often, healthy fears turned pathological in quite unexpected ways. The public could be so unpredictable that it was entirely possible that an effort to promote healthy fear of the disease could go awry, turning quite unhealthy, and so paralyzing people into inaction.

Such concerns went back to the earliest movies released by the ASCC.[88] Like many cultural critics of the early twentieth century, the Society believed that movies had a particular power to incite emotions in their audiences that could overwhelm any rational response to suggestions that they seek medical assistance at the first signs of the disease.[89] It also believed that the new technology was a particularly blunt instrument for addressing individual fears and concerns about cancer. The movie told the same story time and time again to large audiences, but at the end of the show, people went home to their own private fears and concerns. The movie alone could do little to address these personal responses, and so, by omission, it allowed the fears to fester.

88. The cuts and omissions of *Reward of Courage* and *Choose to Live* can be seen as efforts to manage such emotive responses to the movie.

89. For a discussion of similar concerns in Britain about the response of the public to public-education programs, see David Cantor, "Representing 'the Public': Medicine, Charity and Emotion in Twentieth-Century Britain," in *Medicine, Health and the Public Sphere in Britain, 1600–2000,* ed. Steve Sturdy (London: Routledge, 2002), pp. 145–68.

For both reasons, the ASCC envisaged its movies as embedded in a network of other methods of communication that would allow physicians both to combat the pernicious, emotional impact of movies, and to address how the individual should respond to their standardized message.[90] The public health movie was thus part of a broader system that was a hybrid of mass and personal communication: it embraced mass-communication technologies such as the movies, but it also involved individual face-to-face methods of communication, for example between doctor and patient. Thus, cuts of the sort that Frank J. Osborne proposed in *Reward of Courage* (1921) were not necessarily about censoring a message, but about the appropriate place within this system for addressing particular (especially emotive, disturbing) issues. The problem, as others have noted, is that sometimes discussion about Osborne's particular concern—radical surgery—found no place within this hybrid system: not in the movie, nor in the doctor's office.

Concerns that movies might undermine their own message reinforced the ASCC's caution about funding the technology, especially in tight financial times. After 1944, however, such reasons for caution about funding tended to disappear, and the new leaders of the ACS focused greater attention on developing new methods of managing responses to movies: it took a more systematic interest in movie development and production; it recommended cuts and changes where it felt appropriate; it expanded the publication of associated materials, such as guidelines for physicians on how to respond to questions from their movie-going patients; and it also began screening different versions of its movies to assess audience reactions. For example, when the ACS screened different versions of *Time and Two Women* (1957) it found, to its surprise, that audiences reacted more positively to an unexpurgated version of the movie that showed (in animated form) the spreading and bleeding of cervical cancer, than to a shorter version in which the scene was deleted. Nevertheless, it planned more tests—partly to explore the effect of the movie on anxiety feelings, and partly to identify key points that could be used to guide physicians confronted by women with questions about the film.[91]

90. Movies were generally accompanied by lectures, often by a physician who would also be available to answer questions raised by the audience. The ASCC also assumed that family physicians would supplement the movie's message by addressing the particular concerns of individual patients after the show had left town, and the organization provided fact sheets for physicians to help them address such questions.

91. "Testing of the Film, TIME AND TWO WOMEN," *Signals: [ACS] Public Education Newsletter*, 1957, *1* (1): 3–4. See also the citations in n. 87.

If the new masters of the ACS introduced systematic attempts to monitor and manage audience responses before and after the release of a movie, they also gave more attention to efforts to use movies to manipulate the audience psychologically. The psychology of cancer had been a subsidiary theme of cancer movies before 1944. It will be recalled that *Choose to Live* (1940) emphasized the relief that Mary Brown felt on deciding to go to her physician, even before she heard the diagnosis. Few other movies emphasized relief at this stage of the physician-patient encounter; instead, most tended to acknowledge the anxieties that men and women might feel when they detected a warning sign of cancer, when they awaited word on the results of a test, or when they were medically diagnosed with cancer. Relief, in these movies, tended to come at the end of the medical consultation, when, as was often the cinematic case, the patient was presented with a clean bill of health.[92] In the event of bad news, the moment of relief tended to come after the operation when the patient (at least, the one who had sought early treatment) was cured or in recovery. In either case, the aim was to calm audience fears of cancer or its treatment, and so to promote early detection and treatment, trust in physicians, and distrust of quacks. Relief was a key motif of the conversion narrative, which remained popular throughout the 1950s: the consequence of conversion being not only cure, but relief from anxieties about the disease and its treatment.

The cinematic representation of relief may have gained even greater significance in the 1940s and 1950s as a means of counteracting unwanted responses to the ACS's campaigns. In its public-education efforts, the ACS increasingly emphasized the terrible and deadly nature of cancer in an attempt to scare the public into supporting the organization, and into seeking early detection and treatment.[93] Such themes had been a part of cancer-control messages since the creation of the ASCC in 1913, but the ACS stressed them much more aggressively than its forerunner, leading to fears that it might in fact stimulate a paralyzing cancerphobia that could undermine public cooperation. The cinematic representation of relief can thus be seen as a means by which the ACS sought to work against such a possibility. It served to reassure audiences that all could turn out well, whatever their fears of the disease or its treatment: this

92. For example, the relief of near-sighted Mr. Magoo (*Inside Magoo* [1960]) is signified when he begins dancing with a lamp that he believes to be a nurse.

93. Patterson, *Dread Disease* (n. 2), p. 175. For an alternative perspective on the ACS and scare advertising see Charles Falkner, "Do Cancer Drives Create Fear," Bernarr MacFadden's *Health Rev.*, 1950, *94* (3): 30–31, 58–59.

also at a time when movies such as *Time Is Life* (1946) and *Time and Two Women* (1957) began to broach difficult subjects like radical operations that had hitherto been absent from the public-education screens. It also increasingly served to encourage individuals to adopt medically approved techniques that would help them live without the paralyzing fear of cancer. Thus, *Breast Self-Examination* (1950) argued that one of the major reasons for undertaking self-examination was the sense of relief that women felt at *not* detecting a lump: the relief allowed them to put aside their fear in the interval between examinations. Similarly, *Man Alive* (1952) used the cinematic representation of relief as a means of encouraging men to undergo regular medical examinations, and so to live a normal life free from the anxiety of cancer.[94]

Yet relief could be as much a problem as a help. If relief allowed men and women to abandon debilitating fears of cancer, the risk was that it might also prompt them to swing to the opposite end of the emotional spectrum and abandon fear for complacency. *Man Alive* (1952) makes the point: The movie tells the story of Ed Parmlee, who delays seeking medical help when he fears he might have cancer, only to be told by his physician that he does not have it. Ed leaps with exaggerated relief at the news. But when he lands back on earth he is warned by the narrator that while it was foolish to worry day and night about cancer, it is also foolish not to worry at all. Instead, the narrator urges Ed (and the audience) to be on guard, not to let fear make a mess of their lives, and to use common sense. Ed responds by going (with his wife) for the regular check-up that allows him to enjoy life in the period between examinations. Thus, like many movies of the 1950s, *Man Alive* urged individuals to maintain a *healthy fear* of cancer to motivate them to continue routine examinations, even in the absence of any signs of the disease. And then, to ensure that such healthy fears did not turn unhealthy, the movies of the 1950s also sought to promote routine examinations as a means of regulating people's fears of the disease, always in danger of spiraling out of control in the absence of reassurance.

Thus the cycle of fear and its management went on—movies promoted healthy fears to motivate people to seek help, and then promoted routine examinations as a means of regulating such fears. In this celluloid world,

---

94. For accounts of *Man Alive*, see "Film Is Ready for April Use," *ACS Bull.*, 1952, *1* (12): 1, 4; "'Man Alive' Appears in 'Life,'" ibid., *1* (15): 1; "Illinois Theaters Book ACS Film as A Short Subject on Programs," ibid., *1* (17): 3. For a discussion of the gendered messages in this movie and others, see Leslie Reagan, "Engendering the Dread Disease: Women, Men, and Cancer," *Amer. J. Pub. Health*, 1997, *87*: 1779–87.

the routine examination became a means of managing responses to the movies, just as the movie was a means of promoting routine examinations. This entanglement of objectives highlights, on the one hand, the renewed faith in the movie as a means of promoting cancer control in the 1950s, and, on the other hand, the continuance of concerns about the potential of movies to undermine the very messages they were intended to promote. It also highlights a broader historiographic point. As noted in the introduction to this essay, historians have traced an early twentieth-century enthusiasm for movies as a means of educating the public about health issues. But, if this paper has done anything, it has shown that there is another story to tell, of medical anxieties that movies might weaken the public-education messages they were designed to advance by generating excessive fears of disease, and of how such anxieties shaped both the content of the public-education movie, and the enthusiasm for them as public-education tools. Movies might have been touted as an effective means of public education, but they were also feared for prompting the public to ignore the very lessons they were supposed to learn.

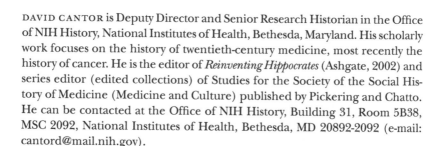

DAVID CANTOR is Deputy Director and Senior Research Historian in the Office of NIH History, National Institutes of Health, Bethesda, Maryland. His scholarly work focuses on the history of twentieth-century medicine, most recently the history of cancer. He is the editor of *Reinventing Hippocrates* (Ashgate, 2002) and series editor (edited collections) of Studies for the Society of the Social History of Medicine (Medicine and Culture) published by Pickering and Chatto. He can be contacted at the Office of NIH History, Building 31, Room 5B38, MSC 2092, National Institutes of Health, Bethesda, MD 20892-2092 (e-mail: cantord@mail.nih.gov).

"For Jimmy and the Boys and Girls of America": Publicizing Childhood Cancers in Twentieth-Century America

GRETCHEN KRUEGER

SUMMARY: This paper examines a collection of images of children printed in cancer education and fund-raising materials distributed by voluntary health organizations, released by public relations departments of specialized cancer hospitals, and featured in popular magazines and newspapers beginning in the late 1940s. Children represented only a small fraction of all persons with cancer, yet they became a key component of the media campaign for the disease. What narratives were embedded in the photographs and profiles? Like the March of Dimes' use of young polio patients to promote their programs, "poster children" were strategically used throughout the mid-to-late twentieth century to advance principles of early cancer detection and prompt treatment; to illustrate or, at times, exaggerate promising biomedical advances in the field; and to elicit emotional responses and donations from a wide audience during the escalation of the war against cancer.

KEYWORDS: cancer, poster child, images, advertising, fund-raising, illness, American Cancer Society

On the evening of 22 May 1948, Ralph Edwards, host of the popular radio program *Truth or Consequences*, introduced his audience to a special guest: "Tonight we take you to a little fellow named Jimmy. We're not going to give you his last name, because he's just like thousands of other young fel-

I would like to thank David Cantor for organizing the "Cancer in the Twentieth Century" workshop, a forum that enabled a small but active community of scholars to share ideas and to form an extended network that has persisted long after the last session of the conference. Such ongoing conversations have strengthened this paper and, consequently, my book manuscript on the history of childhood cancers in America. Both projects have required the able assistance of Thomas Rosenbaum, chief archivist at the Rockefeller Archive Center, Sleepy Hollow, N.Y., and of staff members at the American Cancer Society, Atlanta, Ga.; I am pleased to be able to express my gratitude to these two institutions. Funds to conduct this work were generously provided by Yale University through a John F. Enders Travel Research Grant.

lows and girls in private homes and hospitals all over the country."[1] Without further explanation, the program commenced as Edwards prompted Jimmy to list his favorite Boston Braves players. Members of the team's starting lineup filed into his hospital room one by one, and presented the boy with autographed baseball memorabilia. Jimmy then joined the men in singing "Take Me Out to the Ballgame" on air and received special permission to attend a game the next day—a day designated as "Jimmy's Day" at the ballpark. After his young guest signed off, Edwards told listeners that Jimmy was a twelve-year-old undergoing cancer treatment in Boston. He asked them to contribute money toward a television set for the boy's room and, more generally, to aid "Jimmy and the boys and girls of America."[2] Members of the show's audience responded generously, reportedly donating more than $200,000 to the fund and sending tens of thousands of "get well" cards to Jimmy.[3] By drawing upon child-centered fund-raising strategies pioneered by other earlier voluntary health agencies, the Jimmy Fund and its mission to direct research and treatment toward childhood cancers were launched with overwhelming public support.

In the decades leading up to Edwards's broadcast, a transformation had occurred in American's health: as mortality from common infectious diseases declined, illnesses like heart disease and cancer became leading causes of death in America. In response, the American Society for the Control of Cancer, organized by physicians in 1913, mounted fund-raising and educational efforts through its Women's Field Army to raise public awareness about cancer. The Field Army distributed materials that instructed adults and the elderly about the importance of early detection, the "Warning Signals of Cancer," and the need for prompt treatment by orthodox physicians. By the 1940s, however, childhood cancers had been identified, and cancer-related organizations began integrating the voices, images, and stories of young sufferers into their annual campaigns. Though childhood cancers were rare and differed significantly from cancers commonly observed in adults, children personalized and personified cancer at a time when older patients, their families, and their

---

1. A recording of the original broadcast can be found on the Jimmy Fund Web site at **http://www.jimmyfund.org/abo/broad/jimmybroadcast.asp** (accessed 14 November 2006). See also Saul Wisnia, *Images of America: The Jimmy Fund of the Dana-Farber Cancer Institute* (Charleston, S.C.: Arcadia, 2002), pp. 18–19, for a rough transcript.

2. Wisnia, *Images of America* (n. 1), p. 19.

3. George E. Foley, ed., *The Children's Cancer Foundation: The House That "Jimmy" Built, The First Quarter-Century* (Boston: Dana-Farber Cancer Institute, n.d.), p. 43.

physicians often remained hushed about the dread disease and its grim prognosis.[4]

In this paper I explore the disproportionate use of children in major cancer campaigns mounted by Memorial Hospital for Cancer and Allied Diseases, the Jimmy Fund, the American Cancer Society, and other groups in the mid-twentieth century. What does an analysis of these images and strategies reveal about disease-centered education or fund-raising efforts during this period? Did they reflect changes in cancer research or treatment? What strategies did publicists borrow when incorporating children into cancer campaigns? Historians have harshly criticized mismatches between the depictions of ill children and the lived experience of the disease, such as the "poster children" carefully selected, posed, and displayed by the March of Dimes to promote the possibility of rehabilitation and recovery.[5] Similar arguments can be made regarding the use of young cancer sufferers. Staged photographs of children with cancer—standing side by side with famous personalities, or celebrating holidays in hospital wards—elevated viewers' emotional tie to the cancer cause without informing them of the actual incidence or course of the disease. However, by pairing these sentimental images with frightening captions and text, cancer institutions and associations sent parents a stern warning: *any* child, *every* child, or even *their* child was vulnerable to the threat of this grave set of diseases. This juxtaposition provided evidence for publicists' principal claim—that by supporting basic and clinical cancer research programs, donors could end the loss of young,

4. See James T. Patterson, *The Dread Disease: Cancer and Modern American Culture* (Cambridge: Harvard University Press, 1987), and Susan Sontag, *Illness as Metaphor and AIDS and Its Metaphors* (New York: Doubleday, 1990), for the authors' description of the silence, secrecy, and even shame surrounding cancer and its sufferers. In a recent article, historian Barbara Clow contested this thesis, drawing upon a range of sources that revealed popular and professional views toward cancer in the early twentieth century: Barbara Clow, "Who's Afraid of Susan Sontag? or, The Myths and Metaphors of Cancer Reconsidered," *Soc. Hist. Med.*, 2001, *14*: 293–312, for a full discussion. My purpose in this paper is not to take a stance in the debate, but to suggest that it may be valuable for historians to consider how pictorial evidence from the mid-to-late twentieth century may contribute to the analysis.

5. Historians of polio have been outspoken about the use of children by the National Foundation for Infantile Paralysis (NFIP) to appeal to donors and expand their coffers. Tony Gould, in *A Summer Plague: Polio and Its Survivors* (New Haven: Yale University Press, 1995), attacked the NFIP's use of stories about patients or storytelling by patients to promote its activities. Jane Smith has argued that the NFIP used the pathos of children to manipulate the public to generously support its activities: see Jane S. Smith, *Patenting the Sun: Polio and the Salk Vaccine* (New York: Morrow, 1990), pp. 44, 83, for sample images and a fuller discussion. Naomi Rogers, in the epilogue to *Dirt and Disease: Polio Before FDR* (Rutgers: Rutgers University Press, 1992), p. 172, summarized historians' analyses of the NFIP's methods.

innocent lives from cancer and contribute to the cure of *all* cancers. Such child-centered publicity peaked in the late 1940s through the early 1960s when new chemotherapeutic agents produced the first dramatic remissions in young cancer patients, then reappeared twenty years later when the advent of intensive combination chemotherapy protocols increased long-term survival rates and caused a visible side effect that required no interpretation for viewers—complete hair loss.

Redefining Cancer

During the "Golden Age of Illustration" in the late 1800s, images of children advertised consumer goods,[6] raised support for child-centered health and welfare reforms,[7] and heightened lay awareness of specific diseases both in the popular press and in materials produced and distributed by voluntary health agencies. Newspapers solicited funds for children and families suffering from debilitating or deadly diseases by pairing dramatic accounts with vivid visual media. For example, in 1885 the story of five Newark boys bitten by a rabid dog spread through sustained news coverage in the form of newspaper appeals, published firsthand interviews and political cartoons, and public appearances. Historian Bert Hansen has argued that the publicity surrounding this affair changed lay expectations about medical "breakthroughs" like Pasteur's experimental vaccine and set a pattern for how other scientific discoveries were reported and, perhaps, publicly received.[8] Historian Nancy Tomes has expanded upon Hansen's analysis by using the case study to explore the marketing

6. Companies frequently incorporated depictions of children in their advertisements to promote a wide array of consumer goods, including foods, personal hygiene products, and household cleaning supplies; caricatured drawings of the Romantic child emphasized a direct link between health, sanitation, and the well-being of the entire family. See Nancy Tomes, *The Gospel of Germs: Men, Women, and the Microbe in American Life* (Cambridge: Harvard University Press, 1998); Eileen Margerum, "The Child in American Advertising, 1890–1960: Reflections of a Changing Society," in *Images of the Child*, ed. Harry Eiss (Bowling Green, Ohio: Bowling Green State University Popular Press, 1994), p. 337.

7. Photographers Jacob Riis and Lewis Hine attended to their young subjects' expressions and surroundings to capture realistic images of the "child in peril" on film and to persuade middle-class viewers to support health and welfare reforms. See Anne Higonnet, *Pictures of Innocence: The History and Crisis of Ideal Childhood* (New York: Thames and Hudson, 1998), p. 116, for a discussion of the work of WPA photographers Dorothea Lange and Walker Evans as they used pictures of children to reveal the daily lives of entire families and communities.

8. Bert Hansen, "America's First Medical Breakthrough: How Popular Excitement about a French Rabies Cure in 1885 Raised New Expectations for Medical Progress," *Amer. Hist. Rev.*, 1998, *103*: 373–418.

of disease; the ongoing narrative of the boys' experiences did not simply describe a sequence of events, she insists, but combined "journalism, advertising, and entertainment media" to represent a feared disease.[9]

The profitable triad was skillfully replicated in subsequent health campaigns for other infectious, epidemic diseases such as tuberculosis. In *Gospel of Germs*, Tomes demonstrates that voluntary tuberculosis associations deliberately placed children at the center of their activities: "In their white capes and elaborate hats, they became a sort of human figure trademark. Like the manufacturers of Sun Maid Raisins and Packer's Tar Soap, the anti-TB societies realized, in the words of one Brooklyn worker, that 'children are a very good advertising medium.'"[10] Publicity photographs showed young volunteers, known as Crusaders, canvassing their communities selling Christmas Seals to raise money for local and national TB efforts. Representations of mothers and children on TB posters not only instructed viewers in proper hygienic practices, but also served as advertisements for the group's activities. These methods skillfully extended the association's reach into communities, raised sympathy for the disease's human toll, educated laypersons about prevention, and informed the nation of TB's economic cost—priorities soon adopted by the Public Affairs Department at the Memorial Hospital for Cancer and Allied Diseases in New York City as physicians identified a new threat to child health.

Beginning in the late 1930s and 1940s, as Memorial began to create new services to research and treat children, young sufferers began to dot the institution's publicity and fund-raising materials. In 1933, George Pack and Hayes Martin organized separate clinics in the Mixed Tumor and Head and Neck Divisions to accommodate young patients; the next year, a small pediatric ward with four beds was opened.[11] In 1935, Memorial's Medical Board approved the appointment of Harold Dargeon as consulting pediatrician as a way to emphasize "the concept of a child as a person suffering from a grave illness" rather than a disease-centered approach.[12]

9. Nancy Tomes, "Epidemic Entertainments: Disease and Popular Culture in Early-Twentieth-Century America," *Amer. Lit. Hist.*, 2002, *14*: 625–52, on p. 628.

10. Tomes, *Gospel of Germs* (n. 6), p. 123. Michael E. Teller also briefly described the Christmas Seal campaign in *The Tuberculosis Movement: A Public Health Campaign in the Progressive Era* (Westport, Conn.: Greenwood Press, 1988), pp. 41–42.

11. During Memorial's first fifty years, physicians at the hospital treated children with cancer in the same wards as adults. See George Pack and Robert LeFevre, "The Age and Sex Distribution and Incidence of Neoplastic Diseases at the Memorial Hospital," *J. Cancer Res.*, 1930, *14*: 167–294.

12. Harold Dargeon, "Pediatrics at Memorial Hospital for Cancer and Allied Diseases," 1967, Memorial Sloan Kettering Cancer Center Papers, Rockefeller Archive Center, Pocantico Hills, N.Y. (hereafter MSKCC Papers). The board supported Dargeon and the

By reorganizing its facilities and hiring new staff members, the major cancer hospital acknowledged that children were a distinct population with unique needs. Yet, these initiatives alone did not foster the departmental cooperation required to accurately identify and classify rare childhood cancers.

In 1937, the Pediatric Section of the New York Academy of Medicine sponsored a symposium in which physicians from across Memorial's departments presented cases of cancer in children. In the introduction to *Cancer in Childhood*, the published conference proceedings, coeditors Harold Dargeon and James Ewing (director of Memorial Hospital) summarized the patterns that emerged from the institution's data and compared them to the extant medical literature. They concluded that physicians had previously relied on improper age divisions, incorrect tumor classifications, and small sample sizes when studying cancer in children; consequently, few differences between the cancers that affected children and those that struck adults had been detected. "It is clear," Ewing insisted, "that the conditions of origin and the clinical course of these diseases are so peculiar that they may not be properly compared with any adult tumors, and that this entire subject deserves to be treated as a special department in the descriptive history of neoplastic diseases."[13] In order to keep a quantitative record of cases and a qualitative description of the common tumor types observed in the hospital, the physicians established a Children's Tumor Registry. Statistics drawn from the Registry and other local health records confirmed that pediatric cancers, though rare, were second only to accidents as a cause of mortality in children. This evidence fueled Memorial's child-centered activities and its plans for expansion.

In 1940, Memorial created a seventeen-bed Children's Pavilion, the first facility built specifically to accommodate children with cancer. Articles printed in newspapers and magazines highlighted the Pavilion's "children's corner," an outdoor terrace space that housed a slide and carousel, a classroom designed for young patients who felt well enough to complete schoolwork, and multipurpose areas for working on crafts or singing along to piano accompaniment.[14] Many photographs also showed children

---

Department of Cancer in Children, but critics termed work in the field of pediatric cancer unrealistic and viewed these young cases as hopeless.

13. Harold Dargeon and James Ewing, eds., *Cancer in Childhood and a Discussion of Certain Benign Tumors* (St. Louis: Mosby, 1940), p. 14.

14. Dargeon, "Pediatrics at Memorial Hospital" (n. 12); "First Child-Cancer Ward Functioning in New York," *Newsweek*, 15 January 1940, 1939–40 Scrapbook, MSKCC Papers; *Bridge League Bull.*, November 1939, ibid.

gathered around a large, gaily painted wooden cart overflowing with balloons, plastic toys, dolls, and comic books that was regularly wheeled to the Pavilion and the outpatient clinic by volunteers and members of the Recreation Department staff.[15] In contrast to the few photographs taken of young patients in the early 1930s that depicted bleak hospital rooms and ill children aided by slings or wheelchairs, images released by Memorial's Public Affairs Department in the 1940s featured its expanding medical and social programs for children hospitalized with cancer.[16] By circulating images that focused on young patients who appeared healthy and engaged in familiar routines, a positive message about the specialized hospital's ability to preserve health and conquer disease reached potential donors. However, such images of young victims were exceedingly optimistic at a time when few curative treatments were available.

In some cases, Memorial's Public Affairs Department masked or downplayed physical manifestations of cancer in photographs, yet paired the sentimental images with provocative headlines, captions, or text to amplify their impact and reveal the underlying message the publicity staff wanted to convey to donors. A photograph reprinted in dozens of regional newspapers featured three little boys in bib overalls walking together to the washroom toting toothbrushes, towels, and cups. In another image from the same series, one of the boys perched on a step stool to reach the sink. At first glance, these seemed to be snapshots of children caught in the midst of a simple, daily routine. However, the declaration "Cancer Struck All Three" and the serious warning "Guard those you love from this scourge of childhood" accompanied the photograph in several newspapers.[17] Unlike the "poster children" chosen by the March of Dimes who often wielded braces or crutches to cue the viewer that they were recovering from polio, these children displayed no obvious, outward signs of ill health.

15. E.g., photograph, November 1956, RG 400.1, ser. 4, box 1 Public Affairs—Photos Department (hereafter PA-Photos), folder 48, MSKCC Papers. The caption reflects the tone adopted by the department when describing its services for children: "The toy cart provides a treat for youngsters who must come to the Tower Outpatient Clinic for treatment periodically. Clinic day is party day, and each child gets a gift and refreshments after treatment. The toy cart is stocked and operated by Volunteers. Those children who must stay in the hospital are also treated to parties and recreation activities."

16. E.g., photograph, November 1934, PA-Photos, folder 45. The MSKCC Papers include dozens of photographs from the Public Affairs office. Photographs of the children's ward are filed by categories such as recreation, nursing-aides, Christmas, etc. Unfortunately, only a portion of the photographs are dated or labeled with captions.

17. E.g., *Bloomfield (N.J.) Independent Press*, 1939–40 Scrapbook, MSKCC Papers; photograph, no date, PA-Photos, folder 45.

Such masking techniques were also used in the most common type of publicity photograph—the holiday snapshot. Festivities with lavish decorations provided celebratory backdrops for many photographs as children donned Halloween masks, visited with the Easter bunny, and opened gifts from celebrities dressed as Santa Claus.[18] The caption for one such image read, "An Easter Day party in the Children's Ward of Memorial Center for Cancer and Allied Diseases. People often do not realize that cancer strikes children as well as adults. Yet more children in this country between the ages of 5 and 9 die of cancer than of any other disease."[19] The stark contrast between the joyous scene filled with spring flowers and plush toy rabbits and grim facts about a little-known disease must have shocked viewers who may have been encountering it for the first time. The use of everyday images, grim statistics, and stern warnings alerted parents to this newly recognized menace to child health, but provided little information about the signs of the disease, the limited treatments, its deadly course, or concrete measures that parents could implement. Instead, the staged publicity shots focused attention on the hospital's growing pediatric spaces and services—the means for preserving and restoring children's health.

According to announcements about newly opened facilities or appeals for construction projects, there was a dire need for Memorial's initiatives. In "Children in Danger," an article describing Memorial's new cancer-prevention clinic, a photograph showed two tables of children wearing paper hats and busily working on crafts as they waited for their appointments. The image promoted the idea that the young visitors to the clinic often appeared perfectly healthy, but needed to undergo a complete medical assessment to ensure wellness. The first sentences of the accompanying text, however, described the striking signs of childhood cancers observed by the clinic's medical staff: "One small boy had a persistent swelling on his leg which his careless mother dismissed as a 'bump.' Another child's eyes were strangely protuberant. A third's head changed its size so rapidly he needed a new hat every few months."[20] The contradictory message

18. E.g., Halloween—Children's Ward, stamped as February 1949, PA-Photos, folder 43; Christmas—Children's Ward, 1949, ibid., folder 36; Christmas party, 1945, ibid., folder 31; Christmas—Children's Ward, no date, ibid.

19. Easter Day party, 1949, ibid., folder 40.

20. "Children in Danger," *Newsweek*, 10 March 1947, p. 54. A second photograph showed a family that had benefited from the clinic's services: a smiling boy balanced on his father's knee as his mother crouched beside him. The boy's leg had been amputated, but he appeared to have fully regained his health. Just a year earlier, a promotional photograph published as part of a fund-raising appeal for Memorial had pictured the same boy immediately after surgery: he appeared pale and weak, and a large stuffed rabbit partially masked

conveyed by juxtaposing the image of "normal" children in the waiting room with the graphic descriptions of children's outward signs moved parents to action: only two years after the clinic opened its doors, appointments were filled for a year in advance.

Dramatic, personal stories of young victims and families publicized Memorial's role as a renowned cancer center and, for some, a place of last resort. The story of eight-year-old Dorothy Lewis broadcast the face of childhood cancer and the controversial nature of its treatment.[21] When Dorothy's father, William Lewis, a laborer for the Queens Park Department, refused to allow surgeons to amputate his daughter's leg, a protracted battle had ensued. Physicians insisted that radical surgery was required in order to remove the girl's malignant bone tumor, but Lewis feared the resulting disability. Under increasing pressure from doctors and newspaper readers who followed the story, Lewis agreed to let his daughter undergo weekly radiation therapy at Memorial and, after further complications, permitted physicians at Memorial to amputate Dorothy's right leg nearly a year after her initial diagnosis.[22] The photograph printed in a follow-up article showed Dorothy posed in a chair with her arms wrapped around her favorite dolls. As in many of Memorial's publicity photographs, signs of her surgery and recovery were skillfully concealed.[23]

While some were skeptical of Memorial's invasive approach, the hospital continued to attract children and families from across the country and around the world in the mid-to-late 1940s. A series of newspaper articles described families who had been separated by World War II but were reunited prematurely after receiving childhood cancer diagnoses. In January 1946, a collage of photographs published in the *New York Journal American* featured a picture of a nurse cradling a small infant in her arms. The infant's father, a member of the Navy, had flown from a

---

the space left by the radical operation. The image was one of several included in a spread entitled "Why Memorial Hospital Appeals for Public Aid in Fund Drive," *New York Journal American*, 4 January 1946, 1946 Scrapbook, MSKCC Papers. A comparison of the two images shows how the Public Affairs Department manipulated images of their young patients to fulfill a range of goals.

21. See Gretchen Krueger, "'A Cure Is Near': Children, Families, and Cancer in America, 1945–1980" (Ph.D. diss., Yale University, 2003), for an extended discussion of how patients and families continually negotiated the changing medical management of pediatric cancers during these pivotal years of childhood cancer research and treatment.

22. "Girl Fights Bone Cancer. Father Hoped to Save Her from Being Crippled," *Brooklyn Eagle*, 27 September 1939, 1939–40 Scrapbook, MSKCC Papers. The story was also widely distributed by the Associated Press.

23. "Valiant Is the Word," *New York Journal American*, 11 October 1939, pp. 6–7, 1939–40 Scrapbook, MSKCC Papers.

Pacific base to visit his sick son. Using references to the war in its appeal, the caption read:

> More persons were killed at home by cancer during the war than by bullets and shells in battle. At long last, it seems the public is beginning to realize that cancer is a disease that must be fought militantly with thousands of dollars for research as to its cause and more thousands to arrest in time the disease in victims who have just contracted it.[24]

Later that month, Lieutenant Keith DuBois flew on an Army transport plane from Germany to Memorial Hospital in order to see his eight-month-old son Allan for the first time. Referred by their family physician, his wife and son had traveled from Green Bay, Wisconsin, to New York City for care. DuBois affirmed that it was "wonderful" to see his son, but when questioned further about his emergency homecoming he admitted that "this isn't the way I dreamed about it . . . this isn't the way I wanted it."[25] Following the successful removal of his son's malignant tumor, photographs printed in newspapers across the region showed DuBois dressed in military uniform as he carried his son out of the hospital. The picture suggested that DuBois's battle on the domestic front may also have ended in victory.

Pedro Villegas, father of four-month-old Blanca, flew his daughter from Bogota, Colombia, to Memorial Hospital after discovering a suspicious tumor. Blanca, one of the youngest patients in the Children's Ward, had been in the ward for treatment and observation for more than six months when the Public Affairs Department released a photograph of her first birthday party, replete with flowers, gaily wrapped gifts, and a table full of sweets.[26] As a nurse wearing a gauze mask set a small cake on the tray of Blanca's high chair, she gently curbed the infant's hand from touching the single lit candle. Although the picture included only Blanca, the nurse, and another patient, the caption explained that Blanca's father and many hospital staff and volunteers working on the Memorial Cancer Center Fund Campaign had attended the party for the little girl who had become the "pet" of the unit. Like the arrival of the servicemen to visit their children, the celebration and the girl's plight were explicitly linked to a major fund-raising appeal that was to include not only the construction of the Helena Woolworth McCann Children's Pavilion, but an expansion that included the Sloan Kettering Institute for Cancer

24. "Why Memorial Hospital Appeals for Public Aid" (n. 20).
25. "Officer in from Germany Sees Son First Time in Cancer Ward," *Herald Tribune,* 19 January 1946, 1946 Scrapbook, MSKCC Papers.
26. Photograph of Blanca Villegas, no date, PA-Photos, folder 46.

Research, the James Ewing Hospital, and the Tower Building for Memorial Center outpatients to increase the hospital's overall patient capacity and expand its services.[27] While children with cancer composed only a small percentage of the institution's total patient population, they were repeatedly used to demonstrate Memorial's mission to "accept responsibility for all aspects of the control of childhood neoplasms," to raise money for *all* of Memorial's activities, and, in the 1950s, to vividly illustrate first successes in treating common childhood cancers with experimental chemotherapeutic agents.[28]

Jimmy Captures the Limelight

In the late 1940s, as Memorial developed its child-centered research programs and clinical facilities, the first chemotherapeutic agent effective against acute leukemia (the most common childhood cancer) was evaluated in the laboratory and clinic. Sidney Farber, chief pathologist at Children's Hospital in Boston, observed that daily injections of aminopterin, a folic acid antagonist that disrupted cancer cells' metabolism, induced temporary remissions in ten of fifteen young patients with acute leukemia.[29] Although other clinical investigators initially doubted his results, Farber and many journalists advanced his discovery as a preliminary step in the synthesis and testing of chemical agents for all systemic cancers and solid tumors.[30] As a way to sidestep his critics, Farber looked outside his

27. Despite the major construction projects, Memorial did not have a bed available for every ill child. Children without reservations—even those whose families had traveled long distances—had to be refused admission and were diverted to neighboring hospitals for care.

28. Memorial Center for Cancer and Allied Diseases, *Quadrennial Report, 1947–51* (New York: Memorial Center for Cancer and Allied Diseases, 1951), p. 67. In the 1950s, Memorial integrated children into radio spots and television shows, including appearances on the *Today Show, Conquest* (produced by the American Association for the Advancement of Science and the National Academy of Sciences), and *Medicine U.S.A.—The Living Proof* (produced by the American Medical Association).

29. Sidney Farber et al., "Temporary Remissions in Acute Leukemia in Children Produced by Folic Acid Antagonist 4-aminopteroyl-glutamic acid (Aminopterin)," *New England J. Med.*, 1948, *238*: 787–93. Before the discovery of aminopterin, young patients suffering from acute leukemia died within two months of the onset of the disease.

30. In the 1940s and 1950s, journalists enumerated wartime discoveries and pointed to postwar gains to assure the public that scientists would soon discover "magic bullets" to cure disease. See "Hope for Leukemia," *Newsweek*, 26 April 1948, p. 48, to read a description of Farber's clinical results. Despite such heady predictions and increased public support for research, the promise of a cure for cancer remained largely unfulfilled. See Marcel C. LaFollette, *Making Science Our Own: Public Images of Science, 1910–1955* (Chicago: University of Chicago Press, 1990).

home institution for endorsement of his work—becoming a leader in the American Cancer Society, providing expert testimony at Congressional hearings, and establishing a new fund-raising organization.

By forging partnerships with civically minded groups in the Boston area, Farber established the Children's Cancer Research Foundation (CCRF), a regional platform for expanding the provision of treatment for children with cancer and furthering his own clinical program. In 1947 the Variety Club of New England, an organization of men working in the motion picture and theater business, had pledged $50,000 to establish a Blood Bank and Blood Research Department at the Children's Medical Center in Boston.[31] However, after one of the Club's committees toured the children's cancer ward during a hospital visit and learned about Farber's promising investigations, they joined with the Boston Braves to establish the CCRF. Through the special broadcast of *Truth or Consequences* in 1948, they launched the Jimmy Fund as the organization's fund-raising arm (Fig. 1).

The Fund emphasized its dedication to individual, young cancer sufferers by replicating a strategy pioneered by the March of Dimes—the "poster child." At the kick-off of its annual March of Dimes campaign in 1946, the National Foundation for Infantile Paralysis (NFIP) had introduced its first poster child at a formal White House ceremony. National, regional, and local poster children helped viewers personally relate to polio sufferers and added a sense of immediacy to the threat. Outfitted in crisp dresses and fringed cowboy costumes, accompanied by children's toys or characters, and captured in childlike poses, the posters' subjects were pictured as young, defenseless victims of the disease. "Before and after" images suggested that donations to the March of Dimes directed toward proper rehabilitation programs and disease-specific research would enable children to overcome polio's physical effects and rejoin their peers at play.[32]

Historians of polio have long argued that poster children did not accurately reflect the reality of all sufferers—the diverse ages of those stricken,

31. The Variety Club International had first formed after a group of showmen found an abandoned child in a Pittsburgh movie theater in December 1929. The organization's efforts branched out in many directions, but remained focused on the spiritual, physical, and medical needs of underprivileged children.

32. Franklin Roosevelt created this ideal through his public comments about the disease and the strict control of his physical image in public appearances. Daniel Wilson has shown that illness narratives and correspondence written by polio survivors and their families perpetuated this myth: Daniel J. Wilson, *Living with Polio: The Epidemic and Its Survivors* (Chicago: University of Chicago Press, 2005).

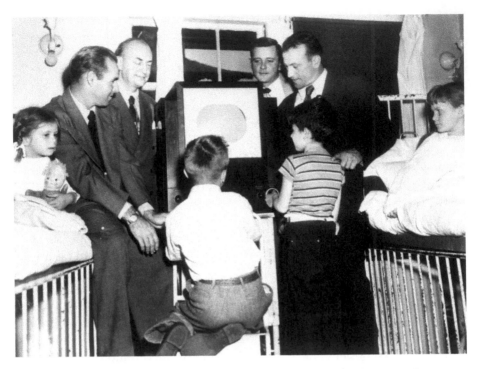

Fig. 2.1. Soon after the broadcast of Jimmy's radio interview, Massachusetts Governor Christian Herter declared the summer of 1948 "Jimmy Fund Time." Baseball-themed "Jimmy Days" were held throughout New England, with Boston Braves players and Variety Club members helping children raise money for a television (above) for the fund's namesake and the Children's Cancer Research Foundation. (Courtesy of the Dana-Farber Cancer Institute, Boston, Mass.)

the severity of paralysis, the grueling rehabilitation routines, and the number of sufferers who never regained full function of their muscles. Rather than disseminating realistic depictions and descriptions of polio and its sufferers, the NFIP has been characterized as a "publicity machine" that utilized "unashamedly sentimental" methods to raise the public's concern about polio and its dangers.[33] The strategy, however, proved to

33. While some parents clamored to have their child selected, other families who had received funds from the organization for the expensive treatment and lengthy rehabilitation expressed reluctance toward participating in the March of Dimes campaigns. One beneficiary recalled, "When I was in both hospitals the National Foundation paid for everything. My parents were not able to pay. So I felt obligated later when everyone wanted stories. They were using me to elicit sympathy so people would part with their money" (quoted in Nina Gilden Seavey, Jane S. Smith, and Paul Wagner, eds., *A Paralyzing Fear: The Triumph over Polio in America* [New York: TV Books, 1998], p. 30).

be a fund-raising tool with broad appeal. Unlike other campaigns that had solicited large donations from a few wealthy patrons, the March of Dimes mounted a citizens' attack on disease. Annual Birthday Balls and appeals made by poster children motivated a broad base of donors who had benefited from the country's economic expansion to devote their spare change to improving the nation's health.[34]

Two years after the March of Dimes introduced its first poster child, the CCRF began planning for its inaugural event. It molded its representative by changing the boy's name from Einar Gustafson to "Jimmy" to protect his privacy and, perhaps, to attach a common boy's name to their efforts. By choosing this pseudonym and playing up his avid interest in the local professional baseball team, publicists created a poster child with all-American attributes and interests.[35] "Jimmy" served several important purposes: he appealed to regional donors, he personified cancer, and he reminded donors that cancer did not spare children. While the original "Jimmy" only participated in the Fund's launch before returning to his family's farm in Maine, the foundation retained its focus on child sufferers by permanently associating his name and a sketch of a boy's profile with all of its fund-raising and promotional activities.

The Jimmy Fund employed a number of visual techniques to illustrate its message that by contributing dollars to biomedical research, a cure for cancer would surely be discovered (Fig. 2). Fund-raising canisters placed at stores and sporting events used the March of Dimes' "before and after" strategy: They pictured a line drawing of a boy in a wheelchair gazing out a window under the query, "I can *DREAM* can't I?" Beneath the plea, a second image displayed the boy's dream of sliding into home base, evading the catcher's efforts to tag him. Overhead, the umpire declared him "safe." Between the two images, the words "Jimmy Fund" were boldly printed to identify the boy's source of hope and recovery. Canisters, movie theater collections, ballpark promotions, and appearances by celebrities

34. A survey of voluntary health agencies made in the early 1940s by the National Health Council studied the growth, organization, and activities of such groups, with the goal of coordinating their efforts under one umbrella. The report noted that new fund-raising strategies aimed to "sell" disease to a broad set of consumers, and that "the picture of the suffering child takes priority over any appeal concerning adults" (Selskar M. Gunn and Philip S. Platt, *Voluntary Health Agencies: An Interpretive Study* [New York: Ronald Press, 1945], p. 219).

35. It is important to note that few of the poster children selected by the March of Dimes or the patients selected by Memorial captured the diverse population of young patients that must have been admitted by the hospital. In one photograph, an African-American child watched television from his bed: Children's Ward Recreation, no date, RG 400.1, ser. 4, box 2, folder 52, MSKCC Papers. Another photograph showed two physicians examining an African-American child: Children's Ward Treatment, ibid., folder 55.

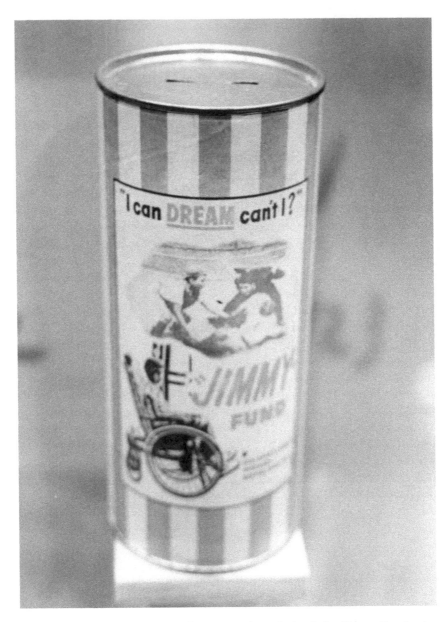

Fig. 2.2. The advent of coin-collection canisters helped the Jimmy Fund raise more than $200,000 by the end of its first campaign season. Several dozen canisters—each labeled with the name of a young patient with cancer—were commonly displayed in the lobbies of movie theaters or passed through audiences by ushers and volunteers before the start of the film. (Courtesy of the Dana-Farber Cancer Institute, Boston, Mass.)

like famed baseball player Ted Williams all prominently featured children in their appeals.[36]

Early donations to the CCRF financed the construction of the Jimmy Fund Building, a modern, technological space for pediatric cancer research and treatment that accommodated children's sizes and needs.[37] At the formal dedication ceremonies in January 1952, Farber and other noted speakers reaffirmed their commitment to a child-centered fund-raising mission, research agenda, and building design. Farber said that he mobilized his staff by framing research projects around "a given patient—a patient with a name, a patient with a personality, . . . the child of parents who are concerned over the welfare of their child."[38] The individual patient who suffered from a particular cancer became the motivation for his research programs and the "total care" model implemented at the facility—a model that emphasized the physical, emotional, and social components of disease as it affected patients and family members. Similarly, the comments made by the dean of the Harvard Medical School emphasized the particular tragedy caused by malignant disease when it affected a young person. He posited that it was the age of the victims that had moved donors to give generously. A third speaker framed the link between the Jimmy Fund and the protection of children in terms of national strength and pride, stating that the people of New England had generously undertaken "this project dedicated to the alleviation of suffering among children and the building of strong bodies and strong minds in true American tradition."[39] The speakers' comments revealed the value of children in America—as individuals, as part of a defined cohort, as family members, and as future citizens. Premature death caused by cancer was a tragedy that deeply affected the family as well as the prospering nation. Rather than simply appending child-focused research and treatment programs to an existing cancer center, cancer in children was now promoted in Boston and New England as a major problem of child health that merited public support and an independent facility.

36. See Wisnia, *Images of America* (n. 1), for a chronological overview of the Jimmy Fund's fund-raising activities.

37. Tom Fleming and Alice Fleming, "Special Report: Cancer in Children," *Cosmopolitan*, August 1963, pp. 52–57, provided a glimpse into the clinical facility in the early 1960s. The waiting room included a merry-go-round and a television set that was mounted within the rugged landscape of a large train set. Tricycles provided kid-sized transportation from the waiting area to the laboratory for blood work. Disney illustrators painted murals of scenes from familiar children's films in hallways and treatment rooms.

38. Foley, *Children's Cancer Foundation* (n. 3), p. 16.

39. Ibid., p. 8.

Wielding the Sword

In the 1940s and 1950s, under the direction of its reorganized board and of Mary Lasker, a society woman and health philanthropist familiar with modern advertising techniques, the American Cancer Society expanded its publicity methods from door-to-door campaigns to annual conventions and appearances, radio spots and articles in popular magazines, and new ACS publications.[40] As part of this proliferation, the ACS added images of child sufferers and young donors to its materials to motivate fund-raising volunteers and inspire benefactors to generously support ACS programs— although the Society's budget and activities focused primarily on adults. Annual ACS fund-raising activities spotlighted young cancer sufferers and survivors to personify advances in cancer therapy through "miraculous" stories of recovery. Unlike medical journal articles that reported minimal or unpredictable improvements in remission rates and overall survival, the ACS selected stories that overstated the efficacy of surgical treatments and new chemotherapeutic agents while downplaying their limitations, side effects, or short duration.[41]

The ACS asked patients to personally appear at annual fund-raising conventions to vividly demonstrate the efficacy of new cancer therapies. In 1953, five cancer patients (two children and three adults) stood on a platform facing the convention attendees as physicians described the course of their cancer treatment. Of the patients, four-year-old leukemia patient Jennifer McCollum garnered the most attention. Treated with aminopterin, the hormone ACTH, and an experimental drug supplied by Memorial, Jennifer's cancer went into remission; her presence on stage thus provided visible proof that chemotherapy prolonged the life of children whose diagnoses had previously equaled an inevitable death sentence. Organizers hoped that her story would inspire those gathered in Chicago to raise the $18 million needed to support the Society's activi-

---

40. See Patterson, *Dread Disease* (n. 4), for a general account of the American Cancer Society and the history of cancer in the United States. Patterson does not discuss children and cancer at length, but includes chemotherapy and its application to acute leukemia in his chapter "The Research Explosion."

41. Medical photographs of young acute leukemia sufferers documented the physical manifestations of the disease, including oral ulcers and uncontrollable hemorrhaging, and illustrated the dramatic cycles of remission and relapse induced by new chemotherapeutic agents: "Leukemia in Children and Adults," *CA: Bull. Cancer Prog.*, 1957, 7 (2): 54. See Daniel Fox and Christopher Lawrence, *Photographing Medicine: Images and Power in Britain and America since 1840* (New York: Greenwood Press, 1988), for a discussion of the camera as a medical instrument to record clinical and pathological findings.

ties in the upcoming year.[42] Two years later, at the ACS national meeting in Cleveland, Ohio, two boys afflicted with cancer were again used to demonstrate gains in research and treatment. Seven-year-old Donald Lewis Marteeney from Kansas City, Missouri, had undergone twenty-one surgeries for neuroblastoma before he was two years old, but had just reached five-year tumor-free survival. Four-year-old Thomas Nagy of Cleveland had been treated with cortisone after his diagnosis of acute leukemia; he relapsed just a few weeks before the meeting, but another treatment with cortisone and aminopterin had successfully induced a second temporary remission and enabled him to attend. In their publicity photograph, the boys stood shoulder to shoulder wielding oversized cancer swords as Thomas held a sign with the year's slogan, "Strike back at cancer, man's cruelest enemy."[43] Neuroblastoma (an aggressive tumor of the nervous system) and acute leukemia (a cancer of the blood and related tissues) differed from the carcinomas commonly found in adults, but some publicists, journalists, and physicians fervently pointed to long-term survival in select young cancer sufferers as models for the control or cure of adult malignancies.

Seven-year-old cancer survivor Leroy Curtis of Denver, Colorado, may have been the ACS's most dynamic young representative of the Society's message of early detection and treatment (which was often a problematic message for young cancer sufferers and their parents). In 1953, a national prize-winning newspaper story published in Denver's *Rocky Mountain News* described the detection of a malignant abdominal tumor at Leroy's first checkup. After surgery and ten months of adjuvant X-ray therapy, his tumor was completely eradicated. By the time he celebrated his fourth birthday with cake, chocolate ice cream, a new cowboy outfit, and a party with the neighborhood children, physicians pronounced him "cured."[44] In 1955, Leroy opened the ACS's annual Crusade by presenting the organization's Sword of Hope to President Dwight Eisenhower. The chairman of the Society's board of directors announced: "We chose Leroy, because we think he is a fine youngster and an excellent example of what can so often be done today to save lives from cancer through early diagnosis and prompt, proper treatment."[45] The event was recorded and widely broadcast on television and in movie theaters across the country. A weekend

42. "A Story-Editorial—Jennifer and the Sword," *ACS Bull.*, 1953, *2* (14): 1.
43. "National Meeting Spurs Enthusiasm for April Crusade," *ACS Bull.*, *4* (11): 1.
44. "Prize Story Depicts Fight for Survival: Quick Action Meant Life to Doomed Boy," *ACS Bull.*, 1953, *2* (23): 4.
45. "White House Ceremony Opens Cancer Crusade," *ACS Bull.*, 1955, *4* (16): 1.

trip to New York City sponsored and staged by the Society put Leroy in the spotlight and highlighted his good health. He visited the children's ward at Memorial Hospital and joined a party for the child patients that included two clowns from the Ringling Brothers, Barnum, and Bailey Circus. He also appeared on several television shows, toured the Central Park Zoo, and spoke about his adventures with a journalist at the *New York Times* newsroom.[46] In 1956, he returned to the National Campaign Meeting in Cincinnati to pose for pictures and star in the afternoon program led by the year's National Campaign Chairman, Ed Sullivan.[47] Referred to as the "one-boy whirlwind" in the *ACS Bulletin*, he opened the show by singing atop a piano. Famous figures, other cancer survivors, physicians, and scientists participated in the conference, but Leroy and his personal experiences with cancer took center stage. Employing the triad of journalism, advertising, and entertainment in its multimedia promotions, the ACS dramatically confirmed that Leroy's health—and his childhood—had been fully restored through early cancer detection and prompt, orthodox treatment. Unfortunately, few other cancer sufferers were as fortunate.

A smaller number of accounts published by the ACS highlighted the dichotomy of helplessness and hopefulness that actually characterized cancer in the 1950s. The same year that Leroy embarked on his ACS publicity tour, the ACS and *Look* magazine produced an informational booklet on cancer for distribution through companies' employee reading racks.[48] In the foreword, Charles S. Cameron, medical and scientific director of the Society, claimed that greater attention to the ACS message as it applied to "cancer, the child killer" would lead to reduced mortality in children. However, the stories of Bobby, Patty, and Linda told in the booklet's pages challenged the plausibility of accurate, early detection and prompt treatment saving young sufferers' lives. Despite parents' efforts to comply with these tenets, children with acute leukemia died within months of diagnosis, and children with other cancers faced uncertain outcomes.[49] Optimism, rather than reality, characterized the depiction of children with cancer in ACS campaigns.

46. "Leroy Curtis on New York Visit Wins Attention for Crusade," *ACS Bull.*, 1955, *4* (17): 4.

47. "Ed Sullivan Has Whirlwind Day at Cincinnati," *ACS Bull.*, 1956, *5* (9): 3.

48. J. Robert Moskin, "Cancer the Child Killer," *Limelight* (published by *Look*), 1955, *2* (6): 2–4.

49. A news brief about Donna Jean Soderberg, poster child for the Leukemia Research Foundation, revealed the true limits of the first chemical therapies: Donna Jean initially responded favorably to ACTH and returned home from the hospital in time to celebrate Easter with her family. Nearly a year later she became resistant to the hormone, and she died shortly afterward. There was nothing that she, her family, or physicians could do to

A Cure Is Near?

Approximately a decade after Sidney Farber participated in Dedication Day ceremonies for the Jimmy Fund Building, Danny Thomas, a performer known for his role on the television program *Make Room for Daddy*, established another institution focused narrowly on the research and treatment of pediatric cancers. Frustrated by the slow pace of progress in the field, Thomas chose a building design modeled on the five-pointed star of St. Jude and named the research hospital after the patron saint of hopeless causes. The first fund-raising brochure pictured the architect's rendering of the proposed building and grounds enclosed within a large, glowing star. Below, a small gathering of children gazed up at the star, their faces bright from its light. One child pointed at the star and the message, "the star of hope for stricken children."[50] Simple sketches of children playing outdoor games like catch, jump rope, and baseball suggested a healthy, active future for children suffering from a set of catastrophic diseases. Utilizing the familiar "before and after" strategy, Thomas illustrated his belief that modern miracles of healing depended on faith in scientific medicine.

Thomas called upon his connections in the entertainment industry to stage large-scale fund-raising events in Memphis, Tennessee, the hospital's home. The first event was an outdoor benefit in a local stadium. Publicity photographs showed Thomas standing in the backseat of a convertible, greeting the audience as he entered the crowded arena.[51] Hollywood and medicine were intertwined as popular musicians, a dance team, and Thomas's costars joined the host as he introduced the program. Less than two weeks later, he spread his appeal nationally by flying to New York for a guest appearance on the television game show *Break the Bank*. During the program, he appealed to children to break their piggy banks and donate a dollar to a new hospital. After personally organizing dozens of fund-raising events, Thomas founded the American Lebanese Syrian Associated Charities (ALSAC) to coordinate activities to cover the hospital's operating costs as it strove to provide free medical care for all of its patients.[52] ALSAC continued to mount major celebrity-themed shows, but

---

slow the rapid progression of the disease. "Leukemia Poster Girl Dies," *New York Times*, 7 May 1950, p. 96.

50. *A Dream Come True: The Story of St. Jude Children's Research Hospital and ALSAC* (Dallas: Taylor, 1983), pp. 46, 47.

51. Ibid., p. 22.

52. *From His Promise: The History of ALSAC and St. Jude Children's Research Hospital* (Memphis: Guild Bindery Press, 1996), pp. 14, 18.

also recruited young volunteers referred to as "Danny's Proud Beggars" to work at grassroots activities like car washes and cake sales, and to carry out door-to-door collections. The "Proud Beggars," like the young TB "Crusaders," used children to make direct contact with donors. While these small-scale projects raised money to cover the hospital's operational costs and to provide free medical care for patients, annual telethons hosted by the Thomas family to benefit St. Jude's patients and programs became their best-known fund-raising activity.[53]

Broadcasts of St. Jude's telethons coincided with major changes in the treatment of childhood cancer. Beginning in the 1960s, the design of effective combination-chemotherapy protocols, the organization of cooperative clinical trial groups, and the refinement of supportive measures like platelet infusions and antibiotic regimens led to prolonged survival for children with cancer. Children were increasingly allowed to leave the hospital and reenter the community for extended periods during outpatient treatment. However, the intensive, toxic chemotherapy regimens frequently caused baldness, a visible side effect or marker of the illness. Pictures of bald children—often wearing colorful hats or headscarves—became the primary image used in annual telethons, promotions for new summer camps built for children with cancer, and other fund-raisers for cancer hospitals.[54] Instead of photographing only "cured" children or those with a healthy outward appearance, cancer organizations now deliberately selected children in the middle of arduous treatment regimens, forcing viewers to consider (and, perhaps, respond to) the consequences of a tragic disease for a patient, the family, and society.[55] The courageous child—one captured in the midst of his or her protracted fight against cancer—became the model patient and poster child.

53. See Paul Longmore, "The Cultural Framing of Disease: Telethons as Case Study," *PMLA*, 2005, *120* (2): 502–8. Longmore points to a telethon aired in New York in 1949 by the Damon Runyon Cancer Fund as the first program produced by a private, voluntary health charity designed to reach the growing audience now accessible through broadcast television.

54. For examples from the Jimmy Fund, see Wisnia, *Images of America* (n. 1), pp. 74, 94, 97, 103; and for those from St. Jude's Hospital, see *From His Promise* (n. 52), esp. unnumbered plates titled "An Album of Hope," pp. 80, 115.

55. For critical scholarship on telethons and disability studies, see the work of Paul K. Longmore, including "Conspicuous Contribution and American Cultural Dilemmas: Telethon Rituals of Cleansing and Renewal," in *The Body and Physical Difference: Discourses of Disability*, ed. David T. Mitchell and Sharon L. Snyder (Ann Arbor: University of Michigan Press, 1997), pp. 134–58.

Conclusion

A *New York Times Magazine* article exploring the increasing corporate involvement in health advocacy acknowledged, "Illness has always been about marketing—long before there were ribbons, there were Jerry Lewis telethons and March of Dimes walk-a-thons."[56] Whether greeting spectators at a dime museum, standing on the White House steps, meeting the starting line-up of the Boston Braves, or posing with their bald heads exposed, children with dread diseases have been used to personalize, publicize, and often exaggerate the threat of disability and disease. As one scholar of modern media and child-centered marketing strategies has argued, "The future, though lacking in detail, was filled with hope and promise—for which children were often the visual clue."[57] In the mid-to-late twentieth century, as the shift toward chronic disease demanded new therapeutic approaches, voluntary health agencies that focused on cancer duplicated earlier child-centered strategies as part of their publicity and fund-raising campaigns. Unlike most adult cancers, acute leukemia and several common childhood tumors responded to drug therapies in observable, measurable ways—thus making young sufferers the ideal subjects for publicists, journalists, investigators, and politicians interested in highlighting advances in cancer research and treatment beginning in the late 1940s and 1950s. Later, heroic accounts and images of children illustrated the possibility of remission and tumor regression as children increasingly achieved long-term survival. However, such efforts continued to be selective in nature, carefully crafting optimistic "cure" or "hope" stories to raise money for cancer research or Ronald McDonald Houses that ignored the negative realities such as the limited gains made in certain pediatric cancers, the high costs of treatment, and the high prevalence of mental and physical disabilities caused by experimental chemotherapy protocols.

Dramatic images and narratives about children with cancer continue to attract attention at the local and national levels. Alexandra Scott, an eight-year-old girl who had been diagnosed with a neuroblastoma at infancy, died in August 2004. Years earlier, she and her family had started Alex's Lemonade Stand to raise money for pediatric cancer research and, specifically, for the two institutions that contributed to her care: Connecticut Children's Medical Center, and Children's Hospital of Philadelphia.

56. Lisa Belkin, "Charity Begins at . . . the Marketing Meeting, the Gala Event, the Product Tie-In: How Breast Cancer Became This Year's Cause," *New York Times Mag.*, 22 December 1996, p. 42.

57. Stephen Kline, *Out of the Garden: Toys, TV, and Children's Culture in the Age of Marketing* (London: Verso, 1993), p. 58.

Widespread news coverage and appearances on popular television talk shows like the *Oprah Winfrey Show* and the *Today Show* had rapidly disseminated her story to local and national audiences, and by the time of her death, Alex and many other young volunteers had raised nearly one million dollars through the construction of lemonade stands in all fifty states, Canada, and France.[58] The obituary by the Associated Press retold Alex's heroic story and included a photograph of the girl tending her drink stand, a simple wooden structure covered with handmade, rainbow-colored signs that asked for a 50-cent donation and informed customers that the profits would benefit pediatric cancer research.[59] Framed by the stand, Alex sported a wide grin and a cocked hat that partially covered her bald head. The jarring disconnect between a neighborhood lemonade stand—a common summertime activity for children—and the serious purpose of Alex's sales drew wide attention to Alex, her grave prognosis, and the ongoing threat of childhood cancers.

While child-focused efforts such as the St. Jude's telethons and the Jimmy Fund continue to the present, the patients' rights movement empowered adults with cancer (and their supporters) to share their personal experiences and critique their care. An increasingly competitive, crowded field of health fund-raising and advocacy has redirected attention away from children and rare childhood cancers, and toward common adult cancers like those of the breast and colon that have responded well to adjuvant chemical and hormonal therapies. While children's faces and tragic stories continue to garner particular attention and spur community action around individual sufferers, the term "poster child" has expanded widely to include spokespersons of all ages. Current fund-raising efforts portray everyday sufferers and survivors bravely battling against cancer and the symptoms that accompany the disease. Famous figures like Lance Armstrong who have suffered from or survived cancer are described and depicted as hero-patients, particularly by pharmaceutical companies heavily involved in cancer-drug development. Katie Couric not only publicly speaks of her husband's death from colon cancer, she leads the charge by televising her own colonoscopy and educational segments. Not only does the American public now expect that all children will survive to adulthood, twenty-first-century health consumers expect scientific medicine to effectively prevent, manage, and eradicate chronic diseases like cancer throughout the human lifespan. It is clear, however, that we must apply

58. See http://www.alexslemonade.org/ (accessed 14 November 2006).

59. "Girl Who Sold Lemonade for Cancer Research Dies at 8," *Seattle Times* (online version), 3 August 2004.

the lessons learned about the use of "poster children"—the myths told through promotional images, the complex goals of the modern hospitals and health organizations, and the exploitation of patients—as health advocacy and marketing expands to include adults and their ills.

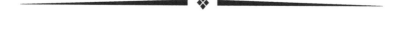

GRETCHEN KRUEGER received the Ph.D. degree from Yale University in 2003. During a three-year postdoctoral fellowship in the Department of the History of Medicine at Johns Hopkins University School of Medicine, she revised several articles based on her dissertation and served as a historical consultant to the American Society of Clinical Oncology. She is currently preparing a book on young patients' and families' experiences of childhood cancer. She is Senior Historian in the Family and Business History Center at Wells Fargo Bank in San Francisco, California (email: gretchen.m.krueger@wellsfargo.com).

Dark Victory: Cancer and Popular Hollywood Film

SUSAN E. LEDERER

SUMMARY: This paper explores the cultural representations of cancer in popular Hollywood films released between 1930 and 1970. These cinematic treatments were not representative of the types of cancer that increasingly afflicted Americans, nor were filmmakers and studios concerned with realistic representations of the disease, its treatment, and its outcomes. As in the "epidemic entertainments" of the early twentieth century that portrayed diseases as cultural commodities, popular filmmakers selectively projected some cancers rather than others, favoring those that were less offensive and more photogenic. Although the characters became weak and died, they did so without gross transformations of their bodies. This paper argues that such representations nonetheless informed American attitudes about cancer and the role of medical research in overcoming the disease.

KEYWORDS: cancer, brain tumor, Hollywood films, Bette Davis, cultural representation of cancer

In 1939 the film actress Bette Davis riveted American audiences, playing a young, willful heiress who stumbles upon the true reason for her frequent headaches and vision problems. In what film critics hailed as "a great role—rangy, full-bodied, designed for a virtuosa, almost sure to invite the faint damning of 'tour de force,'" Davis's character in *Dark Victory* agrees to undergo a brain operation in the belief that it will cure her condition.[1] Although her surgeon knows that the brain tumor will recur, he deceives her. When she artlessly opens her medical chart and reads the death sentence inscribed in the straightforward medical language "prognosis negative," Judith Traherne (Davis's character) realizes

I would like to thank David Cantor, Dorothy Porter, and David Diaz for their thoughtful comments and suggestions for this paper. I also thank the staff of the Margaret Herrick Library, Academy of Motion Pictures Arts and Sciences, Beverly Hills, California.

1. Frank S. Nugent, "Bette Davis Scores New Honors in 'Dark Victory,'" *New York Times*, 21 April 1939, p. 27; Mae Tinee, "'Dark Victory' a New Triumph for Bette Davis," *Chicago Tribune*, 29 April 1939, p. 15.

the ruse. After Judith and her surgeon marry and retire to the country, where he pursues medical research, she once again begins to experience problems in vision. This time, she is the deceiver: she hides her blindness from her husband to allow him to attend a medical conference. Alone in her bedroom, she meets her end bravely. As the camera slowly goes out of focus, her face disappears from the screen.[2]

At first glance, a mainstream Hollywood film about a young woman who dies from brain cancer challenges the conventional historical wisdom about the reluctance to invoke the "C-word" in the first half of the twentieth century. As historian James Patterson and others have argued, early twentieth-century journalists, physicians, and voluntary organizations (the American Society for the Control of Cancer and its successor, the American Cancer Society) crusaded to overcome the popular stigma associated with cancer. Citing the enormous public attention paid to the last days of former president Ulysses S. Grant, who died from throat cancer in 1885, Patterson shows how the slow erosion of public reticence about "the dread disease" continued in the 1940s and 1950s, when magazine and newspaper articles revealed the diagnoses of such prominent individuals as composer George Gershwin (dead from a brain tumor in 1937), ballplayer Babe Ruth (dead from throat cancer in 1948), and athlete Babe Didrikson Zaharias (who died from rectal cancer in 1956).[3] Journalist Ellen Leopold describes how breast cancer moved from "the closet to the commonplace" in the years between 1945 and 1975; drawing on narratives written by women who suffered with breast cancer, she points to the importance of television in the domestication of that disease, especially such female-oriented programs as *The Young and the Restless*, which broadcast the first "fully realized version of a breast cancer saga" in 1974.[4] Yet neither Patterson nor Leopold acknowledges the role that such Hollywood films as *Dark Victory* played in the cultural productions of cancer. Given the salience of Hollywood films in twentieth-century American culture, this is a strange omission. It seems likely that screen portrayals of brain tumors, leukemias, and other cancers coexisted alongside the information provided by voluntary and governmental agencies. The films, cartoons, and other visual materials created by the American Cancer Society and public health departments have received recent historical attention (see

2. Plot descriptions for all films in this essay are taken from the American Film Institute On-Line Catalogue.

3. James Patterson, *The Dread Disease: Cancer and Modern American Culture* (Cambridge: Harvard University Press, 1987).

4. Ellen Leopold, *A Darker Ribbon: Breast Cancer, Women, and Their Doctors in the Twentieth Century* (Boston: Beacon Press, 1999), p. 240.

David Cantor in this volume), but the cinematic portrayal of the disease for mass audiences, especially before President Richard Nixon declared "war on cancer" in 1971, has not.[5]

Based on a survey of Hollywood films identified through the index of the American Film Institute's listings, I argue here that cancer figured more prominently in pre-1971 American screen culture than many commentators have realized. These screen portrayals were hardly representative of the types of cancer that increasingly afflicted Americans in the twentieth century; nor were filmmakers and studios concerned with realistic, factually based representations of the disease, its treatment, and its outcomes. Like the "epidemic entertainments" of the early twentieth century analyzed by historian Nancy Tomes, "malignant melodramas" like *Dark Victory* functioned as cultural commodities.[6] Capitalizing on cultural anxieties but leery of box office "poison," Hollywood filmmakers selectively projected some cancers rather than others. Perhaps not surprisingly, they favored less-offensive and more-photogenic cancers that did not visibly mutilate the characters: the characters became weak and fatigued, and died, but they did so without gross transformations of their bodies. In *Dark Victory*, the tumor that afflicts the heiress remains unseen inside her head and veiled beneath her hair. When the tumor recurs, she experiences a loss of vision, but this does not prevent her gracious and even glamorous deathbed scenes.[7]

Reflecting broader strains in American culture—both popular and biomedical—Hollywood representations of cancer pointed to the research laboratory as the means to conquer the dread disease. In so doing, such representations maintained the activist optimism of voluntary cancer agencies: research dollars would fund laboratories that would then discover new drugs and new techniques to transform the disease into a more manageable entity. The clinical conventions in these films similarly maintained the mainstream medical practice of shielding the patient, whenever possible, from the truth about the grim diagnosis of cancer and the likely outcome. Fear and hope were twinned in such representations, just as they oscillated in the pages and propaganda of the American Cancer Society: fear that the danger signs and symptoms of the disease would be

5. See Leslie J. Reagan, "Engendering the Dread Disease: Women, Men and Cancer," *Amer. J. Pub. Health*, 1997, *87*: 1779–87; Robert Aronowitz, "Do Not Delay: Breast Cancer and Time, 1900–1970," *Milbank Quart.*, 2003, *79*: 355–86.

6. Nancy J. Tomes, "Epidemic Entertainments: Disease and Popular Culture in Early Twentieth-Century America," *Amer. Lit. Hist.*, 2002, *14*: 625–52.

7. See Susan E. Lederer, "Repellent Subjects: Hollywood Censorship and Surgical Images in the 1930s," *Lit. & Med.*, 1998, *17*: 91–113.

detected too late, and hope that the laboratory would deliver the magic bullet against the disease. If these cinematic portrayals of cancer offered limited information about some features of the disease (the nature of a glioma, how it could be surgically removed, how it could recur), they simultaneously perpetuated ideas about the inevitable course of cancer. In several films, for example, the news that an individual has developed cancer serves to rationalize suicide or "mercy killing"; in the context of such films, the cancer diagnosis needs no elaboration, thus naturalizing the idea that death from cancer will be not only protracted and painful, but inevitable. In many Hollywood films, references to cancer were incidental to the storyline; yet they nonetheless confirmed the worst fears of cancer crusaders about the need to counteract such beliefs and to educate and train Americans about the realities of the disease.

As cancer became more visible in twentieth-century American culture, its appearance reflected conflicting and multiple factors. For Hollywood filmmakers, cancer's visibility refracted censorship concerns, commercial viability, and assumptions about audiences. *Dark Victory* and other Hollywood productions enlarged the cultural profile of the dread disease, even as they veiled its physical realities—but like other aspects of American culture, its contours could be traced in the dark.

Counting Cancers

How many Hollywood films before 1971, the year that President Nixon declared "war on cancer," featured the disease, and in what capacity? Radiation oncologist Robert Clark has claimed that only 20 of some 150 Hollywood films with medical themes released between 1930 and 1999 contained cancer themes and only five films featured cancer in the years between 1939 (*Dark Victory*) and 1970 (*Love Story*). The majority of the films he identifies date from the 1990s, including *The Doctor* (1991), in which a surgeon develops laryngeal cancer; *Dying Young* (1991), wherein a young man dies from cancer of the blood; *Phenomenon* (1996), in which a man experiences extraordinary intellectual abilities after he develops a brain tumor; and *Stepmom* (1999), a star vehicle for actress Susan Sarandon, whose character "wearily slouches toward canonization" after she begins to succumb to "terminal cancer."[8] In 2002, sharing his experience as a cancer patient undergoing chemotherapy on the World Wide Web,

8. Robert A. Clark, "Reel Oncology: How Hollywood Films Portray Cancer," www .moffitt,usf.edu/pubs/ccj/v6n5/dept7.htm (2 September 2004). For Sarandon, see Franz Lidz, "In a Higher State of Being (That Is, Dying)," *New York Times*, 10 January 1999, p. 46.

patient Gary Sperling proposed the "All-Cancer Film Festival." Watching "cancer movies," he suggested, provided the opportunity for many lessons. Identifying *An Act of Murder* (1948) as perhaps the first cancer-themed film, Sperling claimed that the film, starring Frederic March as a judge who contemplates mercy killing when his wife is diagnosed with a brain tumor, establishes the "basic cancer movie plot": namely, that a valuable lesson will be learned by witnessing the suffering of a loved one.[9] Both Sperling and Clark offer useful accounts, but they provide too narrow a reading of cancer as it was represented in popular American film before the 1990s. Such films as *Dark Victory*, which centered on the heroine's brain tumor, as well as films in which cancer received only a fleeting reference, offered audiences a form of cultural literacy about the disease, providing information—however flawed—about cancer, its causes, and its outcomes.

But what counts as a cancer movie? How central does the disease have to be to the storyline for it to be considered a cancer movie as such? As the surveys above by Clark and Sperling illustrate, different observers identify the cancer movie in diferent ways. Even within the canonical film reference work, the *American Film Institute Catalog*, the list of films that include a depiction of cancer varies according to the search term employed. Using the keyword "cancer" prduces a list of thirty-three films between the years 1893 and 1970 in which cancer is identified as a subject—ranging from a 1916 silent film *The Closed Road*, which featured a doctor seeking a cure for cancer, to a mostly forgotten 1970 Sidney Lumet film *The Last of the Mobile Hot Shots*, in which the dying scion of an old Louisiana family uses medicinal marijuana before succumbing to cancer.[10] This list does not include *Dark Victory*, which, due to the vagaries of the AFI indexing system, can be located under the subject word "tumor," rather than "cancer," as the principal subject; eighteen films, including *Dark Victory*, can be identified using the keyword "tumor."[11] Of these eighteen, nine revolve around a brain tumor; the tumors in the remaining six films include three in the knee, one in the spine, one nonhuman tumor (horse), and one from a 1904 silent film that is unspecified. Neither the keyword "cancer" nor "tumor" will produce the film identified by Sperling as perhaps the first cancer-themed film; instead, *An Act of Murder* can be located using the

9. See Gary Sperling, All-Cancer Film Festival, **http://slate.msn.com/id/2065895/** (accessed 31 October 2006).

10. The AFI Catalog does not yet include the 1950s.

11. However, three of the eighteen films are related to George Gershwin's real-life cancer, including the bio-pic *Rhapsody in Blue* (1945).

keyword "incurable diseases," which includes films featuring brain tumors, breast cancer, and leukemia, as well as other unspecified fatal illnesses. The key word "leukemia" will also produce some but not all of the above films. Given the variability in the indexing of these films, the precise number of those that feature cancer remains elusive. It seems clear, however, that representations of cancer were considerably more common than commentators have allowed, and that the number far exceeds Clark's identification of twenty films.

Cancer Screening

How did cancer appear in Hollywood films? What aspects of cancer care, recovery, and research received attention from filmmakers and audiences? What kind of knowledge would be available to audiences about cancer?

Before *Dark Victory* in 1939, cancer made few appearances—and when it did appear, it possessed few identifying characteristics and even fewer therapies. In the 1932 RKO picture *Symphony of Six Million*, for example, the father of Jewish physician Felix Klauber falls to the ground; in the next scene the audience learns that his problem is a "tumor of the brain." Despite Felix's reluctance to operate on his own father, he is compelled to perform the surgery. When his father dies on the operating table, the doctor loses his desire to practice medicine. In the 1932 Monogram film *Klondike*, Doctor Robert Cromwell removes a brain tumor from a wealthy local man, and is then tried for his murder after the man lives for only five hours following the surgery. Although he is acquitted, the medical board, believing that he is experimenting on an "incurable invalid," revokes his medical license. Thus, in these two films, the diagnosis of brain cancer requires no special make-up or embarrassingly intimate behaviors; instead it entails dizziness, an operating room sequence, and death. Brain tumors also featured in the 1939 film *The Secret of Doctor Kildare.* In this installment of the popular Kildare series, a young woman whose mother has died from a brain tumor experiences severe headaches and becomes convinced that she has the same ailment. After she becomes the patient of an ersatz nature healer named John Xerxes Archly, young Dr. Kildare sets out to discover the true cause of her symptoms, which include hysterical blindness, and performs a sham surgery to restore her vision.[12]

Dark Victory marked a significant departure from these three films, for the brain tumor was central to the film (and the play of the same name on which it was based). Written by George Brewer, the play debuted on

---

12. All plot summaries are taken from the AFI on-line Catalog.

Broadway on 7 November 1934, starring actress Tallulah Bankhead as the Long Island heiress. Although Bankhead received good notices for her performance, the play proved less than popular: it ran for only fifty-one performances before closing. Yet despite this poor showing, the play interested film producers, notably David Selznick at Metro-Goldwyn-Mayer. When Selznick failed to move ahead with the film, Warner Brothers Studios acquired the rights for a film adaptation. Studio head Jack Warner was reluctant to produce a film about a girl who dies of brain cancer, and producer Hal Wallis shared this reluctance. The screenwriter Casey Robinson recalled how Wallis "turned white" when he heard the plot of *Dark Victory*: "One must remember," Casey explained, "that this was the mid-thirties and that cancer was a dirty word. If someone died, they died of heart failure or some obscure cause."[13] One year later, in 1940, Wallis pursued the cinematic treatment of another disease once considered taboo, receiving special permission from Will Hays and the Hollywood censors (the Production Code Administration) to use the word "syphilis" in the Warner Brothers bio-pic *Dr. Ehrlich's Magic Bullet*.[14]

The willingness to take up the cancer theme as a cinematic subject may have reflected the considerable public attention that the disease received in the late 1930s. In 1937, the United States Congress passed the National Cancer Act

> for the purposes of conducting researches, investigations, experiments, and studies relating to the cause, diagnosis, and treatment of cancer; assisting and fostering similar research activities by other agencies, public and private; and promoting the coordination of all such researches and activities and the useful application of their results, with a view to the development and prompt widespread use of the most effective methods of prevention, diagnosis, and treatment of cancer.[15]

Signed into law by President Franklin D. Roosevelt, the act authorized an appropriation of $750,000 for the construction of a new building in Bethesda and an annual appropriation of $700,000 for cancer research.

The passage of the National Cancer Act coincided with "the first national media blitz" about cancer. Stories about the disease—its prevention, treatment, and the need for research—appeared in a broad array of popular media, from *Good Housekeeping* in June 1936 to an extensive

---

13. Pat McGilligan, *Backstory: Interviews with Screenwriters of Hollywood's Golden Age* (Berkeley: University of California Press, 1986), p. 301.

14. Susan E. Lederer and John Parascandola, "Screening Syphilis: *Dr. Ehrlich's Magic Bullet* Meets the Public Health Service," *J. Hist. Med.*, 1998, *53*: 345–70.

15. *National Cancer Act*, S 2067, 75th Cong., 1st sess.

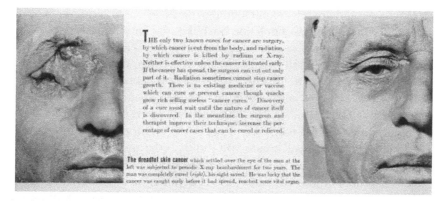

THE only two known cures for cancer are surgery, by which cancer is cut from the body, and radiation, by which cancer is killed by radium or X-ray. Neither is effective unless the cancer is treated early. If the cancer has spread, the surgeon can cut out only part of it. Radiation sometimes cannot stop cancer growth. There is no existing medicine or vaccine which can cure or prevent cancer though quacks grow rich selling useless "cancer cures." Discovery of a cure must wait until the nature of cancer itself is discovered. In the meantime the surgeon and therapist improve their technique, increase the percentage of cancer cases that can be cured or relieved.

The dreadful skin cancer which settled over the eye of the man at the left was subjected to periodic X-ray bombardment for two years. The man was completely cured (*right*), his sight saved. He was lucky that the cancer was caught early before it had spread, reached some vital organ.

Fig. 1. This image from *Life* featured a disfiguring skin cancer "completely cured" by periodic x-ray bombardment. (Source: "Only the Surgeon's Knife or Radiation Can Cure Cancer," *Life*, 1 March 1937, p. 17.)

photo-essay in the popular weekly *Life*.[16] The cover of the 1 March 1937 issue of *Life* featured mice bred for cancer research. Inside the magazine were six large pages of photographs of cancer researchers, radiation devices, a breast biopsy, and a before-and-after photograph of a man whose facial tumor was treated with radiation (Fig. 1). These graphic images of a skin cancer that disfigured the man's face and obscured his vision provoked several angry letters from *Life*'s readers, who branded the display "shocking and repulsive," "horrible and revolting," and "distressing," even though the "after" image showed how effective two years of periodic x-ray bombardment had been in successfully restoring his vision and his health.[17] The photographs may have distressed some readers, but stories (if not images) about radium and "atom smashers" to fight cancer continued to appear in popular magazines and newspapers in the late 1930s and 1940s.[18]

16. Karen Rader, *Making Mice: Standardizing Animals for American Biomedical Research, 1900–1955* (Princeton: Princeton University Press, 2004), pp. 147–49.

17. The article in *Life* was "U.S. Science Wars against an Unknown Enemy: Cancer," 1 March 1937, pp. 11–17. One Burlington, Iowa, reader wrote, "I burned up my copy. . . . I can't imagine anything more repulsive"; A. T. Gordon of Seattle, Washington, wrote, "I tore out the gruesome sheets before anyone could be as shocked as we were." See "Letters to the Editor," *Life*, 22 March 1937, p. 76. See also Susan E. Lederer, "Medicine Comes to *Life*: Photojournalism, Doctors, and Disease" (Paper presented at Yale conference, The Art of Medicine, April 2004).

18. See, e.g., Gerald G. Gross, "10 Grams of Radium Tested Here to Go Throughout U.S.," *Washington Post*, 10 August 1939, p. 4; "Atom Smasher Fights Cancer," *Los Angeles Times*, 10 November 1937, p. 1.

Dark Victory did not offer explicit images of cancerous disfigurement, but one of the things that distinguished both the play and the screenplay was the explicit language of cancer, its symptoms, and its outcome. Although filmmakers expressed concern about the box-office potential for a film about cancer, they did not excise the medical vocabulary of the disease. Consultations with specialists at the Cedars of Lebanon Hospital in Los Angeles, the studio claimed, allowed "scrupulous precision of the medical details."[19] This included references to glioma, carcinoma, and amblyopia. The brain surgeon who will operate on Judith Traherne is initially reluctant to take her on as a patient, since he is planning to give up his practice and go to Vermont in order to research fundamental questions about cancer.[20] As he prepares to leave, he reflects on the lack of information about basic mechanisms in the disease process: "Cells. Brain cells. Why do healthy cells suddenly go berserk—grow wild? Do you know?" he asks a friend; no one knows, he continues: "We call them tumors—gliomas—cysts—cancers. . . . We operate and try to cure with the knife when we don't even know the cause. People put their faith in us because we're doctors."[21] In another scene, when Judith demands to know why she requires a brain operation, the surgeon uses his medical vocabulary, but he also offers a simple analogy in his dialogue with the young heiress:

> Steele: The technical name is glioma.
> Judith: Glioma? It sounds like a kind of plant.
> Steele: Yes—it is rather like a plant—a parasitic one. If it's removed. . . .[22]

Whether the film's doctors label a tumor a "simple carcinoma" or the more arcane "glioma," their language reveals the insidious and uncontrolled nature of the disease; Judith's surgeon, Steele, dismisses her tumor as "a contemptible, meaningless growth."[23]

The word "glioma" was a technical one, but it was a word that newspaper readers in the late 1930s might have already encountered. In 1938, papers in Chicago, New York, and Washington, D.C., published headlines about "glioma babies," explaining that glioma was a cancerous growth that

---

19. Charles Higham, *Warner Brothers* (New York: Scribner's, 1975), p. 137.

20. Vermont was apparently the place to go for medical research: in both Sinclair Lewis's book *Arrowsmith* and the 1931 film version, Martin Arrowsmith goes to Vermont to pursue medical research.

21. Casey Robinson, ed., with an introduction by Bernard F. Dick, *Dark Victory* (Madison: University of Wisconsin Press, 1981), p. 76. Shooting script (1939) available at **http://www .alexanderstreet2.com/afsolive/** (accessed 2 November 2006).

22. Ibid., p. 100.

23. Ibid., p. 111.

spreads along the optic nerve to the brain. Most of the newspaper coverage focused on a Chicago infant, four-month-old Helaine Colan, whose case attracted national attention as her parents debated an operation that might save her life but leave her permanently blinded. An "unofficial jury" composed of nine physicians and three rabbis met "to settle the 'death or blindness' question" that faced the child's family; when the "jury" opted for surgery, the child underwent an operation to remove the cancer and her left eye.[24] In Chicago, where leaders of the city's business, medical, and religious communities weighed in on the question, the *Tribune* published photographs of other child "glioma cases," including Robert Marshall (twenty-eight months old), "who survived the operation for glioma and lives happy, normal life despite glass right eye," and Robert Edmark (twenty-two months old) "doomed by glioma."[25] The *Tribune* also featured photographs of Miss Effa Roach, a "glioma victim," who was able to see eighteen years after surgeons had removed one of her affected eyes.[26]

In addition to reports of children with glioma, newspapers ascribed the deaths of several prominent individuals in the late 1930s to tumors of the brain. In 1935, the widow of a New Rochelle surgeon made the news when she bequeathed her head to neurosurgeon Harvey Cushing. Cushing had performed four surgeries on Mrs. Hans Glogau's brain tumor; in her will, she recorded her hope that "a study of my head after my death may serve the advancement of science."[27] Certainly the most extensively reported brain tumor was the cause of death of the young composer George Gershwin. In July 1937 the creator of *Porgy and Bess*, the man "who made jazz popular," collapsed; as his condition worsened, Johns Hopkins brain surgeon Walter Dandy was contacted by the Coast Guard on board a cruise ship in the Chesapeake Bay and asked to fly immediately to Los Angeles to operate on the ailing composer. Before Dandy's arrival, surgeons from the University of California performed surgery to remove the tumor. Gershwin died several hours following the operation: "Death was due to a cystic tumor of the right temporal lobe of the brain," Dr. Gabriel Seagall informed reporters.[28] In 1938 newspapers reported the deaths of Mabelle Horlick Sidley, heiress to the Horlick malted milk fortune, and

24. "'Jury' to Decide Fate of Baby in Eye Case," *New York Times*, 9 May 1938, p. 19.

25. "2 Little Victims of Glioma—One Lives; One Exists," *Chicago Tribune*, 9 May 1938, p. 2.

26. "Girl Sees Well 18 Years After Removal of Eye," *Chicago Tribune*, 10 May 1938, p. 6, with accompanying photograph of Miss Roach, captioned "Victim of Glioma."

27. "Left Her Head to Science," *New York Times*, 6 October 1935, p. 14.

28. "Operation Fails to Save Life of Famous Composer," *Washington Post*, 12 July 1937, p. 1.

the ex-circus giant, John Aasen Gerthe, both from brain tumors.[29] It was perhaps this spate of brain-tumor-associated deaths that prompted the medical newspaper columnist Logan Clendenning to remind his readers in 1939 that brain tumors were "very rare," and to reassure them that "the treatment of brain tumor today is so generally successful that early diagnosis is imperative."[30]

Women and Cancer

When film critic Frank Nugent reviewed *Dark Victory* for the *New York Times*, he called the film "simply a protracted death scene in which the heroine's doom is sealed almost in the first sequence"; nonetheless, he refused to dismiss it as a species of Hollywood's "emotional flim-flam."[31] More than a "woman's weepie," the film was, in the words of another critic, a story "deeply richly human, its sadness relieved by some bright flashes of humor."[32] Despite these efforts of critics to redeem *Dark Victory*, it undoubtedly was a "woman's film," a genre with its own characteristically unpredictable plot twists, exchanges of dialogue, and stylized conventions of filmic technique (the "happy interlude," the "tragic separation," and so on).[33]

Indeed, the pressbook developed by Warner Brothers Studios explicitly identified the Davis film as intended for female audiences: "*Dark Victory* is definitely a woman's picture and should be exploited as such via the woman's page of your local paper and in cooperation with women's shops"; among other things, the pressbook offered suggestions about the contrasting make-up for Bette Davis and her co-star Geraldine Fitzgerald.[34] As they prepared for the film's release in 1939, some studio representatives continued to worry about the cancer theme and the issue of doom. In the advertising for the film, there was no mention of the brain tumor: the heiress was described as the "victim of a mysterious malady." The publicity (not surprisingly) did not disclose that the heroine becomes blind

29. "Seek Data in Death of Horlick Heiress," *New York Times*, 17 July 1938, p. 16; "Ex-Circus Giant Dies," ibid., 3 August 1938, p. 19.

30. Logan Clendenning, "Today's Health Talk," *Washington Post*, 21 April 1939, p. 18.

31. Nugent, "Bette Davis Scores New Honors" (n. 1).

32. Tinee, "'Dark Victory' a New Triumph" (n. 1).

33. Jeanine Basinger, *A Woman's View: How Hollywood Spoke to Women, 1930–1960* (New York: Knopf, 1993).

34. For the pressbook, see Mary Ann Doane, *The Desire to Desire: The Woman's Film of the 1940s* (Bloomington: Indiana University Press, 1987), pp. 29–30.

and then dies from her brain tumor; instead, it focused on "the love story no woman will ever forget."[35]

If the pressbook avoided the word "cancer," published film reviews did not. Critics in the *Los Angeles Times*, the *New York Times*, and *Life* all explicitly identified the heroine's malady as a brain tumor. Frank Nugent's review described the heroine's brain tumor, the operation, her blindness, and her death.[36] *Life*'s story about the film included pictures of the actor George Brent as the brain specialist who examines her reflexes and eyes and diagnoses a tumor of the brain, pictures of the heroine before her "dangerous operation," and the scene where the doctor "withholds laboratory report which shows her tumor is a malignant type sure to recur."[37]

Producer Jack Warner, the same man who questioned the making of the 1936 film *The Story of Louis Pasteur* ("who wants to see a film about a milk man?"[38]), reportedly had demanded who wanted to see "a picture about a girl who dies?"[39] Large audiences apparently did. The film proved to be both a popular and a critical success, especially with female audiences. When it was held over for a second week at a Washington, D.C., theater, a reporter for the *Washington Post* noted that even a film about "a very sick girl with a brain glyoma that dooms her to an early death" could have "box-office appeal."[40] No doubt the care with which the filmmakers presented the patient's experience with the brain tumor played a role: although the language about cancer in *Dark Victory* was explicit, the representation of the cancer's effects was reassuringly downplayed. After Judith Traherne experiences some difficult headaches, misjudges her horse's approach, and burns her finger without realizing it, she reluctantly agrees to see the specialist and to undergo brain surgery—but fortunately, her surgery requires only minimal shaving of the head and she is able to disguise her operation with chic headwear. Traherne continues to believe that she has been cured, but her doctor, her friend, and the audience know that her time is short. When the cancer recurs, she experiences loss of sight and then a quiet, if glamorous, death (Fig. 2).

35. Matthew Kennedy, *Edmund Goulding's Dark Victory: Hollywood's Genius Bad Boy* (Madison: University of Wisconsin Press, 2004), p. 184.

36. "Screen in Review: Dark Victory," *New York Times*, 21 April 1939, p. 27. See also "Bette Davis' Portrayal in 'Dark Victory' Hailed," *Los Angeles Times*, 8 March 1939, p. A10.

37. "Movie of the Week: Dark Victory," *Life*, 24 April 1939, pp. 31–34.

38. Jerome Lawrence, *Actor: The Life and Times of Paul Muni* (New York: Putnam, 1974), p. 218.

39. Whitney Stine, *Mother Goddam: The Story of the Career of Bette Davis* (New York: Hawthorn Books, 1974), p. 111.

40. "'Dark Victory' Enters Second Week," *Washington Post*, 6 May 1939, p. 8.

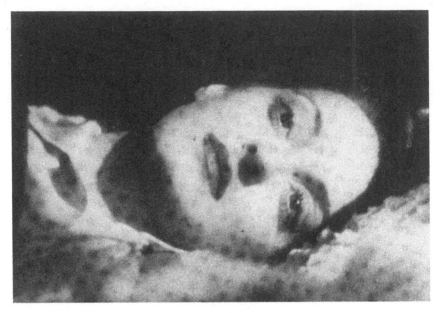

Fig. 2. Judith Traherne's (Bette Davis's) final moments before death claims its "Dark Victory." (Permission to reproduce courtesy of Warner Brothers Studios.)

Gender played a critical role in popular cancer discourse in the middle decades of the twentieth century. Women were instrumental in the funding and organization of the American Society for the Control of Cancer (founded in 1913), and in its reorganization as the American Cancer Society. These organizations targeted women in their propaganda about cancer prevention and cancer treatment. In 1937 the ASCC joined forces with women's clubs across the nation to foster the Women's Field Army, organized to enable women to "fight cancer with knowledge." In the late 1930s, several hundred thousand women belonged to the Field Army and participated in its crusade against cancer. Women attended screenings of films about the importance of self-examination and self-inspection and the responsibility to see the doctor as early as possible if they discovered a lump or any other warning signs of cancer. As the historian Leslie J. Reagan has argued, by the 1950s organizations such as the American Cancer Society recognized the "gendered understanding of cancer" as a problem that required remediation. Many American men, apparently influenced by popular literature about cancer and the efforts of the Women's Field Army, believed that cancer was a woman's disease.[41]

Dark Victory did not feature a cancer that was restricted to women (cervical, ovarian, or breast cancer): brain tumors claimed male, as well as female, lives. But the film's presentation of cancer resonated with gendered conventions about female patients and male physicians in popular cancer narratives. As the historian Kirsten Gardner has noted, such narratives in the late 1930s and 1940s explicitly identified female patients as "good" or "bad," "wise" or "foolish." In the pages of such popular health journals as *Hygeia*, "wise" women examined their bodies, immediately consulted physicians when they found a warning sign, received cancer treatment, and lived to tell their story. Foolish women did not; instead, they ignored the dangers and died. Such depictions "placed a burden on women to detect cancer, implicitly blamed women for late-stage diagnoses, and exaggerated the obvious nature of cancer symptoms."[42] Such depictions, moreover, amplified the moral economy of medical authority.

In 1940, when Bette Davis resumed her film career, Hollywood correspondent Frederick Othman reported that the actress only vaguely resembled "the tired woman who appeared in Dark Victory": he said that Davis's weight had dwindled to 101 pounds when making the picture, but that happily she had rebounded from "skin and bones" to embark on her new film.[43] Although her performance was nominated for an Oscar, Davis did not receive the award, losing out to Vivien Leigh and her role in *Gone With the Wind*. *Dark Victory* dramatically portrayed cancer in a new light, but despite its critical acclaim and popular success, it did not prompt other films that featured cancer so prominently.

Incidental Findings

In the three decades following the release of *Dark Victory*, Hollywood films mostly relegated cancer to the sidelines, but even these lesser roles continued to represent cancer in particular ways for particular audiences. Actor Ronald Reagan, who played a minor character in *Dark Victory*, appeared in a 1942 film, *King's Row*, in which cancer had a small but sig-

---

41. Reagan, "Engendering the Dread Disease" (n. 5).

42. Kirsten E. Gardner, *Early Detection: Women, Cancer, and Awareness Campaigns in the Twentieth-Century United States* (Chapel Hill: University of North Carolina Press, 2006), p. 107.

43. Frederick Othman, "Feeling Great, Bette Davis Back at Work on New Film," *Washington Post*, 21 February 1940, p. 16.

nificant role. The film was based on Henry Bellamann's 1940 novel, which seemed a strange choice for adaptation, for it contained many elements that censors would find objectionable and that audiences might find less than appealing. When Warner Brothers assigned Wolfgang Reinhardt to adapt the book, he informed the producer about the book's "enormous difficulties":

> As far as plot is concerned, the material in *King's Row* is for the most part either censurable or too gruesome and depressing to be used. The hero finding out that his girl has been carrying on incestuous relations with her father, a sadistic doctor who amputates legs and disfigures people willfully, a host of moronic or otherwise mentally diseased characters, the background of a lunatic asylum, people dying of cancer, suicides—these are the principal elements of the story.[44]

Despite these obvious challenges (and attractions), Warner Brothers submitted a script to the Production Code Administration in 1941; Joseph Breen then informed Jack Warner that several elements of the script would have to be substantially altered. In addition to objections about "illicit sex and loose sex," Breen noted that the "mercy-killing of the grandmother" suffering from terminal cancer was not acceptable, and that the portrayal of the sadistic doctor who viciously and unnecessarily amputated Drake's legs (Drake was the character played by Ronald Reagan) would also require alteration.[45] In line with Breen's requirements, the film version includes a depiction of the grandmother suffering from cancer, but she dies without assistance. When Drake is injured, he undergoes a necessary amputation of his legs. In the novel, his character subsequently develops cancer and dies, but this does not take place in the film. In the book, the suffering that cancer brings during the last days of the disease provides the impetus for mercy killing; in the film version, the cancer diagnosis is one that the grandmother conceals from her grandson, thus sparing him the knowledge of her pain, suffering, and imminent death. Thus, one of the things audiences may have gleaned from the film was the deception that cancer required from and for the benefit of family members.

Mercy killing was objectionable to censors in the case of *King's Row*, but it continued to inspire filmmakers. In *An Act of Murder*, for example,

44. Wolfgang Reinhardt to Hal Wallis, 3 July 1940; reprinted in Rudy Behlmer, ed., *Inside Warner Bros. (1935–1951)* (New York: Viking Penguin, 1985), p. 135.

45. Joseph Breen to Jack L. Warner, 22 April 1941, "King's Row," MPAA/PCA Collection, Margaret Herrick Library, Academy of Motion Pictures Arts and Sciences, Beverly Hills, California. Reagan claimed this was his favorite film role; he took the line expressed when he discovers the amputation, "Where's the rest of me?" for the title of his autobiography. See Ronald Reagan and Richard G. Hubler, *Where's the Rest of Me?* (New York: Duell, Sloan and Pearce, 1965).

the diagnosis of cancer brings the issue of euthanasia to the fore. In the film a strict Pennsylvania judge (Calvin Cooke, also known as "Old Man Maximum") learns from the family doctor that his wife is suffering from an incurable disease. While she experiences the classic cinematic symptoms of violent headache, blurry vision, and dizziness, she is not explicitly identified as having a brain tumor, but it becomes clear that she will die in "excruciating pain." Keeping the truth of her prognosis from his wife, the judge, seeing her in agony and distress, contemplates giving her an overdose of the pain medication prescribed by the doctor. The judge is unaware, however, that his wife has learned her diagnosis from papers hidden in his suitcase and has taken an overdose of the medication, and he deliberately rams their car into an embankment. Her death in the accident leads to his prosecution for her murder. An autopsy reveals that the accident did not kill her: she died from the self-administered drug overdose. The judge resumes his position on the bench, promising to consider the heart as well as the head in judging future cases.[46]

Between *Dark Victory* and 1970, cancer continued to make episodic appearances as a plot device in Hollywood films. In 1944 *None But the Lonely Heart* featured Ethel Barrymore and Cary Grant as an impoverished English mother and son. The son learns from a friend that his mother has cancer; he then takes up with London gangsters to make a living. After much heartbreak, his mother succumbs to cancer (the type is not specified) in a prison hospital, leaving her son on his own. Brain tumors continued to be popular with directors. *Crisis* (1950), for example, featured Cary Grant as a neurosurgeon who is forced to treat the unpopular leader of a beleaguered Latin American country who suffers from a brain tumor. Although Grant received coaching for the brain surgery sequence from the UCLA neurologist Tracy Putnam, his character does not perform the surgery when the dictator unexpectedly succumbs to a brain hemorrhage.[47] The 1953 film *My Cousin Rachel*, based on the Daphne du Maurier novel of the same name, featured brain tumors in two characters, a father and son, in nineteenth-century Italy. The

46. The film was reviewed under the title "Live Today for Tomorrow." None of the reviews mentions cancer or brain tumor. Edwin Schallert alludes to the wife's incurable disease: see "Marches Distinguish Mercy-Killing Drama," *Los Angeles Times*, 10 January 1948, p. 23. Mae Tinee describes the wife as "fatally ill": see "Mercy Killing Is Explored in a Grim Movie," *Chicago Daily Tribune*, 9 January 1948, p. B12. For an evaluation of the courtroom scenes, see Paul Bergman and Michael Asimov, *Reel Justice: The Courtroom Goes to the Movies* (Kansas City: Universal Press, 1996), pp. 188–93.

47. The film was banned in Colombia, Peru, and Mexico because it was deemed derogatory to Latin America. See entry "Crisis," AFI Catalog.

1953 *Powder River,* based on the book *Wyatt Earp, Frontier Marshall,* portrayed brain tumors and brain surgery in the Old West.[48]

A brain tumor plays a small but significant role in the 1950 "social problem" film *No Way Out.* In this film, Doctor Luther Brooks (actor Sidney Poitier in his film debut) is the first African American doctor at the hospital. As the doctor on call in the emergency room, he is confronted with a working-class white man and his brother who has been shot by the police in the commission of a robbery. Suspecting that his patient has a brain tumor, Brooks performs a spinal tap. After the patient dies, his brother blames the "nigger doctor" for the death. When the dead man's family refuses to allow an autopsy to confirm the diagnosis of brain tumor, the doctor's career is in jeopardy. Racial tension at the hospital and in the community escalates; Brooks endures such scenes as a white mother screaming "keep your black hands off my boy!"[49] Brooks decides to risk being arrested for the white man's death, knowing that an autopsy will be required. When the autopsy reveals that his diagnosis of brain tumor was correct, he is vindicated. *No Way Out* was condemned by the National Legion of Decency. Censors in Chicago and many major Southern cities refused permission to show the film: some objected to the language of the film, while others objected to the portrayal of a race riot after the doctor is accused. As one commentator noted, the film's portrayal of "the cancerous results of hatred," and not the brain cancer, made it a box office failure.[50]

Medical research and the search for a cure for cancer appeared both in horror films and in more "realist" films. In *The Man with Nine Lives* (1940), a young doctor building on the work of an eccentric scientist (played by actor Boris Karloff) discovers a cure for cancer that involves freezing parts of the body; when the hospital is overrun by desperate people seeking the cure, the young scientist hides out on Crater Island and uncovers the secret of the demented scientist's disappearance. In the bio-pic based on the life of Marie Curie (played by actress Greer Garson), the scientist draws attention to odd burns on her hands; when her physician warns her that the burns may become cancerous, she explains to Pierre Curie that radioactive material may one day be used to treat cancer. (The film ends in

---

48. See entries for individual films in AFI on-line catalog.

49. Lester J. Keyser and Andre Ruskowski, *The Cinema of Sydney Poitier* (San Diego: Barnes, 1980), p. 21.

50. See entry for "No Way Out," AFI Catalog. The censors were concerned about the use of terms such as "nigger," and the portrayal of the riot in the black ghetto (among other things). See Thomas Cripps, *Making Movies Black: The Hollywood Message Movie from World War II to the Civil Rights Era* (Oxford: Oxford University Press, 1993). The film was also banned in the Bahamas until 1955.

1931, therefore bypassing her death from leukemia, which was presumed by many to be the result of her long exposure to radioactive materials.)[51] Much less high-toned was the 1950 "B" movie *Experiment Alcatraz*. In this film, as the title implies, five convicted criminals from Alcatraz "get off the rock" by agreeing to serve in a medical experiment. In a plot inspired by similar experiments at San Quentin Prison, the convicts in the film are injected with radioactive isotopes as part of government-sponsored research on leukemia. When one of the injectees stabs and kills another inmate during the experiment, the research comes to an abrupt end until a crusading young doctor from Oak Ridge arrives to unravel the mysterious death. The film also features a young leukemia patient who offers his own body for experimentation, in order to cure the blood disease.[52]

In most of the Hollywood films before 1970, cancer was a disease that people withheld from their loved ones. In some cases, it is the patient who learns the truth about his or her diagnosis and conceals the news. In *You Came Along* (1945), a former Air Force pilot learns that he has "terminal leukemia." When he goes on a tour to promote War Bonds, he meets and falls in love with a U.S. Treasury agent; he conceals his disease from the young woman, and they marry. His wife then learns from a friend about his disease. When he is sent for treatment to Walter Reed Hospital and he pretends that he has been ordered overseas, she does not challenge him. She later receives a telegram notifying her of his death at the hospital. In *No Sad Songs For Me* (1950), a woman with a young child learns that she has cancer and will live only a few more months. Rather than tell her husband about her terminal condition, she instead finds a woman to take her place as his wife and the mother of his child. The kind of cancer this character suffers is not specified; she experiences no obvious symptoms until the day she becomes weak and asks to be taken to the hospital. She dies off-screen to the stately sounds of Brahms's First Symphony.[53] In the 1968

51. In the AFI entry for *Madame Curie* neither "cancer" nor "leukemia" appears as a principal or additional subject. See Alberto Elena, "Skirts in the Lab: 'Madame Curie' and the Image of the Woman Scientist in the Feature Film," *Pub. Underst. Sci.*, 1997, 6: 269–78.

52. See Susan E. Lederer, "Hollywood and Human Experimentation: Representing Medical Research in Popular Film," in *Medicine's Moving Pictures*, ed. Paula Treichler, Nancy Tomes, and Leslie Reagan (Rochester, N.Y.: University of Rochester Press, 2007).

53. The film was based on the 1944 novel by Ruth Southard, *No Sad Songs for Me* (New York: Doubleday, Doran, 1944). In the novel, Cas goes to see her doctor hoping to learn that she is pregnant; instead, the doctor reads her his findings: "The report was detailed and technical. Cas recognized physiological terms, but the connecting phrases were meaningless. She looked at the X rays. They were blurry and indefinite, like some of the pictures she took of Polly—the kind returned undeveloped. They had no more significance than the words the

film *The Heart Is a Lonely Hunter*, based on the novel by Carson McCullers, Dr. Copeland, a Negro physician committed to Marxism and social justice for his race, diagnoses his own lung cancer, a discovery shared with the mute Mr. Singer. Copeland extracts a promise from Singer that he will not let anyone know that he is dying of cancer. After Copeland's son-in-law is attacked by angry whites and left crippled for life, Singer insists on informing the doctor's daughter about his condition. Singer's mute intervention enables the father and daughter to be reconciled.

In other Hollywood films, family members learn the truth about the patient's diagnosis from the physician and agree to keep the sad news from the patient. This was a pattern set in *Dark Victory* and *An Act of Murder*. When the physician informs the spouse about the diagnosis, the family colludes in keeping the dark secret. In the 1958 film adaptation of Tennessee Williams's *Cat on a Hot Tin Roof*, the terrible screen secret is not Brick's latent homosexuality (all references had to be deleted to conform to the censors) but rather the "Big C," the stomach cancer that plagues Big Daddy. Although his wife and grown children are told the bad news, Big Daddy remains in ignorance, until Brick reveals the true nature of his stomach ailment.[54] In 1970 Gore Vidal adapted another Tennessee Williams play for the screen. On the stage, *The Seven Descents of Myrtle* was a play about a man gravely ill man with tuberculosis, who marries a showgirl in order to provide an heir and thus ensure that the family's decaying Louisiana estate will go to his children rather than his illegitimate, racially mixed half-brother. Among the changes that Vidal made in the screenplay was the alteration of the lead character Lot from a "transvestite homosexual" without any interest in the female sex to a man "impotent" because of his psychological problems. Vidal also altered the character's medical problem from tuberculosis to cancer. Despite these changes, the film, which received an X rating in the early days of the movie rating system, was a terrible flop.[55]

---

doctor was reading. Only 'malignant' made her start, brace herself against the chair. Malignant growth . . ." (p. 6). The doctor tells her she should have come months ago, and now it's too late. "Is it cancer?" she asks. They discuss radium treatments, operations, but she has only nine months to live. Later in the book, she finally tells her husband her diagnosis when she needs to go to the hospital: "Cancer. I'm going to die"; and "It's cancer," she repeated. "Nasty things that sneak up on one without warning. They must be of Japanese origin" (pp. 166–67).

54. See Gene Philips, *The Films of Tennessee Williams* (East Brunswick, N.J.: Associated University Presses, 1980).

55. The X rating had much more to do with the suggestion of a sexual act performed by the white showgirl on her husband's racially mixed half-brother: Gene D. Phillips, "Tennessee Williams's Forgotten Film: *The Last of the Mobile Hot Shots* as a Screen Version of *The Seven Descents of Myrtle*," in Philip C. Kolin, ed., *The Undiscovered Country: The Later Plays of Tennessee Williams* (New York: Peter Lang, 2002), pp. 69–79, on p. 76.

Much more financially successful was the screen tragedy *Love Story* (1970). Jenny Cavilleri, the young Radcliffe graduate who develops a fatal illness, was considerably more sympathetic than the broken-down, mother-fixated Tennessee Williams character. The top grossing film of 1970, *Love Story* presented the tale of the courtship and marriage of a wealthy Harvard hockey player and a scholarship student majoring in music. After their marriage, the young woman consults her doctor about her difficulty in conceiving a child. When the doctor diagnoses a serious (if unspecified) illness, he informs her husband and the two men attempt to keep the news from her as long as possible. She learns the truth about her diagnosis when she is referred to a hematologist for treatment (her disease remains unspecified, but everyone seems to infer that she has leukemia). During her brief illness, Jenny is hospitalized. She looks pale and wan in her hospital bed, replete with her intravenous tubes, but, like Bette Davis in *Dark Victory*, she dies graciously, glamorously, and mercifully quickly. The film does not end with her tragic death from leukemia; rather, it focuses on the reconciliation of her "preppy" husband with his distant, often disapproving patrician father.[56] *Mad* magazine hilariously parodied some of the conventions of screen cancer. In a spoof on *Love Story*, the cancer specialist informs the Ryan O'Neal character, "I'm afraid it's out of our hands." O'Neal's character asks incredulously, "You mean medical science is powerless?" To which the doctor retorts, "What medical science? I'm talking about cinema science."[57]

What can be said of these films and their cancer content? First, there is no linear development in terms of the explicit discussion of cancer: *Dark Victory* was considerably more explicit in many ways than *Love Story* (released three decades later) about the heroine's disease. One of the messages that these screen portrayals reinforced was the death knell sounded by a cancer diagnosis. In *The 13th Letter* (1951), one character, upon receiving a "poison pen" letter informing him that he has cancer, commits suicide rather than face his disease. In the 1945 film *Between Two Women*, cancer is the disease most feared by a young woman who learns that she requires emergency surgery for her "blocked kidney"; despite the fact that she nearly dies from the risky surgery, she is relieved to learn that she does not have cancer. This does not mean that all screen cancers end in death: in *The Young Doctors* (1961), for instance, a young nurse who develops a tumor on her knee reluctantly agrees to undergo amputation

56. See Linda C. Pelzer, *Erich Segal: A Critical Companion* (Westport, Conn.: Greenwood, 1997).

57. Quoted in Lidz, "In a Higher State of Being" (n. 8).

of her leg. (Less fortunate in the film is the young couple whose infant dies when the same pathologist who accurately diagnosed her leg tumor failed to note the baby's Rh blood status.)

Celluloid cancer was very selective. The types of cancers seen most often on screen not surprisingly featured visually acceptable (or at least not disfiguring) conditions. Tumors continued to involve primarily the limbs or the brain, rather than reproductive organs. In *The Last Angry Man* (1959), when a young black thug (Billy Dee Williams in his film debut) is arrested, the aging Dr. Ableman knows that the young man's behavior results from a tumor of the brain (headaches, blurred vision, etc). In Hollywood films, women before 1970 did not suffer breast, ovarian, or cervical cancer, thereby avoiding any suggestion of "unmentionable" anatomies. Similarly, men in Hollywood films did not develop testicular cancer. In only one case does someone (Big Daddy) develop stomach or colon cancer. Although Big Daddy experiences gastric pain and distress, no other symptoms make an appearance. In films before 1970, cancer was a "clean" and apparently nondisfiguring disease that usually ended in death.

Just as cancers were limited in their anatomical scope, so too were the therapeutic weapons against the disease. Although "quack doctors" offered cures, as in *Doctor Kildare's Strange Case*, surgery remained the only reputable course of action—but not even the surgeon's knife could save all sufferers. Finally, the etiology of screen cancer remained obscure. Cigarettes appeared ubiquitously on screen; in one now precious scene from *An Act of Murder*, the physician who informs the judge that his wife has a fatal disease offers him a cigarette to calm him. There was no cinematic association between tobacco and cancer. Although exposure to radiation in the 1940s was recognized as potentially hazardous to health, in 1950s films atomic radiation was more likely to breed gigantic ants (in *Them*, 1954, killer ants the size of city buses emerge near the sands of the Trinity bomb site), gigantic lizards (*Godzilla*, 1954, a 400-foot prehistoric reptile, terrorizes Tokyo), and gigantic leeches (*Attack of the Giant Leeches*, 1959; yes, you guessed it—very large leeches) than it was to cause cancer.[58] Perhaps the one exception to the impact of atomic radiation was *Experiment Alcatraz*, in which the crusading young researcher from Oak Ridge is seen as the potential savior for sufferers from leukemia.

Film was a powerful medium in the years before 1970. In the years between 1916 and 1970, cancer made periodic appearances on screen, contributing to American perceptions of what kind of disease it was, how

---

58. See Spencer Weart, *Nuclear Fear: A History of Images* (Cambridge: Harvard University Press, 1988), pp. 191–94.

it could be treated, how it required more research, and the kinds of outcomes one could expect from cancer. Learning about cancer from the cinema was perhaps a "dark victory," insofar as the collateral messages in the flickering light of movie screens helped shape American expectations about disease, death, and doctors.

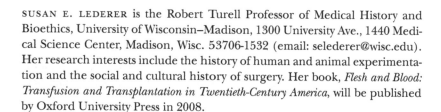

SUSAN E. LEDERER is the Robert Turell Professor of Medical History and Bioethics, University of Wisconsin–Madison, 1300 University Ave., 1440 Medical Science Center, Madison, Wisc. 53706-1532 (email: selederer@wisc.edu). Her research interests include the history of human and animal experimentation and the social and cultural history of surgery. Her book, *Flesh and Blood: Transfusion and Transplantation in Twentieth-Century America*, will be published by Oxford University Press in 2008.

"Cancer as the General Population Knows It": Knowledge, Fear, and Lay Education in 1950s Britain

ELIZABETH TOON

SUMMARY: This article examines British medical debates about cancer education in the 1950s, debates that reveal how those responsible for cancer control thought about the public and their relationship to it, and what they thought the new political economy of medicine introduced by the National Health Service would mean for that relationship. Opponents of education campaigns argued that such programs would add to the economic and organizational pressures on the NHS, by setting in motion an ill-informed, uncontrollable demand that would overwhelm the service. But an influential educational "experiment" devised by the Manchester Committee on Cancer challenged these doubts, arguing that the public's fear was based in their experience with family and friends dying of the disease. The challenge for cancer control, then, was to improve that experience and thus change experiential knowledge.

KEYWORDS: health education, cancer, National Health Service, Great Britain, Manchester Committee on Cancer, Ralston Paterson, "cancerphobia," patient experience, palliative care

Just after the Second World War, gynecologist Malcolm Donaldson set out to convince the British Empire Cancer Campaign (BECC) to expand its prewar program of lay cancer education. Though he chaired the BECC's Educational Committee, Donaldson failed to persuade the organization's

This research has been funded as part of the Wellcome Trust's Constructing Cancers grant to the Centre for the History of Science, Technology and Medicine, University of Manchester. My thanks to archivists and librarians at the National Archives, Kew; Special Collections, the Wellcome Library, London; and the British Medical Association, London. An earlier version of this paper was circulated for the workshop "Cancer in the Twentieth Century," held at the National Institutes of Health, Bethesda, Maryland, 15–17 November 2004. My thanks to the participants at that workshop for their questions and criticisms, and to the *Bulletin*'s anonymous reader for very helpful suggestions. Finally, my greatest thanks to David Cantor and to my CHSTM/cancer project colleagues John V. Pickstone, Emm Barnes, Carsten Timmermann, and Helen Valier (now University of Houston), for their encouragement and critiques.

leaders that a national cancer-education campaign would be worthwhile. Nor would the Ministry of Health accept Donaldson's suggestions, its medical officers arguing that "the time was not ripe for an approach to the general public."[1] When Donaldson managed to recruit allies in the Central Council for Health Education (CCHE), he and they soon found that neither the BECC nor the Ministry would cooperate with them on a national program. Instead, these organizations suggested that lay education about cancer should be left to the initiative of local groups choosing to experiment with it.

To scholars familiar with the history of cancer control, the BECC's and the Ministry's reluctance to create or participate in national educational programs about the "dread disease" might seem odd. In North America, equivalent organizations had just increased their substantial prewar commitment to education, funding national campaigns intended to "fight cancer with knowledge," as the American Cancer Society's motto put it.[2] But in Britain, much of the cancer elite—the clinicians, researchers, public health workers, and government officials who made the disease their business—rejected the idea that they should teach the public about cancer symptoms and treatment. Furthermore, when cancer-education programs were developed and adopted in 1950s Britain, many differed from those in other national contexts: cancer-control organizations elsewhere used the nationally coordinated media "blitz," the big-screen film, and the glossy color pamphlet to get their message across, while British

1. R. Gedling to R. Brain and W. P. Kennedy, September 1949, MH 55/927, National Archives, Kew Gardens, Surrey, U.K. (hereafter NA).

2. On American cancer education, see James T. Patterson, *The Dread Disease: Cancer and Modern American Culture* (Cambridge: Harvard University Press, 1987); Leslie J. Reagan, "Engendering the Dread Disease: Women, Men, and Cancer," *Amer. J. Pub. Health,* 1997, *87*: 1779–87; Barron H. Lerner, *The Breast Cancer Wars: Hope, Fear, and the Pursuit of a Cure in Twentieth-Century America* (New York: Oxford University Press, 2000); Robert Aronowitz, "'Do Not Delay': Breast Cancer and Time, 1900–1970," *Milbank Quart.,* 2001, *79*: 355–86; Kirsten E. Gardner, *Early Detection: Women, Cancer, and Awareness Campaigns in the Twentieth-Century United States* (Chapel Hill: University of North Carolina Press, 2006). A brief comparison of American and British programs is James T. Patterson, "Cancer, Cancerphobia, and Culture: Reflections on Attitudes in the United States and Great Britain," *Twent. Cent. Brit. His.,* 1991, *2*: 137–49. On cancer and disease education in twentieth-century Britain, see David Cantor, "Representing 'the Public': Medicine, Charity and Emotion in Twentieth-Century Britain," in *Medicine, Health and the Public Sphere in Britain, 1600–2000,* ed. Steve Sturdy (London: Routledge, 2002), pp. 144–68; Virginia Berridge and Kelly Loughlin, "Smoking and the New Health Education in Britain, 1950s–1970s," *Amer. J. Pub. Health,* 2005, *95*: 956–64; and Ornella Moscucci's unpublished "Fast-Track to Treatment: Cancer Education in Britain, circa 1900–1948," distributed for *Patients and Pathways: Cancer Therapies in Historical and Sociological Perspective,* University of Manchester, October 2005.

proponents of cancer education devised local efforts, often relying on the humbler media of newspapers and small-group discussions to promote everyday understanding of the disease and its treatment.

What accounts for the British cancer elite's rejection of lay education in the immediate postwar years? And why did strategies for lay cancer education in 1950s Britain differ from those devised elsewhere? Answering these questions helps us see how those responsible for cancer control thought about the public and their relationship to it, and what they thought the new political economy of medicine introduced by the National Health Service (NHS) would mean for that relationship. In the first half of this article I explore the postwar debate over cancer education, examining why opponents of such programs objected so strongly to them. The men and women of the British cancer establishment conceived of themselves as managing the frequently irrational demands of a public they characterized as gullible and emotional, a conceptualization of "the public" that they shared with cancer experts abroad and with other medics at home.[3] But many also believed that the public was *so* irrational about this disease that education—defined as the large-scale mass-media provision of facts about potential symptoms—was counterproductive. What was more, they argued, popular education could only add to the economic and organizational pressures on the NHS, by setting in motion an ill-informed, uncontrollable demand that would overwhelm the services they had labored to establish.

In the second half of the article I examine an influential experiment that challenged existing doubts about cancer education by offering a new model of what cancer education was and what it needed to do. The Manchester Committee on Cancer (MCC) argued that the British public's knowledge came from local, everyday encounters with medical institutions and expertise in their communities. While these proponents of education agreed that the everyday dread of cancer was substantial and frequently irrational, they also argued that the public's fear was understandable and based in reality: it derived from personal experience with family, friends, and neighbors dying of the disease. The real challenge for cancer control, then, was to improve that experience and thus change experiential knowledge, "cancer as the general population knows it." To accomplish this, the Manchester organizers instituted a very different sort of educational program, one that enlisted the voices of everyday Britons and mobilized existing social networks.

3. Cantor, "Representing 'the Public'" (n. 2).

Much Anxious Thought:
What Was Wrong with Lay Cancer Education?

In Britain, discussions about lay cancer education began in the early twentieth century, largely spurred by Charles P. Childe's 1906 book *The Control of a Scourge.*[4] Childe and his allies agreed among themselves and with their international colleagues on a general model of what cancer education was, whom it would address, and what its results would be. First, like others involved in popular health instruction, advocates of cancer education believed themselves to be remedying mass ignorance through the provision of scientific facts, which would then encourage sensible health behavior. Cancer, the medical elite agreed, was the most frightening of diseases, and fear of it could drive otherwise intelligent people into irrational behavior. Cancer education thus needed to bring the everyday Briton to her or his senses—to replace an unthinking fear with a reasoned, appropriate response. Second, women formed the primary audience for cancer education. This grew in part from notions about women's nature and roles: women were said to be more likely to be irrational in the face of cancer, but were also considered more likely to bear responsibility for monitoring their family's health.[5] Third, educators agreed that their focus needed to be the "accessible cancers," those more amenable to early detection by the patient or the general practitioner. Breast and cervical cancer were the most prominent of these, meaning that women seemed to form a disproportionate portion of the population that could be helped by education.

The most powerful assumption about cancer education, though, was that its central message should be that "early cancer is curable." This message, it was thought, would cultivate popular awareness of symptoms that might mean cancer, but would also reduce the public's fear of cancer. If knowledge was increased and fear decreased, the argument went, everyday women and men would present themselves to their GPs as soon as they noticed anything amiss. Any cancer present would be diagnosed at an earlier stage, and its cure would be likelier. In other words, British advocates of lay cancer education endorsed the view that "delay" was their chief foe, drawing on the same discourses as their colleagues elsewhere (but especially in the United States).[6] A few admitted cautiously that earlier diagnosis would not necessarily increase the likelihood of cure for some

4. Moscucci, "Fast-Track to Treatment" (n. 2), pp. 9–10.
5. Reagan, "Engendering" (n. 2); Gardner, *Early Detection* (n. 2), esp. chap. 1.
6. Aronowitz, "'Do Not Delay'" (n. 2); Lerner, *Breast Cancer Wars* (n. 2), pp. 41–60.

cancers and for some individual patients, and even that earlier presentation by patients might not make much of a dent in overall mortality rates. Nonetheless, they believed that a lay educational campaign would, generally, decrease the length of time that patients "delayed" seeking advice after noticing symptoms, which would—again, generally—positively affect the stage distribution of cancers detected, and thereby positively affect cure rates. Other advocates of lay education seem not to have concerned themselves with such complicated caveats. But regardless of how many qualifications they offered to the delay argument, proponents agreed fervently that by increasing the public's knowledge they would demolish a widespread fear sown by equally widespread ignorance.[7]

Nevertheless, much of the British medical community opposed educating laypeople about cancer, and thus relatively little lay cancer education was done in the 1910s, 1920s, and 1930s. As Ornella Moscucci has shown, early twentieth-century opponents of lay education worried that it would foster "cancerphobia," pollute public discourse, and (by facilitating lay knowledge) undermine professional authority.[8] Some local health authorities offered lectures about cancer to lay audiences, but when national organizations like the British Empire Cancer Campaign addressed the public, they did so mostly for fund-raising purposes. In the 1930s the BECC made a formal distinction between fund-raising appeals and education, vesting the latter responsibility in a Propaganda Committee headed by Malcolm Donaldson, a gynecological surgeon at London's St. Bartholomew's Hospital and a National Radium Commission member.[9] Donaldson organized speaker panels in several counties, outfitting local practitioners with "skeleton lectures" to guide their presentations.[10] While the talks were apparently popular and several medics cooperated by giving lectures, the Propaganda Committee was discontinued when the war began.[11]

7. For instance, Ronald W. Raven and Joan Gough-Thomas, "Cancer Education of the Public," *Lancet*, 1951, *258*: 495–96, on p. 496: "the general opinion was expressed that fear of cancer was principally due to ignorance; and, if wise education was given, more patients would consult their doctors at an early stage."

8. Moscucci, "Fast-Track to Treatment" (n. 2), p. 8.

9. David Cantor, "The Definition of Radiobiology: The Medical Research Council's Support for Research into the Biological Effects of Radiation in Britain, 1919–1939" (Ph.D. diss., University of Lancaster, 1987).

10. "Notes for Lord Nathan," 14 September 1954, in SA/CRC/Q.1/3, Papers of the Cancer Research Campaign, formerly the British Empire Cancer Campaign (hereafter BECC Papers), Special Collections, the Wellcome Library for the History and Understanding of Medicine, London (hereafter Wellcome Library).

11. Practical obstacles also intervened, such as wartime paper restrictions.

When the war ended, Donaldson and others expected the BECC to restart its educational initiatives, but the Campaign's leadership responded that it was giving lay cancer education "much anxious thought."[12] They did reconstitute Donaldson's prewar Cancer Propaganda Committee, now renamed the Cancer Education Committee, in 1947; however, this committee was not expected to conduct educational campaigns, but to *consider* whether the BECC *should* conduct educational campaigns.[13] Two years later, the Education Committee proposed that the BECC should expand its lectures on cancer for general practitioners, and should also begin a local "test scheme" of lay education—but the Executive Committee took two years to mull over the proposal, finally announcing that first "the views of all general practitioners throughout the country should be obtained."[14] So along with a booklet urging recipients to become more cancer-conscious in their practice, the BECC sent a questionnaire to all general practitioners in the United Kingdom, asking whether they thought lay education "would be of assistance in securing the earlier diagnosis of cancer, and thereby improving the chances of cure."[15]

While the BECC surveyed the nation's doctors, the Ministry of Health also contemplated lay cancer education, spurred by inquiries from the Central Council for Health Education. This small, quasi-official body had been set up before the war; drawing largely on financial contributions from local authorities, the CCHE produced health-education materials that local authorities could use in their own campaigns, and trained local personnel in educational methods. The CCHE had contacted both the Ministry and the BECC to ask whether they wanted to collaborate on cancer-education materials, but the BECC had declined to respond, instead waiting to see what role vis-à-vis cancer education the Ministry would suggest for the CCHE.[16] Ministry officials expressed their annoyance at the CCHE's push to "do something" despite other bodies' disapproval, and argued that the Council should simply advise local authorities.[17] Producing cancer materials or organizing educational programs,

12. For instance, F. L. Hopwood to F. B. Tours, 24 September 1952, SA/CRC/Q.1/2, BECC Papers.

13. "Notes" (n. 10), BECC Papers.

14. Ibid.

15. F. B. Tours, January 1953, SA/CRC/R.1/4, BECC Papers.

16. Executive Committee Minute 1915, SA/CRC/Q.1/5, BECC Papers.

17. R. Brain, [August 1949]; Gedling to Brain and Kennedy (n. 1); and M. Reed, "Cancer Propaganda," 21 July 1947; all NA MH 55/927. This was part of a larger debate about the CCHE's functions relative to the Ministry of Health. In 1946–47, the Ministry and the Central Office of Information had commissioned, circulated, and revised a script for a lay cancer film, but chose to concentrate on a film for GPs: NA MH 55/910.

the Ministry insisted, was impossible before the National Health Service was fully in place.[18]

In 1949, Ministry officials decided to consult the Central Health Service Council's Standing Cancer and Radiotherapy Advisory Committee (SCRAC) on the matter. Citing the "good deal of propaganda" disseminated by American and Canadian cancer societies, the memorandum noted that Ministry leaders were "very doubtful whether any general approach to the public on these lines would, in this country, be desirable."[19] The SCRAC—composed of leading cancer clinicians and researchers advising the Ministry—debated the issue, and, as internal discussions later revealed, "[they] were, in fact, so divided that they did their best not to give any advice at all."[20] After a few more months the SCRAC agreed that local authorities could undertake educational programs, but implied strong disapproval of any national scheme; the Central Health Services Council endorsed this decision by its Committee. With this guidance, Ministry officials worked to dissuade the CCHE from undertaking anything that could be construed as a national cancer-education program.[21] Finally in early 1951, after much negotiation, the SCRAC agreed it would not object to a CCHE pilot survey on cancer education, although the Ministry made it clear that no government funds would be forthcoming for such a survey.[22] Soon afterward, the SCRAC decided that a national program of lay education was still premature, but that central government (meaning the Ministry) should encourage local authorities and voluntary bodies to explore the effectiveness of such programs.[23]

In late 1952, the Ministry conditionally approved educational "test schemes" and began drafting a circular for local health authorities, suggesting that they avail themselves of the CCHE's model scheme.[24] But before sending out this circular, the Ministry sent it to the British Medical Association's General Medical Services Council (GMSC), asking its opinion on the matter. (Such consultation was common.) The GMSC,

18. "Note for file," 13 September 1948, NA MH 55/927.

19. "Cancer Education: Memorandum by the Ministry of Health," October 1949, ibid.

20. R. Gedling, 9 May 1950, ibid.

21. See the minute by M. R. [probably M. Reed], 19 July 1950, ibid.

22. A. Bavin to R. Sutherland, 9 February 1951, ibid.

23. Standing Cancer and Radiotherapy Advisory Committee, "Minutes of Meeting held 26 June 1952," ibid.; "Central Health Services Council," *Lancet,* 1953, *262*: 295.

24. "Note of meeting," 13 March 1953, NA MH 55/927; "Note of meeting between Mr Malcolm Donaldson and officers of the Department on September 18, 1952," ibid. These memos also discussed the Marie Curie Memorial Foundation's small program of lay cancer education, conducted without much consultation with other organizations.

misreading the circular as a Ministry endorsement of a national lay educational campaign, angrily resolved that it was "doubtful as to the wisdom
of instituting a campaign of this nature," and did not wish to be associated
with such a scheme.[25] The Ministry of Health responded rapidly, assuag-
ing the GMSC's fears with a startling quantity of conditional language:
"We hoped that the draft circular made it clear that local health authorities were simply being invited to explore the possibility of obtaining the
necessary co-operation in order to decide whether to have a local education scheme."[26] Apparently mollified, the GMSC relented, but responded
that "it would wish to be consulted again in the light of experience of the
pilot survey before giving its approval to any general scheme for cancer
education."[27]

Finally, in late August 1953, more than six years after Malcolm Donaldson had started urging all the organizations involved to take up lay cancer
education, the Ministry of Health issued its circular encouraging local
authorities and voluntary bodies to develop exploratory cancer-education
schemes.[28] But enthusiasm for such projects might well have been weak-
ened by the BECC's GP survey, finally published just a month before the
Ministry's circular. More than five thousand practitioners responded,
about one response for every four questionnaires mailed: 2,148 believed
that a program of lay education would be worthwhile, 2,683 thought not,
and 222 qualified their yes or no answers. Campaign spokesman Lord
Horder explained to *Lancet* readers that, given this result, the BECC had
decided to "consider the matter further in the light of this expression of
general-practitioner opinion"—in other words, to do nothing.[29]

Why did lay cancer education cause all this "anxious thought" in the
immediate postwar years? Clearly, much of this caution from all concerned
was a product of the delicate postwar balance between voluntary, official,
and professional groups. In the contentious political stew surrounding
the introduction and implementation of the National Health Service,
all these organizations—the Ministry, the BECC, the BMA, even the
CCHE—were attempting to shore up, reassert, or claim a voice in postwar
medical policymaking. Given the volatile debates at the same time about

25. General Medical Services Committee, "Minutes of the May 12, 1953 meeting," p. 16,
GMSC 1952–53, part 2, British Medical Association Archives, London (hereafter BMAA).

26. Ministry of Health to GMSC, quoted in "Agenda for the July 23, 1953 meeting," p.
33, *GMSC 1953–54*, part 1, BMAA.

27. Ibid., p. 39.

28. Ministry of Health, Circular 18/53.

29. Lord Horder, "The General Practitioner and Lay Education in Cancer" (letter to the
editor), *Lancet*, 1953, *262*: 137.

practitioner remuneration, hospital control, and research funding, it is hardly surprising that even on an apparently tangential matter such as lay cancer education the Ministry wanted neither to offend the BECC or (much worse) the BMA, nor to cede any territory to them. Meanwhile, the relatively powerless CCHE could do little without support from another organization, except to develop some pamphlets and its model scheme for others to use. The repeated emphasis on local schemes also makes sense, given the context: by encouraging local authorities to experiment with lay cancer education, the Ministry could counter the frequent charge that it was overcentralizing the nation's health services. Furthermore, local schemes not only allowed local authorities to display a measure of independence, they shifted the costs and effort of lay education—and the possibility of failure—away from the Ministry.

But these groups' leaders had other reasons for being anxious about lay cancer education, which drew on their assumptions about lay irrationality. Their most common objection (also common in North America) had always been that education would stir up fear rather than eliminating it; now, given the pressures on the new NHS, such fears seemed especially problematic. Claiming that the public was liable to self-diagnosis, opponents of cancer education fretted that a discussion of symptoms would drive "neurotic" Britons to surgeries, while others who might actually have cancer, now paralyzed by fear, would stay away. Worst of all, already harried GPs, overwhelmed by the crowds in their waiting rooms, would be likely to miss some early cancers while giving patients a false and perhaps disastrous sense of security.[30] Ministry correspondence about cancer education repeatedly expressed such concerns; a 1949 memorandum to the SCRAC, for instance, closed by stating that "the number of cases coming up for diagnosis and found not to be suffering from cancer might be increased very substantially," and asking: "Could the hospitals cope with the situation?"[31] By the early 1950s policymakers had realized that NHS costs would be incredibly difficult to rein in. The prospect of Britons' insisting on even more medical attention and diagnostic services, when it was unclear whether these would be certain to lower cancer mortality, must have been a frightening one. It was far better, the Ministry and the

30. SCRAC members also pointed out that bed shortages remained acute and waiting lists long: "Minutes of Meeting held 26 June 1952," NA MH 55/927.

31. "Cancer Education: Memorandum by the Ministry of Health" (draft, October 1949), ibid. See also Gedling to Brain and Kennedy (n. 1): "From the Minister's point of view the problem resolves itself largely into whether, if some propaganda of the kind suggested by Dr. Donaldson is done, there will be diagnostic and treatment facilities available for those who hearken to it."

BECC agreed, to teach GPs how to look for cancers *before* educational campaigns encouraged fearful Britons, newly empowered by a health service that was free at the point of delivery, to demand medical attention. The Ministry and BECC thus channeled their efforts into improving GPs' diagnostic skills through educational materials for practitioners rather than the public.

Advocates of lay cancer education made rebutting the arguments about cancerphobia and its implications for health services a priority. First, they claimed that, when conducted in other countries, cancer education had not sowed fear. Some cited the experience of health authorities in places like Massachusetts, where cancer education had been under way for several years. Others tried to sway opponents with home-grown proof. Malcolm Donaldson, for instance, administered a questionnaire to the middle-class clubwomen who attended his lectures, and they responded that the lecture had "relieved my mind," rather than "increased my worry."[32] Some educational advocates even argued that crammed waiting rooms were inevitable, as was the occasional neurotic or hypochondriac. As the team behind a Sheffield "pilot trial" of early detection insisted, "the problem is not that of cancerphobia specifically, but the vastly greater one of neurosis generally."[33] It was the medical profession's responsibility, they concluded, to allay the public's cancer fears, not dismiss them.

Equally substantial were concerns that lay cancer education might further pressure overburdened GPs, at a time when the ire of many general practitioners—whether directed at consultants, Ministry of Health administrators, or demanding patients—was palpable. Many medical professionals believed that the NHS threatened the GP's status, for the GP no longer seemed an independent professional who owned his or her practice and conducted it according to his or her druthers. The initial levels of remuneration that the NHS provided to GPs were lower than expected, and the increase in paperwork and patient load was sizeable. The 1952 Danckwerts Award partly settled pay issues, but the nation's GPs and the organization that claimed to speak for them, the BMA, remained concerned about workload.[34] Understandably, then, the organizations considering cancer

32. Malcolm Donaldson, "Lay Education in Cancer" (letter to the editor), *Lancet*, 1953, *262*: 199.

33. J. Walter and E. C. Atkinson, "Early Cancer Detection and Education: A Pilot Trial," *Brit. Med. J.*, 1955, *1*: 627–30, on p. 630. See also "Educating the Layman: Hunterian Society's Debate," *Lancet*, 1948, *252*: 820.

34. Charles Webster, *The National Health Service: A Political History* (Oxford: Oxford University Press, 1998); David Morrell, "Introduction and Overview," pp. 1–19, and Charles Webster, "The Politics of General Practice," pp. 20–44, in *General Practice under the National*

education did not want to get on the wrong side of the nation's general practitioners—at least, not over this subject. This also explains why the organizations concerned were careful to claim that they were considering the GP's opinion. When advocates of cancer education set out to disprove the "crowded surgery" argument, they needed to reassure two audiences at once: reluctant GPs, and their equally reluctant leadership.

Another pervasive objection, less clearly articulated but frequently invoked, centered on the form that lay education might take. Many in the cancer elite seemed to think that lay cancer education meant an "American-style" campaign, which they insisted was unsuitable for Britain. Usually they failed to explain what they meant by "American-style" education, but it was the American Cancer Society's mass-media campaign they disliked. BECC and Ministry of Health leaders had long been doubtful of such efforts generally, and their opposition crystallized after a delegation representing Britain's cancer establishment toured North American research, clinical, and organizational centers in 1948. One delegate, Stanford Cade of Westminster Hospital, seemed equivocal about the ACS's educational work, writing: "It has rendered cancer a reality to the man in the street."[35] Others, including Brian Windeyer of the Middlesex Hospital and F. B. Tours, the BECC's secretary-general, were less measured. Windeyer, an internationally respected radiotherapist, objected strongly to what he saw as a constant emphasis on fear. Tours wrote almost wistfully of the great sums of money the ACS had raised, but then criticized the "glaring" posters and advertisements that constantly reminded Americans of cancer's death toll.[36] At the tour's end, Cade, Windeyer, Tours, and their leader, Lord Horder, agreed that what they saw as a "strident" appeal to fear, while it might succeed in the United States, was wrong for Britain. Cementing their rejection of the American approach was a statistic that they found especially alarming: cancer-detection clinics in the United States had waiting lists of up to eight months, because Americans had taken the gospel of early detection to heart.[37] The ACS might have viewed this fact as an unfortunate but temporary sequela of success, but the British visitors took it as an indictment of not only the approach, but also its execution.

Health Service, 1948–1997, ed. Irvine Loudon, John Horder, and Charles Webster (London: Clarendon Press, 1998); Elston Grey-Turner and F. M. Sutherland, *History of the British Medical Association*, vol. 2: *1932–1981* (London: British Medical Association, 1982), chap. 5.

35. Stanford Cade, in "Report of a Visit to Canada and the United States by a Delegation from the British Empire Cancer Campaign, July 1948," [issued 25 March 1949], p. 13, PP/FGS/E.30, F. G. Spears Papers, Wellcome Library.

36. F. B. Tours, ibid., pp. 102–3.

37. Ibid., pp. 13 (Cade), 41 (Windeyer), and 102–3 (Tours).

These objections to the ACS's approach—that its appeal to fear would not work on the other side of the Atlantic, and that it might cause even more problems than it solved—featured in almost all discussions of cancer education over the next decade. Though they never articulated what they thought constituted the British national "character," the nation's elite clinicians and health officials maintained that using fear to spur Britons to action was unsuitable.[38] Even the enthusiastic Donaldson admitted that "in America it is put across in the wrong way."[39] Neither the opponents nor the proponents of lay cancer education had hard evidence regarding whether the high-visibility, hard-sell approach they identified with American campaigns would succeed or fail in the British context. Certainly they made no reference to formal, structured assessments of the British mindset, such as Mass Observation or other social surveys. Rather, they—like many of those engaged in health education in the first half of the twentieth century, on both sides of the Atlantic—relied on assumptions about the nature of a public they thought they knew well enough. Given these objections, if cancer education were to be accepted as valid, it would have to prove its merit in terms that made sense to the cancer elite.

This attitude toward education illustrates a key difference between the British cancer elite and the Americans whose work they observed and analyzed: American cancer workers seem to have decided fairly early on that education would cut delay, which would reduce cancer mortality, and then to have gotten on with it—from the early campaigns of the 1920s, through the increased activity of the late 1930s, to the full-scale media onslaught of the late 1940s. Robert Aronowitz suggests that the delay argument had a "self-evident" rationale, and its American advocates were relatively unconcerned with collecting "robust data" to support the argument.[40] Indeed, it was well after these educational initiatives began that some American investigators collected statistical evidence intended to prove education's value, suggesting that an apparently improving stage distribution and growing overall presentation rates were at least partly a result of educational activities.[41] By contrast, the British cancer elite demanded that proof *before* they would start a broad cancer-education campaign, and even then they remained skeptical: even the most positive assessments

38. Lerner, *Breast Cancer Wars* (n. 2), pp. 64–67.

39. "Report on the Special Meeting of the Chelsea Cancer Committee," 12 January 1950, p. 8, NA MH 55/927.

40. Aronowitz, "'Do Not Delay'" (n. 2), p. 358.

41. Guy F. Robbins et al., "The Significance of Early Treatment of Breast Cancer: Changes Correlated with the Cancer Education Programs of 1940–1955," *Cancer*, 1959, *12*: 688–92; Aronowitz, "'Do Not Delay'" (n. 2), p. 380.

of American cancer campaigns, for instance, still concluded that health education's effects were "imponderable" and nearly impossible to prove statistically.[42] In the end, finding proof that such campaigns could work in Britain would fall to the organizers of an "experiment" offering a very different approach to both education and the public.

Rethinking Knowledge, Fear, and Ignorance: The Manchester Educational Experiment

The Manchester Committee on Cancer (MCC) began its educational experiment in the early 1950s, having done independent fund-raising for cancer research and other publicity activities in the northwest since the 1920s.[43] The interest in cancer education in this group was led by Ralston Paterson, the radiotherapist director of the Christie Hospital and Holt Radium Institute. Admired for his organizational skills, Paterson designed some of the first randomized controlled trials in cancer therapy. He also stressed the importance of statistical investigation as a tool for assessing practice, an orientation that informed his approach to cancer education. His team included Jean Aitken-Swan, a Christie social worker, and John Wakefield, the MCC's executive officer.

The Manchester team's "experiment" simultaneously drew on some common assumptions about cancer education and tested others. The group began with the proposition that the problem to be solved was delay, especially women's delay in seeking medical attention for what would turn out to be breast or cervical cancers. These experts also presumed that while the object of a cancer-education campaign was to dispel fear, education itself, if incorrectly undertaken, might *spread* fear instead. As a result, the Manchester group described much of its plan in terms of what it would *not* do. Their work would not be negative, they claimed, and they would especially avoid what they termed "the lurid 'This might happen to you' approach."[44] Nor would they stress "cancer signs," as was common

---

42. "Cancer Education and Earlier Diagnosis," [probably 1953], NA MH 55/927. See also Richard Doll to Neville Goodman, 13 August 1953, ibid.; R. W. Scarff to F. L. Hopwood, 16 March 1954, SA/CRC/Q.1/3, and correspondence regarding H. H. Bentall, "Cancer Education," January 1956, SA/CRC/Q.1/4, BECC Papers.

43. Eileen Magnello, *A Centenary History of the Christie Hospital Manchester* (Manchester: Christie Hospital, 2001), pp. 46–47.

44. Ralston Paterson, C. Metcalfe Brown, and John Wakefield, "An Experiment in Cancer Education," *Brit. Med. J.*, 1954, *1*: 1219–21, on p. 1219; John Wakefield, "Cancer Education in Practice," in *Education of the Public Regarding Cancer: Report of Conference Held at B.M.A. House, 24 January 1957* (Central Council on Health Education, 1957), pp. 29–35, on p. 30, NA ED [Ministry of Education] 50/693.

in North American cancer education; instead, potential symptoms were described as "abnormal" and thus as a reason to consult a doctor. The group would not oversell its message by making broad claims like "cancer is curable," or even "early cancer is curable." Finally, the Manchester experiment would not take what MCC leaders called "the grand approach with large audiences and spectacular publicity," but would proceed through informal talks to small groups, short items in local newspapers, and short pamphlets.[45]

Especially distinctive were the steps that Paterson's group took to devise this experiment so that its results would be as statistically convincing as possible. Before launching the campaign, the MCC commissioned large social surveys of women in Manchester city, Salford, and Stockport, while Christie personnel conducted in-depth interviews with cancer patients and their family members.[46] These surveys promised a baseline assessment of the population, allowing the group to have a measurable sense of what exactly had changed in the meantime, presumably at least partly due to the educational program. While others involved with cancer education used opinion polls to judge the state of public knowledge, they tended to rely on national surveys rather than local ones, and it is unclear whether they used the surveys to measure the effects of particular programs.[47] The Manchester group, by contrast, expected surveys and interviews to explain "why women put off seeking advice for symptoms which they suspect to be cancer."[48]

As expected, the questionnaire demonstrated that women of all social classes considered cancer the most alarming disease. But what was both troubling and illuminating, the Manchester team decided, was that a substantial proportion of the women surveyed (from half to three-quarters) believed that cancer was *never* curable.[49] This contrasted with the two-thirds

45. Paterson, Brown, and Wakefield, "Experiment" (n. 44), p. 1219.

46. This was actually two surveys: one of 1,200 women, specifically about cancer, and another of 1,200 women questioned at the end of a mass radiography survey conducted by commercial canvassers and health visitors. See Ralston Paterson and Jean Aitken-Swan, "Public Opinion on Cancer: A Survey among Women in the Manchester Area," *Lancet*, 1954, *267*: 857–61, on p. 857.

47. By the mid-1950s the Manchester group and the Canadian Cancer Society used the same questionnaire to facilitate international comparisons: Ralston Paterson, "Why Do Cancer Patients Delay?" *Can. Med. Assoc. J.*, 1955, *73*: 931–40.

48. Paterson and Aitken-Swan, "Public Opinion" (n. 46), p. 857.

49. Fifty percent of the women responding to the cancer survey said they believed cancer could never be cured, while women responding to the same question at the end of the tuberculosis survey were more pessimistic: 55% of those asked by health visitors said cancer could never be cured, while 74% of those asked by commercial canvassers said so. The obvious conclusion,

of Americans surveyed who said that cancer could be cured.[50] Further questioning turned up another important finding: for some cancers, the problem was not one of ignorance. Only 40% of those surveyed thought that "a show of blood or discharge ten years or so after the change of life" might mean cancer. However, nearly 40% ranked a painless lump in the breast as the most alarming of a number of symptoms (including "constant cough" and "losing weight"), and 83% of those said that their alarm was because it was a sign of cancer.[51] Most revealing, though, were the responses from the open-ended questions included in the survey. Even among women in the "average +" group who held "presumably the most enlightened opinion," the pain and apparent incurability that they associated with cancer worried them the most:

> "The dreadful pain that one automatically associates with cancer."
>
> "The pain is so terrifying."
>
> "The suffering is so intense and usually so long drawn out."
>
> "It always seems to prove fatal."
>
> "The widespread idea that they can't do anything about it."[52]

This pessimism, the Manchester group agreed, was the chief problem that lay education needed to address.

Detailed interviews conducted with cancer patients and their families seemed to support these conclusions. Social worker Jean Aitken-Swan interviewed 239 women and 75 men who were Christie patients or their relatives.[53] The results, Aitken-Swan and Paterson argued, demonstrated that two distinct problems accounted for delay, for the patients interviewed (or described by relatives) fell into two distinct groups, with different behavior patterns regarding symptoms and medical advice. Some patients were judged to be genuinely ignorant: they did not know what their symptoms might mean. "Not-knowing," as Aitken-Swan and Paterson put it, accounted for their failure to suspect cancer and thus consult medical professionals. Sometimes this was because the symptoms were less commonly associated with cancer, or seemed related to recent pregnancies or previous health problems. This explained most delay in cases

---

though the Manchester team did not draw it, was that women felt more comfortable admitting this pessimism to commercial canvassers than to potentially judgmental health visitors.

50. Paterson and Aitken-Swan, "Public Opinion" (n. 46), p. 858.

51. Ibid., p. 859.

52. Ibid., p. 860.

53. These interviews seem not to have survived.

of cervical, skin, and mouth cancer.[54] By contrast, many patients "knew" perfectly well that their symptoms might mean they had cancer. Some who "knew" sought medical attention quickly, especially younger patients who seemed more inclined generally to consult medical professionals. But a significant remainder of patients "knew" but delayed more than three months, sometimes more than a year; these patients, then, formed "the main challenge to any public education project."[55] Many—especially breast cancer patients—presented themselves for diagnosis and treatment only when their symptoms became too problematic to manage or when relatives forced them to.

What, then, accounted for why some people who "knew" chose to act and others chose to delay? Differences in intelligence did not explain it, as IQ testing showed. The answer, Aitken-Swan and Paterson suggested, was fear—and the defensive psychological reactions that sometimes arose from it, such as denial, suppression and rationalization, and fatalistic acceptance. But the fear was not always of the cancer per se, but of what these patients associated with it: invalidism, hospitals, doctors, treatment, and, especially among older patients, anxiety about dependency, "of 'being sent away' and losing their rooms or houses. So much depended on their keeping going, and they saw no hopeful outcome if they let themselves get into the hands of the hospitals."[56] Interview excerpts quoted by Aitken-Swan and Paterson illustrated this:

> One timid, elderly lady said, "That's the God's truth, and I wouldn't tell you a lie. It was just that I was frightened I'd be sent away. I couldn't help it."[57]

The Manchester group believed that these reactions were problematic, sometimes citing others who claimed that delay was evidence of psychological pathology.[58] Nevertheless, their publications maintained

---

54. Jean Aitken-Swan and Ralston Paterson, "The Cancer Patient: Delay in Seeking Advice," *Brit. Med. J.*, 1955, 2: 623–27, on pp. 623–24.

55. Ibid., pp. 624–25.

56. Ibid., p. 625. This resembles the attitude found by Lucinda McCray Beier's studies of health in working-class Lancashire communities: Beier, "Expertise and Control: Childbearing in Three Twentieth-Century Working-Class Lancashire Communities," *Bull. Hist. Med.*, 2004, 78: 379–409; Beier, "'We Were Green as Grass': Learning about Sex and Reproduction in Three Working-Class Lancashire Communities," *Soc. Hist. Med.*, 2003, 16: 461–80.

57. Paterson, "Why Delay?" (n. 47), pp. 933–34.

58. See, e.g., J. G. Henderson, E. D. Wittkower, and M. N. Lougheed, "A Psychiatric Investigation of the Delay Factor in Patient to Doctor Presentation in Cancer," *J. Psychosom. Med.*, 1958, 3: 27–41, cited by John Wakefield, "A Co-operative Scheme of Public Education about Cancer," *Brit. J. Clin. Pract.*, 1961, 15: 165–67.

a relatively sympathetic tone. For instance, in 1957 John Wakefield told prospective educators:

> Fear of cancer seems to dwell on a deep emotional level; and any scheme to alleviate fear must therefore try to influence this same primitive level of emotion. People must be convinced that they and their families will be better off if they act in the way we urge them. This is no easy task. For almost all the evidence before them confirms people in their belief that cancer is a distressing, painful and inevitably fatal disease for which doctors can do little.[59]

While he referred to the fear of cancer as a "primitive" emotion, Wakefield here, as always, reminded medical professionals and other educators that everyday people had rational reasons for dreading cancer. He also insisted that

> the divergent paths of learning of speaker and audience have created a gap that [the speaker] must try to bridge. He may think his audience of cotton operatives very ignorant of elementary matters of medicine; but to them he will seem no less of an ignoramus on the intricacies of cotton spinning.[60]

Such statements highlight a difference between this approach and the usual rhetoric deployed by North American and British advocates of cancer education: the latter portrayed the audience for instruction as an ignorant, irrational mass in need of expert guidance; while the Manchester group described an audience of unschooled but not necessarily unintelligent everyday people who acted reasonably, given the evidence available to them.

This perception was at the heart of the Manchester group's assessment of what was at stake in cancer education. The problem facing them was not public ignorance of cancer symptoms, but the public's knowledge of the disease's all-too-frequent consequences. As Paterson had argued, "One could almost say axiomatically that every adult woman knows what a *lump* in the breast *may* mean."[61] Rather, the problem was the widespread fear of what would happen if one had cancer: pain, suffering, dependency, and death. And, the Manchester group pointed out, the public's pessimism about cancer had a "very substantial justification," for "over *all* the cancers taken together, death is still a much more common outcome than cure, and the manner of death is, by and large, often as distressing as can be."[62] Aitken-Swan's interviews with families of deceased cancer

---

59. Wakefield, "Cancer Education in Practice" (n. 44), p. 32.

60. John Wakefield, *Cancer and Public Education* (London: Pitman Medical Publishing, 1962), p. 26.

61. Paterson, "Why Delay?" (n. 47), p. 934 (emphasis in original).

62. Ibid., p. 935.

patients showed how many patients in the terminal stages of cancer were unable to obtain admission to the hospital where they had initially been treated, or to any hospital at all. Some patients had attentive GPs who visited regularly, and their families were usually satisfied with the care the patient had received—but other families argued that their GP had lost interest in the patient once it was clear that the patient was dying. The family members knew very well what the terminal patient experienced, as in many cases they had borne the chief responsibility for nursing.[63] "This," Aitken-Swan and Paterson wrote, "is cancer as the general population knows it—unpleasant, incurable, and rejected."[64] So pervasive was this experiential knowledge that it had "a direct bearing on the public's lack of confidence in what can be done for the cancer patient," and "lack of confidence in the efficacy of any treatment" accounted for delay.[65]

Paterson's group argued that their approach to lay education—a quiet but incessant barrage delivered through already-established community networks—was the best weapon against such a "climate of fear."[66] They chose three boroughs—Bury, Rochdale, and Oldham—surrounding Manchester city proper, with a largely working-class population of 620,000. After explaining the plan to hospital staff, BMA branches, and medical officers of health, Wakefield contacted local organizations—civic groups, women's clubs, church groups, political party branches, cooperative guilds, pensioners' associations, and even sports clubs—to schedule talks during routine meetings. He also visited the editors of the twelve local newspapers that covered the target area, to "ensure the accurate reporting of meetings and to avoid unfortunate sub-editing."[67] Speakers were drawn largely from the Christie Hospital's staff, although Wakefield himself frequently filled in. Meanwhile, the local newspapers reported

63. Jean Aitken-Swan, "Nursing the Late Cancer Patient at Home: The Family's Impressions," *Practitioner*, 1959, *183*: 64–69.

64. Aitken-Swan and Paterson, "Cancer Patient" (n. 54), p. 627. This reiterated what a 1952 survey found: a substantial proportion of dying cancer patients were dependent on family, friends, and neighbors for care, and many were aware that they had been "sent home from hospital to die" (Joint National Cancer Survey Committee of the Marie Curie Memorial and the Queen's Institute of District Nursing, *A Report on a National Survey Concerning Patients with Cancer Nursed at Home* [Marie Curie Memorial, April 1952], p. 25, SA/QNI/P.1/5, The Queen's Nursing Institute Collection, Wellcome Library). See also Noémi Tousignant, "Exposing Relief: Place, Cancer Pain and Appropriate Care for the Dying in Britain, 1950–1980" (M.Sc. thesis, University of Manchester, 2001).

65. Aitken-Swan and Paterson, "Cancer Patient" (n. 54), p. 627.

66. Wakefield, "Co-operative Scheme" (n. 58), p. 166.

67. Paterson, Brown, and Wakefield, "Experiment" (n. 44), pp. 1219–21, on p. 1220; Paterson, "Why Delay?" (n. 47), p. 936.

on the talks given at local meetings, aided by a condensed version of the lecture mailed to them afterward. And as a follow-up to the lectures, the MCC mailed copies of two pamphlets (on breast and on cervical cancer) to each group's secretary about two weeks after the talk was given. Although Wakefield later admitted that this approach did not directly reach "the apathetic and the unclubbable," it did, he argued, reach into the heart of the community, creating "a considerable 'scatter-effect,' an outward-spreading ripple of enlightenment . . . potentially one of the most powerful of all [influences] in changing existing attitudes."[68]

This emphasis on low-key, everyday efforts to change community attitudes and beliefs from within even produced a new form of cancer education: the voices of former sufferers themselves. After observing the "dramatic" impact on a group when a member testified how she had been cured of cancer, Wakefield and his colleagues took to tape-recording the stories of everyday residents of the community and playing them at other meetings. Here Wakefield invoked one of the few social analysis texts that would guide the Manchester group's educational experiment, or at least the only one the group ever cited: Richard Hoggart's chapter on "Them" and "Us" in *The Uses of Literacy: Aspects of Working-Class Life*.[69] Allowing an everyday person to take the stage, Wakefield insisted, was remarkably effective, for "her words were accepted without any of the reserve accorded to the claims of someone outside the group, the unvoiced and perhaps unconscious suspicion that they are being 'told the tale.'"[70] Cured-cancer clubs in the United States were intended to attract media attention; by contrast, the Manchester group used recognizably local voices to tell convincing stories about cancer treatment directly to the public.

Did it work? By the late 1950s, the Manchester group argued in print that their educational interventions had succeeded, albeit in a limited way. To assess progress, they examined changes in public opinion in their target area, as measured against public opinion in a "control" area (Preston, Blackburn, and Wigan); analyzed trends in delay compared to those in control communities; and conducted interviews to see whether the campaign had changed individual patients' behavior. The surveys returned mixed results, although the team tried to portray them in a generally positive light. When asked in 1957 if cancer was curable, a much greater proportion of women surveyed in the experimental area responded that it was (55%), compared to women from the control area surveyed at the same time (46%) and

68. Wakefield, *Cancer and Public Education* (n. 60), pp. 23, 24.
69. Richard Hoggart, *The Uses of Literacy: Aspects of Working-Class Life* (London: Chatto and Windus, 1957).
70. Wakefield, *Cancer and Public Education* (n. 60), p. 27.

women from the area adjacent to the experimental zone four years earlier (36%).[71] Furthermore, a greater proportion of women surveyed in the target area now seemed to believe that early treatment increased the chances of a cure (71%). These results were statistically significant, and seemed convincing that the educational program had produced, "though in modest degree only, a real change in public opinion."[72]

Nevertheless, other measures suggested that the experiment's success had been limited. For instance, a slightly greater proportion of women in the control area correctly identified the "first signs" of cervical and breast cancer than did women in the experimental area. The skeptic, Paterson's team admitted, could interpret this as "implying that in an area where there has been five years of cancer education there is rather less knowledge about the symptoms than in the control area."[73] Not surprisingly, the Manchester group took a more positive approach, arguing that the goal had *not* been to teach women to identify cancer symptoms; rather, they had stressed significant symptoms only when they could have "linked this with the emphasis that 'these do not necessarily mean cancer by any means—they merely mean that you should see your doctor and be examined.'"[74] The group also put a positive spin on the fact that only 8% of women surveyed in the experimental area had heard of talks on cancer being given: after all, they pointed out, only 11% actually belonged to a women's group, so by their (questionable) reasoning, eight of every eleven members of such groups had been reached. Rather than using this finding to indict their choice of campaign focus, the Manchester group concluded that they simply needed to expand their efforts, perhaps through factory lectures.[75]

But while women's opinions had apparently shown some evidence of change, the important question remained: had women with this "improved outlook on the curability of some cancers and on the value of early treatment" acted on this?[76] Here the Manchester team brought out their own statistics drawn from the Christie Hospital, where, they pointed out, "the great majority of [Manchester-area] patients with breast and cervix cancer . . . are sooner or later referred."[77] There did seem to be

71. Ralston Paterson and Jean Aitken-Swan, "Public Opinion on Cancer: Changes Following Five Years of Cancer Education," *Lancet*, 1958, *272*: 791–93, on p. 791.

72. Ibid., p. 792.

73. Ibid.

74. Ibid., pp. 792–93

75. Ibid.

76. Ibid., p. 793.

77. Jean Aitken-Swan and Ralston Paterson, "Assessment of the Results of Five Years of Cancer Education," *Brit. Med. J.*, 1959, *1*: 708–12, on p. 709.

a small but steady improvement in the numbers of cancer patients who had sought medical attention for their symptoms less than a month after noticing them, from 28% in 1950–51 to 38% in 1954–55. This improvement was not quite, but "very nearly" statistically significant, and no such improvement was visible in the control area.[78] Furthermore, the proportion of women with breast and cervical cancer who "presented" while in stages I and II seemed to have risen, from 55% to 64% of breast cancer patients and from 50% to 70% of cervical cancer patients. Interviews with patients likewise turned up equally suggestive but not conclusive results. A relatively large number of patients from the experimental area recalled having heard about the campaign's talks (28%) or having read articles in the local papers about these talks (35%). And many of the women who "took immediate action" in response to a symptom of breast cancer—in other words, who consulted a physician within a month—cited the campaign as the main factor motivating them. In fact, 36 of the 211 breast-cancer patients in the "immediate action" group attributed their action to the campaign.[79]

In the end, Paterson and his team claimed limited success for their educational campaign. They argued that there had been "a change in opinion and action," especially for breast cancer, even though that change was "extremely gradual" and "effected through a minority of the women reached."[80] This, they admitted, could be attributed to "an overall improved attitude to 'doctoring' and an increased willingness to seek advice for all abnormal or disturbing symptoms."[81] But the team also felt that, given their own "stringent" measures of success, they might have to continue education for a longer time in order to produce substantial results, and they indicated that they might consider a slight change in tactics: while talks had apparently been more influential than newspaper articles in shaping behavior, they clearly did not reach as large an audience as expected. (Not long after the initial experiment was finished, the MCC sent a "Mobile Information Unit" staffed with nurses to visit offices, stores, and factories.) Finally, the group hit on a more interesting conclusion: they might accept that the number of women whose attitudes and behavior would be affected by an educational campaign would be small. However, Aitken-Swan and Paterson concluded, perhaps this minority could be convinced to influence their fearful sisters, since "the advice and

78. Ibid., p. 709.
79. Ibid., p. 711.
80. Ibid.
81. Ibid., p. 712.

persuasion of friends" was said to be the second most important factor in convincing women with symptoms to seek medical advice.[82]

Conclusion

The Manchester approach to lay cancer education satisfied many critics among the British cancer elite that education could be valuable, and Paterson and Wakefield soon became de facto experts on the subject, frequently consulted by the Ministry of Health and others. (Wakefield even became chair of the International Union Against Cancer's Educational Committee.) Cancer education itself, however, remained a relatively low priority for the Ministry and other groups until the 1960s. As Virginia Berridge and Kelly Loughlin show, it was not until the link between smoking and lung cancer was established that British health organizations embraced national advertising-style cancer-education campaigns.[83] Meanwhile, the MCC continued experimenting with cancer education locally, in hopes of demonstrating its value nationally. In the 1960s and 1970s, they and a similar group in nearby Merseyside produced more social-scientific evaluations of women's knowledge and practices regarding cancer, using these analyses to judge the efficacy of local programs. Together with the published reports of the Manchester group's 1950s work, these are good sources for documenting everyday British women's ideas about cancer and its treatment. Most popular media of the period seem to have discussed cancer in terms of high-tech research accomplishments and gleaming new facilities. By contrast, surveys and interviews such as the Manchester group's hint at how cancer (and chronic and terminal diseases generally) fit into the social landscape of everyday Britons.

The discourse about public cancer education offers us insight into the concerns of the cancer elite about postwar medical care. We have seen how discussions about an "irrational" public stood in for concerns about how, or even whether, the public could be convinced to use health services wisely—that is, according to the goals set out by medical professionals and health planners. Much of the postwar British cancer elite shared with North American counterparts what we might call a "deficit" model of education, assuming that the problem facing cancer authorities was the ignorance and irrationality of the everyday Briton. But knowledge, they feared, would in this special case simply exacerbate public fears, by encouraging worried women and men to seek attention from a system

82. Ibid.
83. Berridge and Loughlin, "Smoking" (n. 2).

that was organizationally unprepared for them and already struggling to control costs. In such a climate, it was perhaps inevitable that the cancer elite would demand evidence that lay education could be made to work in Britain before they would risk carefully negotiated organizational relationships and restricted resources.

By contrast, the Manchester group's reconceptualization of lay cancer education and the problems it was meant to solve was surprisingly well suited to the contentious medical economy of postwar Britain. By avoiding discussions of specific symptoms, it released proponents of lay cancer education from the charge that they encouraged self-diagnosis; furthermore, it argued (optimistically) that the public could be taught to use health services in a rational way. Indeed, perhaps the most interesting aspect of the Manchester team's approach to cancer education was that it redistributed the burden of action among the public to be educated, the educators who spoke to them, and even the experts responsible for organizing cancer services. After all, if educators hoped to sell the good news about cancer to the public, they needed cancer centers, hospitals, and specialists to do the good work that would make the positive results of "modern" treatment visible. In a world where cancer sufferers still all too frequently died painful and lonely deaths, the Manchester group admitted that it would be slow and difficult to change the average experience of cancer, and thus the average person's understanding of it. Although the educational experts remained in charge of that effort, what made the Manchester experiment unique was the degree to which its leaders were willing to look to everyday Britons—if only temporarily—to understand their version of "the truth about cancer."

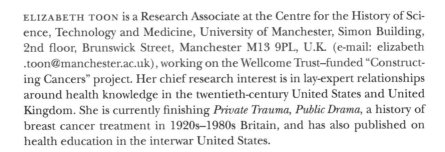

ELIZABETH TOON is a Research Associate at the Centre for the History of Science, Technology and Medicine, University of Manchester, Simon Building, 2nd floor, Brunswick Street, Manchester M13 9PL, U.K. (e-mail: elizabeth .toon@manchester.ac.uk), working on the Wellcome Trust–funded "Constructing Cancers" project. Her chief research interest is in lay-expert relationships around health knowledge in the twentieth-century United States and United Kingdom. She is currently finishing *Private Trauma, Public Drama*, a history of breast cancer treatment in 1920s–1980s Britain, and has also published on health education in the interwar United States.

Part II / Therapeutics

The "Ineffable Freemasonry of Sex": Feminist Surgeons and the Establishment of Radiotherapy in Early Twentieth-Century Britain

ORNELLA MOSCUCCI

SUMMARY: In 1924 the London Committee of the Medical Women's Federation was instrumental in establishing a clinic for the purpose of investigating the radium treatment of cervical cancer. The scheme was later to evolve into a hospital, the Marie Curie, where adherence to the methods developed in Stockholm served to establish radiotherapy as an alternative to surgery in cancer of the cervix. This article examines the women's contribution in the light of feminist and professional struggles over the relative merits of surgery and radiotherapy. It argues that radiotherapy was an issue of special interest to women surgeons, not only because of the long history of feminist opposition to gynecological surgery, but also because it could widen women's access to the medical profession in the face of male exclusion from training posts and honorary appointments at voluntary hospitals.

KEYWORDS: radiotherapy, radical abdominal hysterectomy, women surgeons, cervical cancer, Marie Curie Hospital

I wish to thank David Cantor, Aileen Clarke, Virginia Berridge, and John Pickstone for comments on an earlier draft of this paper. The research has been funded by the Wellcome Trust.

Introduction

Historians have recognized the part played by medical women in the establishment of radiotherapy in Britain.[1] The Marie Curie Hospital, the first special hospital for the radium treatment of cancer, grew out of a clinic established in 1924 by the London Committee of the Medical Women's Federation (MWF). Staffed entirely by medical women, the institution became famous for its outstanding success with the radium treatment of cervical cancer at a time when radical surgery was still regarded as the mainstay of treatment in "operable" cases. By the late 1930s the hospital had expanded its work to include rectal and breast cancer. It treated some seven hundred in-patients annually in thirty-nine beds, with facilities for radium and X-ray therapy, hostel accommodation for out-of-town patients, and up-to-date pathological and research laboratories.

In this article I reexamine the women's contribution in the light of the debate over the relative merits of surgery and radiotherapy. Central to this story was the contemporary concern with cervical cancer. The leading cause of female cancer death in Britain between 1840 and 1940, it had been the focus of therapeutic intervention since the last quarter of the nineteenth century with the development of both vaginal and radical abdominal hysterectomy. The latter, a procedure usually associated with the name of Ernst Wertheim, was by 1920 the treatment of choice for cervical cancer, despite widespread public and medical anxiety about its high mortality and "mutilating" consequences. It was partly because cervical cancer was an exclusively female disease, partly because of the long history of feminist opposition to gynecological surgery, I argue, that radiotherapy for cervical cancer became an issue of special interest to women surgeons, many of whom were active in the suffrage movement and in various campaigns to improve women's health. In addition, radiotherapy offered medical women career opportunities that were not readily available within the male-dominated field of surgical practice. A marginal specialty, it could accommodate female outsiders in the face of male exclusion from training posts and honorary appointments at major voluntary hospitals. Gender politics, in other words, were a significant dimension of the debate over the value of radiotherapy for cervical cancer. Exploring women's contribution is thus important in order fully to

1. Caroline Murphy, "A History of Radiotherapy to 1950: Cancer and Radiotherapy in Britain, 1850–1950" (Ph.D. diss., University of Manchester, 1986), chap. 5, pp. 25–31; Mary Ann Elston, "Run by Women, (Mainly) for Women: Medical Women's Hospitals in Britain, 1866–1948," in *Women and Modern Medicine*, ed. Lawrence Conrad and Anne Hardy (Amsterdam: Rodopi, 2001), pp. 73–107, on p. 90.

appreciate the broader political and social forces that shaped cancer care in early twentieth-century Britain.

Surgeons Ascendant

The leading cause of cancer death among British women until 1940, for much of the nineteenth century century cervical cancer inspired dread in doctors and patients alike. When John Williams, professor of midwifery at University College London, delivered the Harveian Lectures for 1886, he stated that no apology was needed for making this disease the subject of his talks: "The frequency with which it is met, its irresistible progress, the horrible sufferings which it entails upon its victims, the utter helplessness of medicine in its presence, and its fatal character, all alike join in demanding a careful study of its insidious onset, and destructive habits."[2] In Alban Berg's 1917 opera *Woyzeck* the subject of cancer of the womb was introduced by a short musical sequence constructed around the note B, which came to symbolize death throughout the opera.[3]

Attempts to treat cervical cancer by amputation and hysterectomy were made at the beginning of the nineteenth century, but they rarely eradicated the disease, and the fearful, often fatal hemorrhages that attended the treatment served to discourage further attempts. As the obstetrician Charles West remarked in 1858, "the supposed triumphs of surgery in cutting short the disease . . . were, for the most part, purely imaginary; and the trophies once displayed in our museums are now generally put out of sight, as the mementoes of a pathological blunder and a needless operation."[4] Cauterization in the "early" cases (i.e., where the cancer did not extend beyond the limits of the uterus) and palliation for the more advanced were thus standard practice in Britain for much of the nineteenth century.

In the last quarter of the century, however, the pendulum began to swing the other way and surgeons began to take a decidedly more interventionist approach to the disease. Amputation of the cervix was reintroduced for the early cases, while the development of abdominal surgery made it possible to tackle the more advanced cases by extirpating the uterus. The first attempts in this direction were made in the late 1870s

2. John Williams, *Cancer of the Uterus: Being the Harveian Lectures for 1886* (London: Lewis, 1888), p. 1.

3. Patrice Pinell, *The Fight against Cancer: France 1890–1940* (London: Routledge, 2002), p. 1.

4. Charles West, *Lectures on the Diseases of Women* (London: Churchill, 1858), p. 395.

by Wilhelm Freund, a German gynecologist who pioneered a procedure involving the removal of the uterus and parametrium. The purpose of Freund's hysterectomy was twofold: first, to root out the disease by removing not only the cancerous tissue, but also a good margin of apparently healthy tissue (hence the term "radical operation"); second, to extend the field of operability. But the dreadful mortality that attended Freund's abdominal hysterectomy (70 percent) caused widespread opposition, leading to the development of a vaginal procedure attended by a lower mortality (about 10 percent on average by 1889).[5] A further evolution of the method involved the introduction of episiotomy to widen the vagina so as to facilitate the excision of a larger portion of the parametrium, and the isolation of the ureters. The Viennese gynecologist Friedrich Schauta used this technique in 1901 to develop his own method, which involved the removal of a cuff of vagina together with the uterus.

During the 1890s, the belief that cervical cancer spread centrifugally along the lymph nodes provided the impetus for the development of radical abdominal hysterectomy. The model for this procedure was the radical mastectomy operation popularized by William Halsted in the early 1890s. Halsted advocated the removal of the breast, the larger of the two chest wall muscles, and the axillary glands in one piece, to prevent both the dissemination of cancer cells and local recurrence.[6] Reasoning by analogy, some surgeons and gynecologists criticized vaginal hysterectomy on the grounds that it could not deal with the problem of lymphatic spread. They argued that only the removal of the pelvic nodes, as well as the ovaries, the fallopian tubes, the uterus, and the healthy tissue around it could prevent recurrences. This extensive surgery is not viable unless an abdominal operation is performed. It is far easier to remove the upper portion of the broad ligaments with the fallopian tubes and ovaries in abdominal hysterectomy than when the operation is performed from below. Furthermore, the operation permits the removal of the lymph nodes lying on the iliac vessels, which is impossible by the vaginal route.

Radical abdominal hysterectomy was a German-American innovation: German from Freund who originated the abdominal route, and American

5. Frederick John McCann, *Cancer of the Womb: Its Symptoms, Diagnosis, Prognosis, and Treatment* (London: Frowde, 1907), pp. 86–87.

6. Samuel James Crowe, *Halsted of Johns Hopkins: The Man and His Men* (Springfield, Ill.: Thomas, 1957); Barron H. Lerner, *The Breast Cancer Wars: Fear, Hope and the Pursuit of a Cure in Twentieth-Century America* (Oxford: Oxford University Press, 2003), pp. 17–27. On the development of radical surgery, see Gert H. Brieger, "From Conservative to Radical Surgery in Late Nineteenth-Century America," in *Medical Theory, Surgical Practice: Studies in the History of Surgery*, ed. Christopher Lawrence (London: Routledge, 1995), pp. 216–31.

from the surgeons who developed it. In 1895 Emil Ries of Chicago was the first to show, by experimenting on dogs and cadavers, that a radical operation on the lines of Halsted's mastectomy was feasible; and in the same year John G. Clark, a colleague of Halsted's at Johns Hopkins Hospital, performed it on a living woman.[7] He was followed by Howard Kelly, also of Johns Hopkins, who perfected the method of dissecting the ureters from the region around the growth. Clark subsequently reported twelve cases of radical abdominal hysterectomy, though the technique used in each varied slightly: in some he had removed the lymph nodes, in others the parametrium and part of the vagina.

Total abdominal hysterectomy was subsequently standardized and popularized by the Austrian gynecologist Ernst Wertheim. A student of the legendary pioneer of abdominal surgery Theodor Billroth, Wertheim worked with the gynecologist R. Chobrak in Vienna and in 1891 he became first assistant to Friedrich Schauta. When he was appointed head of the Department of Gynecology at the Bettina Pavilion of the Elisabeth Hospital in Vienna, Wertheim obtained his own operating facilities and he then began to develop an extended abdominal operation for the treatment of cervical cancer. Wertheim's procedure was essentially a modification of the abdominal hysterectomy devised by Ries and Clark. Its distinguishing features were the thorough removal of the cellular tissue around the uterus, and the clamping of the vagina beneath the cancer (this was aimed at isolating the growth before removal, so as to avoid the risk of "infecting" the healthy portion of the vagina with cancer cells). Wertheim did not initially remove the lymph nodes as a routine; however, he subsequently became convinced that lymphatic involvement was a feature in the majority of cases, so he extended the procedure to include the pelvic glands.[8]

Wertheim claimed that his chief motive was to offer hope to those women who were "shut out from life" because of advanced carcinoma, but the high mortality from the operation was a cause for concern to many of his contemporaries. The fiercest criticisms came from feminists, who

7. John G. Clark, "More Radical Method of Performing Hysterectomy for Cancer of the Uterus," *Johns Hopkins Hosp. Bull.*, 1895, *6*: 120. For an account of the early history of this procedure, see Victor Bonney, "Wertheim's Operation in Retrospect," *Lancet*, 1949, *1*: 637–39; Howard Kelly, *Operative Gynecology*, 2d ed, 2 vols. (New York: Appleton, 1909), 2: 468–69.

8. "A Discussion on the Diagnosis and Treatment of Cancer of the Uterus" (leading article), *Brit. Med. J.*, 1905, *2*: 689–704. The gynecological profession was sharply divided on the question of lymphadenectomy: many doctors thought that the breast/cervical cancer analogy was wrong. See, e.g., McCann, *Cancer of the Womb* (n. 5), p. 96.

linked the development of "mutilating" operations with male violence, the uncaring attitudes of practitioners, and the use of animals in laboratories. Many feared that indifference to the sufferings of animals would encourage a loss of humanity: the suspicion was that it could be animals first, and women and workers next.[9] But gynecologists themselves had their doubts about radical abdominal hysterectomy. A British critic, the gynecologist Frederick McCann, remarked in 1907: "unless temporary or permanent benefit can be promised to the patient, it is not justifiable to subject her to a prolonged and dangerous operation which cannot completely remove the disease, more especially as the palliative operations and methods of treatment give considerable relief in the advanced stages of the disease and are less dangerous."[10] McCann was echoed by William Japp Sinclair, who roundly condemned the extended radical abdominal hysterectomies as "homicidal vivisections, which nothing hitherto advanced in their support appears to palliate, much less to justify."[11] Similar concerns were voiced in France and the United States.[12]

Such views need to be placed in the context of the evolution of British gynecology from about 1800 onward. Throughout the nineteenth century the specialty was dominated by practitioners who aspired to be gentlemanly physicians and spurned surgery as a lowly occupation, beneath the dignity of educated medical men. By the end of the century, however, the status of surgery was on the rise, and the younger men and women who were entering the profession had fewer prejudices against operative treatment. At the same time, the process of specialization was attracting surgeons to the field of gynecology, bringing to an end the conservative phase that had dominated its practice since the late eighteenth century. Wertheim's operation was caught in the cross-fire between the older generation of obstetric physicians on the one hand, and the younger generation of surgeons and obstetricians with surgical aspirations on the other.

The turning point in the fortunes of the extended abdominal hysterectomy in Britain came in 1905, when Wertheim introduced his method at an epoch-making meeting of the British Medical Association. At this

9. Ornella Moscucci, *The Science of Woman: Gynaecology and Gender in England, 1800–1929* (Cambridge: Cambridge University Press, 1990).

10. McCann, *Cancer of the Womb* (n. 5), p. 89.

11. William Japp Sinclair, "Carcinoma in Women, Chiefly in Its Clinical Aspects," *Brit. Med. J.*, 1902, 2: 321–27, on p. 325.

12. See Herbert Spencer, "A Discussion of the Measures to Be Recommended to Secure the Earlier Recognition of Uterine Cancer," *Brit. Med. J.*, 1907, 2: 431–40; Pierre Darmon, *Les cellules folles: L'homme face au cancer de l'Antiquité à nos jours* (Paris: Librairie Plon, 1993), p. 220.

meeting the eminent surgeon impressed his audience with claims that 30 percent of the cases treated by his procedure were free from recurrence after five years, as against the 10 percent or less obtained by simple abdominal or vaginal hysterectomy. Furthermore, he asserted that his operation was applicable to just over 50 percent of all cases of carcinoma of the cervix, instead of the 10–15 percent that was the limit of the lesser procedures. Wertheim had had thirty deaths in his first one hundred cases, but by the time he read his paper the operative mortality had fallen to 7 percent.[13]

Wertheim's operation was pioneered in Britain by abdominal surgeons: Cuthbert Lockyer of London's Samaritan Free Hospital, and Victor Bonney and Comyns Berkeley of the Middlesex Hospital. They were later joined by obstetricians like William Fletcher Shaw of Manchester, who founded the Royal College of Obstetricians and Gynaecologists in 1929. Bonney and Fletcher Shaw in particular continued to champion Wertheim's method during the 1920s even as the new techniques of radiotherapy challenged the dominance of surgeons in cancer therapy. Bonney saw surgery as the key to the rise in status of gynecology. A stalwart supporter of the Royal College of Surgeons, he wanted to maintain gynecology within the broader sphere of surgery, and he was determined that radiotherapy should remain the handmaiden of surgery.[14] But it should not be assumed that Bonney was insensitive toward women's feelings about gynecological surgery—indeed, one of his main claims to fame was the development of a conservative operation for uterine fibroids (myomectomy) at a time when hysterectomy was the standard treatment for the condition. "Apart from its physical value," he once commented, "the womb has for most women a sentimental value which, however illogical, cannot be lightly dismissed."[15] Bonney's views may have been influenced by events in his private life: in 1905 his wife had a hysterectomy for fibroids, and the couple was childless.

New Weapons, New Hopes

Although radical abdominal hysterectomy was "running the gauntlet of an animated professional criticism" in the early 1900s, few gynecologists

13. William Fletcher Shaw, "Wertheim's Hysterectomy for Carcinoma of the Cervix," *Lancet*, 1927, 2: 538.

14. Geoffrey Chamberlain, *Victor Bonney: The Gynaecological Surgeon of the Twentieth Century* (New York: Parthenon, 2000).

15. Ibid., p. 46.

questioned the propriety of surgical treatment.[16] "That cancer of the uterus is a hopeless and uniformly fatal disease is a proposition that has been true in the past through the whole period of human history during which the disease has been known," wrote the obstetrician Arthur Lewers in 1902:

> But the position is now entirely altered, since we now know that, if only cases are recognised in an early stage, a fair proportion may be permanently relieved by operation. . . . Hence it may be hoped that in the future suspicious symptoms will lead to prompt and thorough investigation, since at all events a diagnosis of cancer of the uterus in an early stage is now by no means equivalent to the diagnosis of a fatal disease.[17]

The problem for gynecologists was that many patients presented with disease that was too far advanced for operative treatment. Thus when X rays and radium were discovered, hopes were immediately raised that irradiation techniques might be beneficial in the "inoperable" cases. It was the apparent success of X rays and radium with both benign and malignant skin conditions that led to the application of the healing rays to less accessible tumors in the body's natural cavities: the mouth, the nose, the throat, the rectum, and the uterus. In 1903 Pierre Curie suggested that the advantage of radium over X rays was that it could be applied accurately to the place requiring treatment when contained in a fine tube.[18] This brought radium into the range of surgical treatments, attracting the attention of surgeons. By October 1903, a design for an aluminum tube to enable the insertion of radium into a tumor had appeared in the *Archives of the Roentgen Rays*, the first British radiological journal.[19]

While attracting widespread medical and public interest, the use of various sources of radiation in the treatment of cancer was initially viewed with suspicion by the medical profession. X-ray therapy was associated with the fringe practice of medical electricity, while radium therapy had its roots in heliotherapy, spa treatments, and the use of cauteries. The removal of cancer by cauterization was one of the oldest procedures in medicine, but by the early 1900s surgery had become the treatment of choice and any therapy that challenged the orthodoxy was branded as quackery.[20]

---

16. Kelly, *Operative Gynecology* (n. 7), 2: 468.

17. Arthur H. N. Lewers, *Cancer of the Uterus* (London: Lewis, 1902), p. 1.

18. Murphy, "History of Radiotherapy" (n. 1), chap. 3, p. 34.

19. Founded in 1896 under the title *Archives of Clinical Skiagraphy*. See Murphy, "History of Radiotherapy" (n. 1), chap. 2, p. 10.

20. See, e.g., Ernest F. Bashford, "Cancer, Credulity and Quackery," *Brit. Med. J.*, 1911, *1*: 1221–30.

In Britain the first reports of X-ray and radium therapy for gynecological disease began to appear in the early 1900s. In 1904 the *Journal of Obstetrics and Gynaecology* (founded in 1902) first described attempts to treat cancer of the vagina and of the breast by X-ray therapy, but the results were said to be disappointing.[21] In 1905, the obstetrician John Shields Fairbairn commented: "so far, nothing has been proved of the value of the rays as a therapeutic measure."[22] In the second edition of W. Playfair and T. Allbutt's *System of Gynaecology*, published in 1906, the gynecologist Amand Routh, of London's Charing Cross Hospital, wrote of testing the effects of radium in a case of inoperable cancer of the cervix: he had observed a marked reduction in symptoms, but the growth had continued to spread in the deeper tissues.[23]

By 1913 there was mounting evidence of radium's palliative effects in inoperable cases. In the first report of the London Radium Institute, founded in 1911 at the instigation of King Edward VII, it was stated that a total of thirty-nine cases of cancer of the uterus had been treated during the first year of activity of the institution: three patients had been discharged apparently cured, nineteen were "improved." Hayward Pinch, the medical superintendent, remarked that "in cases of inoperable malignant disease in this situation radium will often bring about results which cannot be attained by any other known method of treatment. . . . The rate of growth is checked, sometimes completely arrested, and the surrounding infiltration and induration are so much lessened that in a few instances cases previously declared to be inoperable become operable"; he noted, however, that the treatment was rarely curative: "though it may, and often does, check the rate of growth, yet in most cases dissemination will sooner or later occur, and the disease spread to parts beyond the effective range of radium."[24] Leading surgeons sought to damp down expectations. The rapid rise and demise of wonder cures such as Robert Koch's much-hyped tuberculin remedy twenty years earlier engendered an attitude of caution. As the surgeon Henry T. Butlin observed in 1909, "Berlin did a fine business while the craze lasted, but many of the patients spent more than they could afford to do on a treatment which was purely experimental, while

21. S. Sloan, "Report of the Glasgow Obstetric and Gynaecological Society," *J. Obstet. & Gyn.*, 1904, *5*: 309.

22. J. S. Fairbairn, "Röntgen Rays in Obstetrics and Gynaecology," *J. Obstet. & Gyn.*, 1905, *7*: 367–68, on p. 368.

23. Amand Routh, "Minor Uterine Operations," in *A System of Gynaecology*, ed. Thomas Allbutt and W. Playfair, 2nd ed. (London: Macmillan, 1906), p. 809.

24. A. E. Hayward Pinch, "A Report of the Work of the Radium Institute," *Brit. Med. J.*, 1913, *1*: 149–65, on p. 153.

others died miserably in hotels and lodging-houses"; British practitioners should not send patients to Paris for radium treatment merely in the hope that it might "do some good."[25]

Gynecologists' enthusiasm for X rays and radium therapy nonetheless rose during the 1910s, stimulated by the growing realization that radical cancer surgery had reached its limit. "The last card in the operative treatment of malignant disease appears to have been played," wrote Victor Bonney in 1915: "The hope that in the future more searching and safer means of cure than the scalpel and the dissecting forceps may be discovered is growing brighter."[26] Radiotherapy at first found a place in the treatment of inoperable cases, both as a palliative and as a means of extending the field of operability. After the First World War, surgeons began to use radium and X rays postoperatively in an attempt to diminish the tendency to recurrence.

A major change in philosophy was evident by the early 1920s, when advocates began to suggest that radiation alone could be used in operable cases. In 1920 the *British Medical Journal* argued that the treatment of cervical cancer by radium therapy should no longer be confined to inoperable cases: "More modern methods . . . together with a better appreciation of dosage and its effects, are undoubtedly pointing in the direction of radium therapy in earlier cases—even in those which are operable."[27] Advocates of Wertheim's hysterectomy were unconvinced, but increasingly during the 1920s the achievements of surgery were challenged by radiologists and gynecologists themselves. Enthusiasm for irradiation among surgeons rose sharply after 1925, prompting talk of a "boom of radium."[28] A notable convert was Comyns Berkeley, Bonney's associate at the Middlesex: he established a radium clinic at the Lambeth Hospital in London, and in the late 1920s he became a member both of the first National Radium Commission and of the League of Nations Commission on Radium.[29]

According to advocates, the main advantage of the new technique was its very low mortality compared with radical abdominal hysterectomy (approximately 2 percent in 1933, compared with an average death rate

25. Henry T. Butlin, "On Radium in the Treatment of Cancer and Some Associated Conditions," *Lancet*, 1909, 2: 1411–14, on p. 1414.

26. Victor Bonney, "A Review of Modern Gynaecological Practice," *Lancet*, 1915, 2: 1283–89, on p. 1285.

27. "Radium Therapy" (leading article), *Brit. Med. J.*, 1920, 1: 644–45.

28. A. E. Barclay, "The New Importance of Radium," *Lancet*, 1929, 1: 1061–62, on p. 1061.

29. For a biography of Berkeley, see Sir John Peel, *The Lives of the Fellows of the Royal College of Obstetricians and Gynaecologists 1929–1969* (London: Heinemann, 1976), pp. 69–72.

of 15.3 percent for Wertheim's operation).[30] Furthermore, radiotherapy was said to reduce the amount of "mutilation" to a minimum. This was a key point for the champions of irradiation, since the fear of operation and mutilation was widely regarded as a major cause of delay in treatment. Radiation therapy had none of the disadvantages of surgery; hence, it could help reduce delay and boost sufferers' chances of a cure.

From the point of view of the patient, the added attraction of radiotherapy was that it was less disruptive of ordinary daily activities than major abdominal surgery. One of the factors that contributed to the popularity of the Erlangen deep X-ray method in the 1920s was that the treatment could be completed in a short time and on an outpatient basis, thus enabling continuation of paid employment. When the gynecologist Louisa Martindale decided to adopt the Erlangen method in 1922, she found that the treatment appealed to many "doctors, headmistresses and other professional women as well as others who disliked to face an operation involving hospitalisation and a long convalescence, and—what to some is a serious matter—the loss of the uterus."[31]

Treatment with X rays or radium was not an easy option, however. Exhaustion, severe anemia, nausea, and sterility were the norm after a course of treatment with the deep X-ray therapy favored by Martindale, until it was realized that the inhalation of the noxious gases produced by the apparatus was an important factor in the causation of X-ray sickness. Proper ventilation and the removal of the apparatus from the treatment-room helped reduce the side effects of the treatment, but by the 1930s the search for ever more powerful X-ray machines was provoking renewed anxiety about the method. Radium researchers and medical physicists themselves deplored the "gigantism" of the new high-voltage apparatus and the "subjugation" of the patient to the machine, arguing that in their desire for X rays of greater penetrating power, radiologists were losing sight of the most important principle of successful treatment: "Primum non nocere."[32]

Meanwhile, radium therapy had become increasingly invasive with the development of surgical techniques aimed at opening the tumor to the

30. "Radiotherapy in Cancer of the Cervix" (leading article), *Brit. Med. J.*, 1933, 2: 243–44.

31. Louisa Martindale, *A Woman Surgeon* (London: Gollancz, 1951), p. 115. On the reception of the Erlangen method in Britain, see Paul D. Serwer, "The Rise of Radiation Protection: Science, Medicine, and Technology in Society, 1896–1935" (Ph.D. diss., Princeton University, 1978).

32. Helen Chambers and Sidney Russ, "Principles of Radiological Treatment and Their Bearing on Hospital X-ray Organization," *Brit. Med. J.*, 1935, 2: 9–11.

radium—the so-called surgery of access. Frans Daels's intrapelvic method, for example, involved incisions through the pelvis and blunt dissections of tissues followed by the insertion of radium containers directly into the growth. "Radio-surgery" was a response to those surgeons who claimed that radiotherapy could not deal with the lymphatic glands, but the insertion of needles did increase the risk of septic infection, which was one of the most common causes of death after radiotherapy.[33]

Turf Wars

As the new radiation techniques found a niche in cancer therapy, questions arose as to who should determine and carry out the treatment. The problem was usually formulated in terms of effectiveness and expertise, but the underlying issue was one of control. Who was to have jurisdiction over the cancer patient? In Britain, X-ray therapy was developed mostly by radiologists working in medical electricity departments, and gynecologists showed little interest in the technique. As Louisa Martindale noted in her autobiography, published in 1951, it was not surprising that in England the method had never been popular among the surgeons: "A surgeon is naturally anxious to treat the patient himself," she wrote, "and it was not the British custom to equip gynaecological clinics with their own X-ray facilities."[34] Martindale was unusual in being one of the first gynecologists in Britain to use X rays in her own practice. A fluent speaker of German, in 1913 she heard about the promising results that Professors Bernhard Krönig and Karl Gauss were obtaining with radiation therapy and she went to Freiburg to learn the techniques; what she saw impressed her so much that on her return to England she invested in an X-ray machine and began to treat certain benign conditions of the uterus, and cancer of the breast. By the early 1920s she was experimenting with the Erlangen method, which she had seen demonstrated in Professor Ludwig Seitz's department. Martindale's view was that the clinician responsible for determining and carrying out the treatment should be the gynecologist rather than the radiotherapist. This was because of the gynecologist's diagnostic expertise: "Careful and accurate diagnosis," she observed in her autobiography, "is the main factor in obtaining success and, for this reason, it was held in Freiburg that the treatment should be carried out by the gynaecologist in an X-ray therapeutic department attached to a

33. Septic infections were attributed to previous operative treatment. See "Radiotherapy in Cancer of the Cervix" (n. 30), p. 243.
34. Martindale, *Woman Surgeon* (n. 31), p. 115.

gynaecological clinic."[35] Martindale realized that the high fees charged for gynecological operations provided a strong incentive to surgery. Anxious that financial considerations might bias her judgment, she resolved to adopt the policy already implemented at Freiburg and charge the same fee for a hysterectomy as for X-ray treatment.

The question of control in radium therapy was more complex than for X-ray treatment. Some radiologists used radium as well as X rays, but most radium therapy was carried out by surgeons, gynecologists, dermatologists, and laryngologists; most importantly, surgeons controlled the insertion of radium into tumors. When the first specialized radium institutes in Britain were established, tensions arose over the control of cases. How could referring practitioners and specialists protect their professional and financial interests? The solution adopted at the London Radium Institute was to set up a complex hierarchical structure of tasks and responsibilities aimed at reducing the impact of the institution on the private practice of referring doctors. As the chairman of the Institute's medical committee, the eminent surgeon Sir Frederick Treves, explained in a letter to Hayward Pinch, it was desirable that he should limit "as far as possible" his responsibilities with regard to the patients admitted to the Institute: "It rests with you to indicate the specific treatment by radium to be employed . . . to see that the treatment by radium that is recommended is carried out. . . . For that treatment you are responsible."[36] Diagnosis was, however, the responsibility of the referring doctor: no patient, whether necessitous or well-to-do, was to be admitted without a certificate from the practitioner, who thus retained his or her right to determine the therapy. In difficult cases, a third party was to be called in. Necessitous cases were to be seen by a member of the Honorary Staff, but a paying patient's own doctor could choose any consultant. If Pinch was invited to choose a consultant, the patient would have to pay a fee, no matter where the consultation took place. Furthermore, when the methods of treatment required specialized skill, as for example in the insertion of radium into the uterus, Pinch was to hand over the patient to the appropriate specialist. The surgical manipulations required in such cases were free of charge for gratuitous patients; in all other cases a separate fee was payable directly to the specialist. Commenting on these arrangements, the *Lancet* remarked: "Sir Frederick Treves's letter is so simple and clear a document that it might well be framed and hung in the corridors of the institute, if only to convince everyone that

35. Ibid., p. 114.
36. "The Radium Institute," *Brit. Med. J.*, 1911, 2: 302–4, on p. 302.

the institute cannot be made use of to put fees into the pockets of any specially selected members of the medical profession."[37]

The radium-therapy boom of the 1920s prompted the first attempts to discourage the entry of "inexpert" practitioners into radium therapy. Mounting public concern about the safety of radiation lent weight to the argument that radiology should be placed in the hands of experienced workers.[38] Radiologists and surgeons with a special interest in radiotherapy were united in condemning empiricism in radiotherapy: "We see surgeons and gynaecologists rushing across to Brussels and elsewhere and, after a week of observation, returning as experts, writing up a few cases, and imagining that they are advancing scientific progress," wrote scornfully the radiologist A. E. Barclay in 1929; in Barclay's view, expert knowledge of radium and X rays was of far greater importance than expert surgery (which he alleged was a "comparatively simple matter" in the surgery of access): "The expert who controls the treatment should be the man who has expert knowledge of the most potent weapons—i.e., radium and X rays. . . . Till we realise that it is surgery and not radiation treatment which should now be regarded as the refuge of the destitute we shall not progress."[39]

At the same time, advocates of radiotherapy sought to rebut the criticisms leveled by those surgeons who professed skepticism about the value of radium. One of the most vocal critics was Victor Bonney: the eminent surgeon had no truck with those who argued that the "purely operative" treatment of cervical cancer could no longer compete with irradiation in term of success. In an article published in 1930, Bonney strongly deprecated

> as altogether premature the appeals that have been made to the younger generations of gynaecological surgeons not to embark on the operative treatment of cancer of the cervix, but instead to take up radium therapy, the present estimate of whose value in this connexion is founded solely on figures from abroad. Not until the results of reliable workers in this country are available shall we be in a position to properly appraise its effects, for it does not follow that the same measure of success attending a method of treatment in one country is necessarily attained when it is carried out in another country.[40]

37. "The Radium Institute," *Lancet*, 1911, 2: 396–99, on p. 396.

38. See Murphy, "History of Radiotherapy" (n. 1); David Cantor, "The MRC's Support for Experimental Radiology during the Inter-War Years," in *Historical Perspectives on the Role of the MRC: Essays in the History of the Medical Research Council of the United Kingdom and Its Predecessor, the Medical Research Committee, 1913–1953*, ed. Joan Austoker and Linda Bryder (Oxford: Oxford University Press, 1989), pp. 181–204.

39. Barclay, "New Importance of Radium" (n. 28), p. 1062.

40. Victor Bonney, "Surgical Treatment of Carcinoma of the Cervix," *Lancet*, 1930, *1*: 277–82, on p. 282.

William Fletcher Shaw also expressed concern about the lack of British statistics. "It is," he wrote in a letter published in the *British Medical Journal* for 1927, "surely not asking very much of British radiology to publish statistics on, at any rate, a five-year basis."[41] The Manchester gynecologist had been using radium applications to increase the field of operability since the early 1920s, but he drew the line at the suggestion that radiation therapy should become a substitute for surgical excision in operable cases.[42]

In order to rebut these criticisms and distance themselves from the bulk of surgeons who took up radium therapy, advocates deployed the rhetoric of science, arguing for the establishment of separate institutions, staffed by experienced workers, in which methods could be tried, tested, and standardized. According to the gynecologist Malcolm Donaldson, one of the British pioneers of radium therapy for cervical cancer, the number of cases of malignant disease admitted to the general hospitals was not large enough to support systematic research programs, and most of the cases were distributed among clinicians who had no interest in research anyway: "Clinical research needs a great number of beds and a special organization, which I maintain is not possible in any general hospital."[43] As well as centralization and specialization, Donaldson recommended the establishment of a hierarchical system of management in which teams of workers would be subordinate to a fully qualified director of research. A key medical concept in the interwar period, the notion of teamwork was seen as an antidote to the old style of competitive individualism in medical practice: "Competition may have its merits in many walks of life," wrote Donaldson in 1933, "but co-ordinaton and co-operation are far more important to the advancement of medical science."[44]

Yet the logic of centralization did not necessarily entail the subordination of the surgeon to the radiologist. It could be argued that surgeon and radiologist were equal partners in a relationship, since one could do

41. William Fletcher Shaw, "Treatment of Cancer by Radium" (letter), *Brit. Med J.*, 1927, 2: 1244.

42. As radium enthusiasts pointed out, the case for radical hysterectomy also rested largely on foreign statistics. See G. E. Birkett, "Treatment of Cancer by Radium" (letter), *Brit. Med. J.*, 1928, 1: 75. For an account of the surgery vs. radiotherapy debate in France, see Pinell, *Fight against Cancer* (n. 3), pp. 115–23. The development of radiotherapy services in Canada is discussed by Charles R. R. Hayter, *An Element of Hope: Radium and the Response to Cancer in Canada, 1900–1940* (Montreal: McGill-Queen's University Press, 2005).

43. Quoted in Cantor, "MRC's Support" (n. 38), p. 190.

44. Malcolm Donaldson, "A Suggestion for the Organization of Clinical Research in Cancer," *Brit. Med. J.*, 1933, 1: 68–69, on p. 69. On the concept of teamwork in medicine between the two world wars, see Steve Sturdy and Roger Cooter, "Science, Scientific Management, and the Transformation of Medicine in Britain, c. 1870–1950," *Hist. Sci.*, 1998, 36: 421–66.

in one sphere what the other could not do. As the *British Medical Journal* commented in 1933, the surgery of access demanded specialized skills that were outside the radiologist's sphere of expertise: "*At first sight* the impression is that we are dealing with an essentially simple procedure which demands no special surgical or gynaecological qualifications."[45] At the same time, one needed to realize that the surgery of access was "only a means to an end," namely, the "efficient distribution of the radiations from the radio-active material in the containers"; this was a "physical problem of no small complexity," which demanded specialist skill and expertise: as the techniques of radiotherapy advanced, no surgeon or gynecologist could hope to acquire the necessary know-how simply by attending a short course in "radium surgery."[46] There were thus strong arguments for teamwork in the delivery of radium therapy: "Co-ordination, co-operation, and permanency of specialist staff are certainly not least among the essential conditions for success," the journal observed.[47] The *Lancet* agreed that the development of the surgery of access pointed to one conclusion: "even in the new era the radiologist and surgeon must work together."[48] Taking the argument further, the journal argued for the unification of surgical and radiotherapeutic tasks: "most efficient of all will be the man who can combine surgical with radiological technique in his own repertory."[49]

It is against this background that we must now consider the Medical Women's Federation initiative. Originally established as a clinic in 1924, by 1929 the MWF's scheme had evolved into a thirty-bed hospital entirely staffed by medical women. Its work was to play a key role in establishing radiotherapy for cervical cancer, demonstrating the value of a rational "scientific" approach to the new radiation therapies.

The MWF's Cancer Committee

The MWF's research scheme was the brainchild of pathologist Dr. Helen Chambers, the first cancer researcher employed by the Medical Research Council (MRC) at the Middlesex Hospital Cancer Research Laboratories. Chambers's links with the Middlesex and the MRC were significant. The Middlesex had the longest tradition of specialized cancer work, and the strongest tradition of radium research: it was the first hospital to appoint

---

45. "Radiotherapy in Cancer of the Cervix" (n. 30), p. 243 (emphasis added).
46. Ibid.
47. Ibid., p. 244.
48. "Radium for Cancer" (leading article), *Lancet*, 1928, *1*: 973–74, on p. 973.
49. Ibid.

a medical physicist, and the original beneficiary of the radium acquired in 1919 by the Medical Research Committee, the predecessor of the MRC, from surplus government stock.[50] In the 1920s the MRC played a key role in promoting clinical research into the medical uses of radium. As David Cantor has shown, the chief objectives of this work were to overcome surgical resistance to radium therapy, and to discourage the entry of inexpert surgeons into the field.[51] Chambers's initiative served to further both of these objectives.

Chambers's association with the Middlesex Hospital went back to 1908, when she won a newly founded scholarship in cancer research. Chambers, who already held a part-time appointment at the Royal Free Hospital as assistant pathologist, worked in collaboration with Sidney Russ, the physicist and radium expert who was later to become the first secretary of the MRC's Radiology Committee. Between 1911 and 1913 they produced a series of articles on the biological effects of radium, which established Chambers's reputation in cancer research.

In 1915 Chambers resigned her appointment at the Royal Free Hospital in order to become pathologist to the Endell Street Military Hospital in London. At the end of the war she was one of the first to receive the Order of the Commander of the British Empire, and when the Endell Street Hospital closed, she returned to full-time cancer research with Professor Russ at the Middlesex Hospital.[52] Although her main line of research was the induction of cancer immunity, using in particular small doses of X rays, she was enthusiastic about the possibilities of radium therapy, especially in the treatment of cervical cancer. In February 1924 she gave an address on radium therapy to the monthly meeting of the London Association of the MWF, in which she drew attention to the value and shortage of radium. She suggested that a body of medical women might cooperate in a study of one specific aspect of cancer therapy; an exploratory committee was immediately formed, with Dr. Chambers and four gynecological surgeons as members. The committee included a number of practitioners who had been active as feminists, suffragists, and champions of women's health: Miss Maud Chadburn, founder of the South London Hospital for Women; Lady Florence Barrett, later to become Dean of the London

50. See Murphy, "History of Radiotherapy" (n. 1), chap. 5, pp. 14–18.

51. Cantor, "MRC's Support" (n. 38).

52. Biographical data on Helen Chambers are drawn from her obituaries: *Lancet*, 1935, 2: 228–29; *Med. Women's Fed. Quart. Rev.*, Jan.1935, pp. 58–61. Chambers's work on cancer immunity produced meager results, and in MRC circles there was some skepticism about the clinical applicability of the research. See Walter Fletcher to George Newman, 15 December 1923, National Archives (NA), London, FD 1/2037.

School of Medicine for Women; Lady Grace Maud Briscoe, physician to the Shoreditch Maternity Centre; and Louisa Martindale, founder of the New Sussex Hospital for Women. Miss (later Dame) Louise McIlroy, the first professor of obstetrics and gynecology at the Royal Free Hospital, and Miss E. Bolton, surgeon at the Elizabeth Garrett Anderson, also joined the committee as co-opted members.[53]

As a first step, it was decided to investigate the effects of radium therapy in carcinoma of the uterus. The choice of this cancer was not accidental. As we have seen, evidence from foreign centers suggested that radiotherapy was a viable alternative to surgery in the treatment of cancer of the cervix, yet many British surgeons still doubted that radiation could supplant Wertheim's hysterectomy. A well-designed clinical trial had the potential to generate reliable statistics about the value of radium therapy in British practice, thus providing ammunition against the stalwarts of operative treatment.

Quite apart from the potential utility of the research, there were special reasons why the investigation should have been of interest to the members of the Cancer Committee. Cervical cancer was undoubtedly an issue that medical women could claim as their own. For a start, the etiology of cervical cancer was bound up with two major women's causes: the prevention of venereal disease, and the reduction of the risks of childbearing. Earlier in the century suffragists and women doctors like Louisa Martindale had claimed that carcinoma of the cervix was one of the consequences of gonorrheal infections brought home by promiscuous husbands.[54] The supposed connection between venereal disease and cancer served to highlight the penalty that women paid for male depravity, providing an argument against the double standard of sexual morality and the "enslavement" of women within marriage. As the question of maternal mortality and morbidity climbed to the top of the political agenda in the 1920s, medical attention shifted onto obstetric injury as a cause of cervical cancer. High rates of maternal death raised questions about the standards of obstetric care, suggesting to feminists that society was failing to appreciate women's key role as childbearers. The high incidence of cervical cancer reflected the general neglect of women's social and biological functions, implicitly demonstrating the need for reforms aimed at improving the material conditions of women's lives.[55]

53. Helen Chambers, "The Marie Curie Hospital," *Med. Women's Fed. Newsl.*, March 1930, pp. 19–23.

54. Michael Worboys, "Unsexing Gonorrhoea: Bacteriologists, Gynaecologists, and Suffragists in Britain, 1860–1920," *Soc. Hist. Med.*, 2004, *17*: 41–59.

55. See, e.g., Sylvia Pankhurst, *Save the Mothers* (London: Knopf, 1930), p. 46.

The ideology of medical women's mission to other women came into play with regard to the diagnosis of cervical cancer. Since the second half of the nineteenth century, the case for women doctors had rested largely on the claim that women could provide medical and surgical care that did not violate women's modesty. Women's aversion to intrusive medical examinations was widely blamed as a cause of delay in the treatment of cervical cancer, so this was clearly an area where women's otherwise unmet health-care needs would be best served by medical women. In a wartime fund-raising pamphlet for the Marie Curie Hospital, writer Vita Sackville-West emphasized the special role that medical women could play in cancer care as friends and confidantes to their patients:

> [The hospital] exists to minister to peculiarly feminine ailments; and no one but a woman can know what they mean. They are ailments, which touch her in the most instinctive, primitive recesses of her being. . . . But if she knows she can go to a hospital where she meets with nothing but the indefinable freemasonry of sex; meets only other women who, though doctors, are speaking the same intimate language as herself; women to whom no revelation is novel, even the most secret fears and shyness and atavistic complexes—then her reluctance [to seek medical advice] may be modified and the danger taken before it is too late.[56]

Sackville-West also drew attention to the value of radiotherapy as a humane, woman-friendly alternative to "mutilating" surgery, deftly exploiting the long history of public concern over the treatment of charity patients in public hospitals. During the nineteenth century, fictional exposés of hospital practice had helped generate the belief that charity patients were being utilized as human subjects for vivisectionist experiments, fuelling working-class distrust of hospitals and surgical practice.[57] Sackville-West alluded to these anxieties in order to drum up support for the Marie Curie Hospital:

> Fear of the surgeon's knife is a serious deterrent, but the application of radium appears to suggest no alarm. It is easy to see the extreme importance of this factor. . . . It must be recalled that many of the patients come from the poorer quarters of London, patients to whom "the orspital" meant a bewildered and helpless dread, but who delivered themselves over to the care of *this* hospital the more willingly for the knowledge that their poor bodies were not going to be

56. Vita Sackville-West, *The Marie Curie Hospital*, 1947, p. 20, Contemporary Medical Archives Centre (CMAC), Wellcome Library, London, SA/MWF/C.41.

57. Anne L. Scott, "Physical Purity Feminism and State Medicine in Late Nineteenth-Century England," *Women's Hist. Rev.*, 1999, 4: 625–52; Moscucci, *Science of Woman* (n. 9), pp. 124–25.

carved up while they lay under the arc-lights unconscious and without defence. On the contrary, they were going to find it a time of comfort and relaxation such as they had never known before in a hard-working life.[58]

This emphasis on medical women's mission to the poor should not be taken as implying that the MWF's venture was untainted by considerations of professional success. Medical women had been quick to see that the new field of radiation therapy and medical electricity could enhance their employment opportunities at a time when de facto sex discrimination placed serious constraints on their careers. As radiologist Mary Magill observed in 1925, medical women could no longer afford to ignore any branch of medicine, least of all radiology:

> The special hospitals, staffed entirely by women, need women radiologists to take charge of their X-ray departments; women practitioners look for women radiologists to whom they can send their patients; and women patients do, in the majority of cases, prefer that opaque meals and similar unpleasant proce-dures should be conducted by women. Those who, for any reason, temperamen-tal or otherwise, feel that pure clinical work is not for them, may well consider the enormous possibilities offered by radiology and electro-therapeutics.[59]

From cancer research to radiography, the appeal of the new radiation techniques was compelling.

In 1925, the MWF's Cancer Committee invited Dr. Elizabeth Hurdon to become research officer of the project. A graduate of The University of Toronto, English-born Elizabeth Hurdon was well qualified to undertake the work. After studying at the Johns Hopkins Hospital under William Osler, she had taken up a post as associate in gynecology at the Johns Hopkins University and collaborated with Howard Kelly in the publica-tion of two important textbooks.[60] Most importantly, under the "Big Four" of the Johns Hopkins Hospital Hurdon had gained a wide experience of teamwork. She was thus capable of organizing the scheme along the lines already suggested by Donaldson and others, as an integrated organiza-tion managed by a consultant expert.[61] Once appointed to the position of director, Hurdon became the linchpin of the scheme. The MWF's project gave participating gynecologists responsibility for carrying out the treat-ment, but the dosage and technique were determined by the Committee. The Director transported the radium to the four participating hospitals

58. Sackville-West, *Marie Curie Hospital* (n. 56), p. 20.

59. Mary Magill, "The Practice of Radiology and Electro-Therapeutics for Medical Women," *Med. Women's Fed. Newsl.*, July 1925, pp. 21–26, on p. 21.

60. See Elizabeth Hurdon's obituary, *Brit. Med. J.*, 1941, 2: 299.

61. Sturdy and Cooter, "Science, Scientific Management" (n. 44).

(the South London Hospital for Women, the Elizabeth Garrett Anderson Hospital, the Royal Free Hospital, and the New Sussex Hospital) in turn, attended the insertion of the radium, advised the dosage, and kept in touch with the patients, following up each case and making records.

The research had the approval of the MRC's Radiology Committee, and from 1925 onward it was included in its research program. Quite apart from Chambers's links with Sidney Russ, the view that cancer of the uterus was a "female" concern played a crucial role in securing the Committee's support. As Walter Fletcher, the MRC's first secretary, explained in 1925 to George Newman, the chief medical officer to the Ministry of Health, "these women are dealing with cancer in women, and in so far as this radium is concerned, chiefly with cancer of the womb. . . . of all the radium jobs, this seems the most appropriate for women to tackle, for obvious reasons."[62] What he feared, however, was that the women's scheme might become a new "campaign." Fletcher had opposed the establishment of the British Empire Cancer Campaign (BECC) two years earlier, partly on the grounds that it would divert much-needed funds away from established research bodies; to his mind, the MWF's project posed similar dangers.

Fletcher's fears were to prove unfounded. The MWF's appeal collected very little money, and in the end it was the BECC that funded Hurdon's salary.[63] The BECC also loaned the 500 mg of radium that the MWF needed to initiate the project. In order to elaborate the technique to be followed, Hurdon toured radium therapy centers in Europe and America collecting information and comparing methods of treatment. On her return the Committee agreed to adopt the technique developed by James Heyman at Stockholm's Radiumhemmet, which involved the intracavitary insertion of radium in three separate applications, two weeks apart.[64] The first patient, an elderly woman with advanced cervical carcinoma, was treated by Louisa Martindale at the New Sussex Hospital in September 1925. In the next three years, more than three hundred patients were treated at the four women's hospitals concerned. Dr. Hurdon attended every operation.

By 1929, 322 cases had been treated, and of these only 68 were operable. The Cancer Committee had adopted the five-year surgical "cure" as the gold standard of successful treatment; hence, no definite claim could be made about the value of the therapy. The results were said to

62. Fletcher to Newman, 3 April 1925, NA, FD 1/697.
63. Fletcher to BECC secretary, 4 August 1925, ibid.
64. The aim was to damage malignant cells by the first dose, and to destroy all cancer cells by the succeeding applications, thus enabling the vascular connective tissue to recover in the intervals. See Elizabeth Hurdon, *Cancer of the Uterus* (Oxford: Oxford University Press, 1942), p. 53.

be "encouraging," however. According to Helen Chambers, 90 percent of the operable cases were free from all the signs of cancer, while all the inoperable cases were "materially benefited." Most of the deaths were attributed to "asthenia due to internal metastases"; only one death had occurred as a direct result of the treatment.[65] The statistics provided by Chambers also indicated significant changes in treatment patterns at the four participating institutions. Between 1925 and 1927, eighteen cases had been referred for recurrence after operation; by 1928 the number of such cases had dropped to two: "This is accounted for by the fact that most of our women surgeons do not operate at the present time on cases of cervical cancer, but prefer to treat them at a Radium Clinic," Chambers explained.[66]

The evolution of the clinic into a central hospital closely reflected the Radiology Committee's growing support for the centralization of radiotherapy in a few specialist institutions. By the late 1920s, advocates of radium therapy had become disillusioned with providing the general hospitals with radium for research purposes. The difficulties highlighted by members of the Radiology Committee included a paucity of beds for cancer research, poor record keeping and follow up, and inefficient use of radium.[67] Writing in 1930, Helen Chambers claimed that a shortage of beds for treatment, the inefficient use of radium owing to the time lost in transit, and the problem of following up cases in the absence of a central out-patient department were the main factors that had led to the establishment of the Marie Curie Hospital in 1929. "By this time," she added,

> it was generally recognised that Radium therapy was a highly specialised field of work which should only be undertaken at a Centre designed and equipped for the purpose. No one should use Radium who had not had special training. It was realised that the success of the treatment depended entirely upon careful dosage and technique and that the co-ordination of an organised team was essential.[68]

The new hospital was opened in London's Hampstead district under the direction of Elizabeth Hurdon. It had thirty beds, both public and private; an operating theater; and a pathological laboratory. The medical staff consisted of seventeen surgeons, five physicians, a pathologist, and a radiologist, backed up by a "scientific advisory council" that interestingly included Walter Fletcher and three members of the MRC's Radiology

---

65. Chambers, "Marie Curie Hospital" (n. 53), p. 21.
66. Ibid., p. 22.
67. See Cantor, "MRC's Support" (n. 38).
68. Chambers, "Marie Curie Hospital" (n. 53), p. 20.

Committee: Sidney Russ, Sir Cuthbert Wallace, and Professor E. H. Kettle. Marie Curie was most interested in the project and was pleased to allow her name to be given to the new hospital.[69]

In the previous century, the women-run hospitals had attracted support from titled ladies and upper-class married women philanthropists. In the late 1920s, the list of subscribers to the Marie Curie Hospital still included wealthy philanthropists, but in addition it boasted prominent feminists such as Margaret Bondfield, the Labour MP; Lady Rhondda, proprietor of the liberal feminist paper *Time and Tide*; and Millicent Fawcett, former president of the National Union of Women's Suffrage and younger sister of Elizabeth Garrett Anderson. Also represented were campaigners for women's welfare like Eleanor Rathbone, the Family Allowance pioneer, and women doctors themselves; indeed, the largest donation (£10,000) came from Dr. Elizabeth Courtauld, a distant relative of the textiles manufacturer Samuel Courtauld.[70] The medical women's cause was championed by the *New Statesman*, the Fabian Socialist weekly founded in 1912 by Sidney and Beatrice Webb. Writing under the pseudonym "Lens," eugenicist doctor Caleb Saleeby, a Fabian socialist and friend of George Bernard Shaw, hailed the Marie Curie Hospital as a new beginning in cancer therapy. An enthusiast for radium, Saleeby vehemently criticized the "monstrously selfish, arrogant, obstructive and anti-social record of the surgeons in this country as a body in respect of the radiation of cancer," arguing that "wherever radium is available, the ghastly and deadly operation of panhysterectomy should be condemned as malpraxis."[71] Saleeby welcomed the medical women's plan to extend radium therapy to the treatment of breast cancer, as advocated by surgeon Geoffrey Keynes: "Let us rejoice that, at last, after thousands of years, mankind may begin to say, *Exit* the surgery of cancer."[72] Saleeby's strongly worded articles were condemned by the medical press as "mischievous claptrap," but they did succeed in raising a neat sum for the new hospital.

The hospital expanded in the 1930s with the addition of an adjoining building in 1933, the provision of apparatus for deep X-ray therapy in 1934, and the establishment in 1937 of a research laboratory equipped to house animals for work in experimental pathology.[73] As a tribute to Helen Chambers, who had died of breast cancer in 1935, the new

69. "The Marie Curie Hospital," *Lancet*, 1934, 1: 527–28.

70. See NA, FD 1/697 for a list of early supporters.

71. Lens (pseud.), "The Marie Curie Hospital," *New Statesman*, March 1929, p. 692.

72. Ibid.

73. In the light of feminists' traditional opposition to vivisection, this was an interesting development. It deserves further examination.

research facilities were named after her. By the outbreak of the Second World War the initial investigation on the use of radium for carcinoma of the cervix had been extended to the treatment of inoperable cancers of the breast. A statistical analysis of cases of uterine cancer treated at the hospital since its foundation showed that the five-year survival rate in the early cases was 83 percent, and 30 percent in the more serious cases. Writing in 1951, Louisa Martindale attributed the good results to the treatment protocol, which included strict asepsis and the application of radium by fully trained surgeons, on patients who were deemed to be fit for the treatment.[74] In addition, she highlighted both the significance of gender and the importance of teamwork: "The director is always present with her advice and co-operation. Indeed there is much to be said for the Marie Curie Hospital woman surgeon, not only because she is consulted by the patient earlier in her case, when the symptoms are only slight, but because she agrees to follow out a certain technique and is meticulous in its application."[75]

Conclusion

Contemporary male gynecologists recognized the key role that cervical cancer had played in the establishment of radiotherapy. Thus Frank Cook, writing in 1954, stated: "To quote Malcolm Donaldson (1933): 'Gynaecology was the realm in which radium therapy was first used to any great extent; and in this field it still has its greatest value.' It has more recently been said with a considerable degree of truth that the history of radiotherapy of cervical cancer well represents the history of radio-therapy as a whole."[76] Cook singled out the Marie Curie Hospital for special mention, emphasizing the statistical reliability of its results and the benefits conferred to innumerable patients.

Underlying this success story was a unique combination of professional and ideological factors that had served to make radiotherapy for cervical cancer a "woman's issue." Medical women's entry into the field was motivated by long-standing traditions of service to other women, especially those less fortunate than themselves, but it also served as a strategy

74. Martindale, *Woman Surgeon* (n. 31), pp. 209–10. See also Hurdon, *Cancer of the Uterus* (n. 64), p. 67.

75. Martindale, *Woman Surgeon* (n. 31), pp. 209–10.

76. Frank Cook, "The Progress of Radio-Therapy in Gynaecology," in *Historical Review of British Obstetrics and Gynaecology 1800–1950*, ed. J. M. Munro Kerr, R. W. Johnstone, and Miles H. Phillips (Edinburgh: Livingstone, 1954), pp. 382–89, on p. 383.

for professional advancement at a time when a career structure based around specialist hospital appointments was gradually crystallizing within British medicine.[77] While die-hard male surgeons sought to preserve the preeminence of operative treatment for cervical cancer, women surgeons found in radiotherapy a means of asserting their commitment to compassionate cancer care.

ORNELLA MOSCUCCI lectures in history at the London School of Hygiene and Tropical Medicine, Keppel Street, London WC1E 7HT, U.K., where she also runs the seminar series organized by the Centre for History in Public Health. Her research interests include subjects relating to cancer, women's health, and women medical practitioners. Her most recent projects concern the prevention and treatment of gynecological cancer in Britain from 1860 to 1948, and a history of the MRC childhood leukemia trials. Ornella Moscucci is a member of the Executive Committee of the Society for the Social History of Medicine, and the Society's representative on the editorial board of *Social History of Medicine* (e-mail: Ornella.Moscucci@lshtm.ac.uk).

77. Elston, "Run by Women" (n. 1), pp. 90–93.

Contested Cumulations: Configurations of Cancer Treatments through the Twentieth Century

JOHN V. PICKSTONE

SUMMARY: The treatment of cancer through the twentieth century may be seen as the successive addition of modalities: first surgery; then radiotherapy, especially between the world wars; and then chemotherapy, from the 1960s. This paper explores some of the systematic differences between the modalities, and how these additions were negotiated in different countries, with different long-term consequences for the development of services and specialization. It focuses chiefly on the United Kingdom and the United States, the former exemplifying a centralized health polity, and the latter, liberal markets combined with large and crucial postwar inputs from government. The differences between health polities were especially important for interwar radiotherapy, which in its centralized form appeared as paradigmatic of the analytical/rationalizing mode in modern medicine. Chemotherapy exemplified a more inventive and experimentalist mode that became common after World War II, and that, through the practice of trials, shaped the new subprofession of medical oncology. The interactions of the modalities, at various levels, are modeled as *contested cumulations* showing strong *path dependency*. The paper ends by reviewing the present situation, especially for Britain, and by underlining the relevance of history.

KEYWORDS: cancer treatments, ways of knowing, specialization, contested cumulations, path dependency, national differences

This paper is a product of the Wellcome Trust project on the history of cancer in the United Kingdom since ca. 1940, on which I am fortunate to work with Carsten Timmermann (recalcitrant cancers, and treatments), Helen Valier (blood/lymph cancers and research/clinic), Elizabeth Toon (breast cancer and public understandings), and Emm Barnes (pediatric oncology and educational material for children). I am also grateful to several colleagues elsewhere—especially David Cantor, Gretchen Krueger, Gerald Kutcher, Ilana Löwy, and Patrice Pinell—for both information and suggestions. I would like to thank many helpful archivists in the United States and the United Kingdom, and I am especially indebted to my Manchester colleagues at the Christie Hospital, Emeritus Professor Derek Crowther and Dr. Ron Stout, for generously sharing their knowledge and perspectives.

164

This paper originated in reflections on the present divisions of specialist labor in cancer hospitals and regional cancer centers in Britain—between medical oncologists who practice chemotherapy, and clinical oncologists who practice radiotherapy with chemotherapy (and who used to be called radiotherapists). This division of labor is similar to that in Swedish cancer hospitals, but substantially different from most of Europe where the doctors who give radiotherapy do not also give chemotherapy, and especially from the United States where medical oncology is a common specialty in community hospitals and office practice as well as in cancer centers and cancer hospitals. And of course, there is a third major party: the surgeons, again differing in organization and their means of advancing practice. The three modalities developed successively, through a long series of professional negotiations; the pathways and the results differ between countries.

Here, then, was an opportunity to see how new modalities had been added to old, in contested cumulations, and how different national patterns could be explained in part through path dependency. But it was also a chance to explore the different structures of practice, knowledge, and politics that characterized each of those modalities, and that may characterize aspects of scientific medicine more generally.[1]

Modes of Medicine, Contingency, and Path Dependency

In a series of publications, I have tried to develop models of "ways of knowing" and "ways of working" as elements, or ideal types, from which the complex practices of science, technology, and medicine may be said to be compounded. In such configurational models, historical change is usually a matter of contested displacements (rather than successions):

1. Cancer history has benefited of late from a series of excellent review articles that build on each other, and that include treatment as well as research: David Cantor, "Cancer," in *Companion Encyclopedia of the History of Medicine*, ed. W. Bynum and R. Porter (London: Routledge, 1993), pp. 536–60; Ilana Löwy, "The Century of the Transformed Cell," in *Science in the Twentieth Century*, ed. J. Krige and D. Pestre (Amsterdam: Harwood, 1998), pp. 461–78; Patrice Pinell, "Cancer," in *Medicine in the Twentieth Century*, ed. Roger Cooter and John Pickstone (Amsterdam: Harwood Academic, 2000), pp. 671–86; Jean Paul Gaudillière, "The Cancer Century," in *The Cambridge History of Science*, vol. 6, *The Biomedical and Earth Sciences since 1800*, ed. Peter Bowler and John V. Pickstone (New York: Cambridge University Press, forthcoming). For another example of how history may allow doctors to appreciate the contingencies of divisions between specialisms, see Jeffrey P. Baker, "Historical Adventures in the Newborn Nursery: Forgotten Stories and Syndromes," in *Clio in the Clinic: History in Medical Practice*, ed. Jacalyn Duffin (New York: Oxford University Press, 2005), pp. 105–15, esp. pp. 107–9.

new modes of knowledge and practice come to articulate with previous modes, and these articulations are evident at various scales from the level of "case histories" up to that of "big pictures." I have argued that *analysis* (with its correlate of rationalized production) and *experimentalism* (correlated with systematic invention) were the modes of knowledge and action most characteristic of science, technology, and medicine over the last two centuries.[2]

Here, I will suggest that radiotherapy, as developed in the centralized, specialist institutions that epitomized the medical modernity of the interwar decades, was paradigmatically analytical in its forms of work. Radiotherapy institutes included a variety of scientists and technicians as well as doctors; they standardized their therapies and accumulated statistics (about almost all their cases) at a time when most clinicians relied on individual judgments about individual patients. To be sure, cancer chemotherapy, when it developed after World War II, was also highly "scientific" by the standards of contemporary medicine elsewhere; but chemotherapy relied on new kinds of clinical trials—on the experimentalism that had grown from research laboratories, and especially from the testing of new antibacterial remedies. (Indeed, the word "chemotherapy" then covered all these antibacterials as well as the anticancer therapeutics to which the term would later become restricted.) In some senses (for cancer and more generally), experimentalism built on analysis, but the ways of working were different: trials were about using chemical novelties, or inventions, on particular groups of patients. I will suggest that these meta-level differences accentuated the problems of articulation and accommodation when new modalities were added to older ones.

But having sketched the model, and to avoid misunderstandings, I should next mark out the limits of the paper. First, I note that the three therapeutic modalities that are my central concern are but part of the story of cancer treatment, even for recent decades. The analytical-rationalizing and the experimentalist-inventing modes of medicine were always and necessarily accompanied by other ways of knowing—for example, attention to the *natural history* of disease and a concern with *meanings* of the disease to patients as well as to doctors. Practitioners were not just rationalizers or systematic inventors, they also exercised *craft* skills and *rhetorical* devices, even when they were also analyzing and experimenting.

2. John V. Pickstone, *Ways of Knowing: A New History of Science, Technology and Medicine* (Manchester: Manchester University Press, 2000; Chicago: Chicago University Press, 2001); Pickstone, "The Biographical and the Analytical," in *Medicine and Change: Innovation, Continuity and Recurrence*, ed. I. Löwy (Paris: Libbey, 1993), pp. 23–48.

Thus, for example, a fuller account of radiotherapy would include its own symbolic meanings and rhetorical powers; and it would also include the ways in which radiotherapy changed the "natural history" of cancer and its public presence and emotional charge.[3]

Second, I want to clarify my chronological starting point. This is not a full historical narrative of the increasing complexity of cancer therapeutics; for that, we would need to explore how long-standing "bedside" understandings of cancer articulated with mid-nineteenth-century pathological anatomy, and both modes with the new surgery of the late nineteenth century. We would need to explore how some cancers came to be regarded as operable, and how surgical interventions changed customary clinical histories. But in this sketch of twentieth-century cancer therapeutics, I simply take surgery as the first of the main three modalities. In its dependence on the understanding of cancers as local lesions of tissues, modern surgery may be seen as analytical; but the conditions of research and practice in surgery were substantially and persistently different from those in radiotherapy, mainly because, whatever the anatomical models, the industrialization of surgical equipment, or the proliferation of ancillary specialists, the practice of operative surgery has remained essentially craft-based.

And then a third note, to justify the focus on the three main modalities when cancer also involved the many other kinds of medical, nursing, and technical work that have become common in recent medicine—including specialized diagnostic methods and screening, the control of side effects or of pain, physiotherapy, palliative care, psychological treatments, cancer education and prevention.[4] But here our focus is on the interactions of the destructive measures aimed at the cancer itself, and for (relative) simplicity I largely exclude hormonal treatments and later biological treatments.

3. In Pickstone, *Ways of Knowing* (n. 2), there are historical chapters on the meanings of nature and artifacts, and on natural history as a tradition; both are treated as constitutive of "science, technology, and medicine" generally.

4. See Rosemary Stevens, *Medical Practice in Modern England: The Impact of Specialization and State Medicine* (New Haven: Yale University Press, 1966); Stevens, *American Medicine and the Public Interest* (New Haven: Yale University Press, 1971). For paramedicals, see Gerry Larkin, "Health Workers," in *Companion to Medicine in the Twentieth Century*, ed. Roger Cooter and John Pickstone (London: Routledge, 2003), pp. 531–42. A major work appeared too late to be used here: George Weisz, *Divide and Conquer: A Comparative History of Medical Specialization* (New York: Oxford University Press, 2005). See also the articles edited by Patrice Pinell in "La spécialisation de la médécine, XIX–XX siècles," *Actes de la recherche en sciences sociales*, 2005, *156–57*. For professional jurisdictions more generally, see Andrew Abbott, *The System of Professions: An Essay on the Division of Expert Labor* (Chicago: University of Chicago Press, 1988).

Surgery, radiotherapy, and chemotherapy were seen as weapons variously attacking the cancer. One might even take the armamentarium argument further: there is also a characteristic addition *within* some modalities. This is most obvious for recent chemotherapy, which commonly involves cocktails of drugs, and perhaps different cocktails used in sequence.

This cumulation of medical weaponry focused on a single site seems especially characteristic of cancer treatment, and so too are the international differences that have resulted from the differential development of the modalities. Where one mode was developed in a particular way in a particular context, then future "additions" to the system were also likely to be different—not just because the contextual differences may have continued, but because the effects of old contexts had been built into the system.

Yet, as we explore what economists call this "path dependency," we also need to take account of the countertendencies. Cancer doctors themselves have often been aware of the historical paths and the contingencies built into the treatments they used. And for that reason, from the interwar years, they advocated *teamwork*, in part to try to ensure that the treatment given did not depend on which specialist the patient happened to see first, or which therapeutic specialism was best developed in that particular hospital. Such teamwork, like the multidisciplinary protocols that are now common, may perhaps be seen as a way of limiting history—as producing schedules by which all suitable patients can be treated, whatever their circumstances and wherever they are cared for. Yet, inevitably, to some extent, all such efforts are themselves historically rooted: the forms of teamwork, like the patterns of referral and of treatment, are also shaped by histories.

To be sure, the world of cancer therapy is now global and full of evidence-based protocols that claim international validity. Specialists from many countries attend the big American meetings, and these societies see themselves as international in their reach.[5] In most countries, the government, the professional communities, and perhaps the medical businesses, produce guidelines on practice which are meant to standardize across their domains. But for all the information now flowing between sites and nations, cancer services and treatments continue to differ between places because of their different histories, and especially the different relative histories of the three professional modalities.

5. See the ASCO and ASTRO Web sites.

The Locations of Cancer Surgery

As Patrice Pinell has well shown for France, it was the development of anti-septic and aseptic surgery that established the curability of some kinds of cancer.[6] Of course, cancers had been removed before, but at huge imme-diate risk to the patient. When mortality rates for surgery improved, one could at least assess the proportion of operated cancer cases who survived longer than had been expected without the operation.

Cancer surgery expanded after ca. 1870 both within "general surgery" and in the largely surgical nascent specialties of urology, ENT, and gyne-cology. Though gastrointestinal cancers remained in general surgery (and stomach cancers remained a major killer through the mid-twentieth century), in all the new specialist fields cancers were a major part of the operative work. For patients in cities, served by specialists, cancers of the cervix and uterus mostly "belonged" to gynecologists, those of the mouth and throat to ENT surgeons, and so forth.

This organizational story of cancer surgery seems simple in outline and fairly similar across most countries. Until recently, few surgeons defined themselves primarily as cancer surgeons—they were "regional" surgeons first and cancer surgeons second. Surgeons usually worked "alone" and did not require hugely expensive equipment. But there are national dif-ferences, especially since World War I, partly because surgery then had to articulate with other modalities, notably radiotherapy. In France, Swe-den, and Britain, the institutions or hospital departments for cancer that were established or developed between the wars were usually dominated by radiotherapists or pathologists. Most surgery was in general hospitals rather than special cancer centers, unless it was especially complicated and required close association with other specialists.

But in the United States, cancer hospitals, though often started as charities for the incurable, seem to have been dominated from before World War II by surgeons who rode the waves of cancer philanthropy and the powerful cancer-education programs that were characteristic of the United States.[7] In the 1920s the Memorial cancer hospital in New York was led by a pathologist, James Ewing, and a surgeon, Henry Janeway, who together developed radiotherapy as an independent modality; but by World War II the use of radium and therapeutic X rays had become ancillary either to surgery or to diagnostic radiology. After World War II,

---

6. Patrice Pinell, *The Fight against Cancer: France, 1890–1940* (London: Routledge, 2002).

7. James T. Patterson, *The Dread Disease: Cancer and Modern American Culture* (Cambridge: Harvard University Press, 1987), pp. 137–70.

the wartime advances in antibiotics, anesthetics, blood transfusions, and other forms of patient support were seen as expanding the scope of cancer surgery—sometimes, again, at the expense of radiotherapy. Barron Lerner has well shown how American cancer treatment in the 1940s and 1950s was epitomized by heroic surgery, not least at the Memorial whose alumni led the American Cancer Society.[8]

One of the latest, and richest, specialist cancer hospitals was the hospital planned in Texas in 1941 as a state cancer hospital and research facility, and drawn to Houston by a matching grant from the legacy of M. D. Anderson.[9] Gilbert Fletcher, a French émigré, was recruited to create a radiotherapy department, which claimed to follow European practice; but in the eyes of at least one well-placed commentator, the doctors who shaped the M. D. Anderson Hospital (MDA) "ended up imitating the Memorial Hospital of New York in its division of clinical work prior to the indications for treatment"[10]—which suggests that patients were primarily assigned to the surgeons. Certainly the director and surgeon-in-chief, R. Lee Clark, was a national figure in the American College of Surgeons, especially in its efforts to define the requirements for hospital cancer centers.[11] The MDA could have chosen another method, which they had in fact observed closely at the Ellis Fischel Cancer Hospital at Columbia, Missouri, where Juan del Regato, a young Cuban with advanced Parisian training, ran the radiotherapy and had about seventy beds—but that was a state hospital for indigents.[12]

Some postwar surgeons were keen to develop laboratory programs—for example, Owen Wangensteen with the physiologist Maurice B. Visscher at Minneapolis.[13] But generally, if we may borrow the industrial model of research and development (R&D), surgical analyses and technical novelties were more like D than R; they were not conspicuous as discoveries,

8. Barron H. Lerner, *The Breast Cancer Wars: Hope, Fear, and the Pursuit of a Cure in Twentieth-Century America* (New York: Oxford University Press, 2001), pp. 69–91.

9. *The First Twenty Years of the University of Texas M. D. Anderson Hospital and Tumor Institute* (Houston: University of Texas M. D. Anderson Hospital and Tumor Institute, 1964). For information on the MDA, I am also indebted to Helen Valier and Emm Barnes.

10. Juan A. del Regato, "The Unfolding of Therapeutic Radiology in the United States: A Participant's View and Autobiographical Essay," in del Regato, *Radiation Oncologists: The Unfolding of a Medical Specialty* (Fairfax, Va.: Radiology Centennial, 1993), pp. 197–209, on pp. 201–2.

11. See R. Lee Clark papers at the McGovern Archive, Houston, Tex., esp. ser. 4.

12. Del Regato, *Radiation Oncologists* (n. 10), pp. 201–2.

13. See Leonard G. Wilson, *Medical Revolution in Minnesota: A History of the University of Minnesota Medical School* (Minneapolis: Midiwiwin Press, 1989).

or as requiring institutional reconfigurations.[14] Surgery is still the main treatment for many kinds of cancer, and in the last three decades some surgeons have specialized in cancer; some may be involved in biopsy tests, even for cancers that are then treated by other kinds of specialist. But for all its therapeutic importance, surgery has usually been the dispersed, individualized base on which, or against which, other kinds of cancer specialist would organize. Without ignoring the difference between academic surgery and practice in the medical market, we may refer to the characteristic organization of surgery as "liberal." Though surgery is based on an analytical understanding of the body, and it long relied on "case series," its systematic use of experimental statistics dates only from the 1970s; and except perhaps in Soviet Russia, "surgical labor" has proved hard to divide. As we shall now see, in some places, and especially for the surgical insertion of radium, radiotherapeutics followed that liberal model, even when centralized, rationalized facilities were being promoted elsewhere.

Radiotherapeutics and Surgery: The Liberal Model

Radiotherapy seems to be the modality in which national differences became most apparent and institutionalized; indeed, it is the modality that has been most definitive of *cancer* services in Britain and Europe. But neither radium nor X-ray therapy was peculiarly identified with cancer until after World War I (except in the sense that they could *cause* it). It is across a range of diseases that we must first explore the relations of the new modality to the old.

It was through actions on the skin that X rays and then radium were chiefly recognized as local medical agents (beyond the visualization role of X rays). Both were usually seen as acting like cauteries or caustics—as "burning" the skin. As such they were conceptually related to surgery, but also to the chemical caustics that had long been used against superficial cancers. Partly because *some* skin cancers proved easily tractable (or, like rodent ulcers, were defined out of "cancer"), they tended to become part of dermatology (and marginal to cancer), along with conditions such as ringworm. At the start of the twentieth century in Manchester, the Cancer Pavilion experimented with X rays and, when disappointed, passed its machine to the skin hospital. After the Great War, when a Radium Institute was established in Manchester, its first radiotherapist had been

14. For comparisons and relationships of industrial and surgical research, see Thomas Schlich, *Surgery, Science and Industry: A Revolution in Fracture Care, 1950s–1990s* (Basingstoke: Palgrave, 2002).

a dermatologist, but he began to work chiefly on cancers of the mouth and womb; skin cancers were left to the skin hospital.[15] Before World War I, and beyond the skin, as it were, X rays and radium were used chiefly for palliation—for shrinking inoperable tumors and relieving pain. We tend to forget this "biographical" dimension, but it radically changed the "natural history" of cancer and its social meanings. As Caroline Murphy pointed out, the foul, suppurating cancers were now rarely seen—though radiotherapy could also produce disfigurations. Cancer, for the most part, came to be a dissolution of the body.[16]

Surgery was already the established remedy for accessible cancers, and other treatments were now added into the space labeled "inoperable." They were envisaged as palliative, as a possible means of extending "cautery" beyond the scalpel's reach, or perhaps as avoiding surgical "mutilation." The Manchester Radium Institute had been promoted by a prominent ENT surgeon in the hope of extending the range of "operations" for cancer of the mouth and larynx, and avoiding the chopping out of the tongue and other parts; indeed, such procedures were successfully developed in the 1920s and 1930s.[17] At the Middlesex Hospital in London, the surgeon who helped develop radium for uterine cancer did so on inoperable patients, but it worked well enough that he came to offer "operable" patients a choice of therapy. He had learned his radium treatment from Sweden, and so did the women doctors of the Marie Curie Hospital in London who established radium as the preferred treatment for cervical cancer.[18] For breast cancer, the addition of radiotherapy to surgery owed something to redefinitions of the surgically acceptable. Geoffrey Keynes, a cultivated British surgeon who opposed the radical mastectomy and encouraged radiotherapy, viewed the Halsted operation as a "horrible mutilation."[19]

Inasmuch as radium extended the range of surgery, its use could be seen as an extension of the practice of surgeons who specialized in ENT

---

15. Caroline Murphy, "Cancer and Radiotherapy in Britain 1850–1950" (Ph.D. diss., University of Manchester, Faculty of Technology, 1986), p. 326.

16. Caroline Murphy, "From Friedenheim to Hospice: A Century of Cancer Hospitals," in *The Hospital in History*, ed. Lindsay Granshaw and Roy Porter (London: Routledge, 1989), pp. 221–41.

17. Eileen Magnello, in association with the Wellcome Unit for the History of Medicine, University of Manchester, *A Centenary History of the Christie Hospital, Manchester* (Manchester: Christie Hospital NHS Trust, 2003), pp. 23–35.

18. See Ornella Moscucci, "The 'Ineffable Freemasonry of Sex': Feminist Surgeons and the Establishment of Radiotherapy in Early Twentieth-Century Britain," in this issue.

19. Lerner, *Breast Cancer Wars* (n. 8), pp. 33–37.

or gynecology, just as it proved an extension of dermatology. For hospital *in*patients more generally, the surgeons "owned" many of the beds and so "naturally" controlled the treatment. To some extent, that logic of body-site specialization was indeed followed, especially for brachytherapy— treatment by the insertion of radium needles. The radium needles were easily portable, they required surgical insertion, and they were not hopelessly expensive. They could be part of the practice of a specialist surgeon or gynecologist—and so they commonly were, perhaps especially in the United States, where the use of radium was not regulated by the state and where the American Radium Society was dominated by surgeons.[20]

In this liberal model, all significant hospitals had surgical radium-therapy; X-ray therapy was an annex to diagnostic radiology, and radiologists did not control beds. In other countries, including Britain, this liberal model was also used, but the extent of the practice is not well documented. Because it was not specially "organized" or much linked with research, it is not well known; it followed the customary divisions between (internal) medicine and surgery, extending the latter, as it also extended the paraclinical practice of radiology.

The Centralized Model of Cancer Services

However, radium and intensive X rays were not "ordinary" therapies. Both were dangerous, especially in the hands of doctors with little understanding of radioactivity; and they were very expensive. The price of radium varied considerably over the interwar period, as demand fluctuated or new sources were discovered, but for a cancer hospital to acquire an amount sufficient for curative and palliative treatments required substantial special charity funding and/or government support. Radium was one of the first medical technologies funded by public appeals, and by the 1920s, in some regions and countries, specialists in radiotherapy were developing schemes for centralized treatment and research.

In the centralized model, all radium treatment and most X-ray treatment was to be given in specialist regional or national institutions which might also be responsible for major cancer surgery. In such institutions, pathologists, diagnostic radiologists, radiotherapists, and surgeons would all be experts on *cancer* and its treatment. They would work in teams, along

20. Carl R. Bogardus, "Intersociety, Government, and Economic Relations," in *Radiation Oncology*, ed. R. A. Gagliardi and J. F. Watson, vol. 3 of the X-ray Centenary History volumes of the American Radiological Society (Fairfax, Va.: Radiology Centennial, 1996), pp. 201–29, on p. 218.

with physicists and statisticians and special nurses. The institution would have research laboratories and there would be close collaboration between researchers and clinicians. All patients would be treated by agreed regimes and entered into the statistics by which the regimes could be evaluated. Here was a model of medical modernism, based on analysis and rationalized production—though supplemented by individualized care "beyond the cancer," as it were.[21] It gained additional plausibility from the widespread interwar concern with cancer mortality. As deaths from acute infectious disease continued to decline, cancer became a major public health disease, alongside tuberculosis, and cancer "prevention" came to mean early treatment in the hope of preventing death.

In no country were all the elements of the centralized model realized together, but they remained an ideal to which hospital service planners continually had reference, through to the present—for example, the current plan for improving cancer services in Britain.[22] I do not mean to suggest that planners deliberately went back to old plans; or that they were always aware of the models as realized in key institutions, though this would usually be the case. Rather, the stress on centralization, a multiplicity of special skills, teamwork, and statistics was a model that came naturally to experts in institutions throughout the twentieth century, whether the object for reform was a hospital service, a factory, a research laboratory, or a city government. It was a very general model based on analysis and rationalization.

France and Sweden as Models

The nearest approach on paper was the plans in France, after the Great War, for regional cancer centers that would include surgery. These, as Pinell has shown, derived from wartime medical organization and from the direct links between wartime organizers and clinicians, scientists, and social elites; they were partly financed by charity, especially initially, but most of the support came from the state. The high profile of cancer arose in part from the public health perception of increasing incidence, in part from French pride in radium and the Curies, and from a link with that other temple of Gallic scientific medicine—the Pasteur Institute; in part, too, from the perception that other countries were getting ahead of

21. See Pickstone, *Ways of Knowing* (n. 2), esp. pp. 181–82; Olga Amsterdamska and Anja Hiddinga, "The Analytical Body," in Cooter and Pickstone, *Medicine* (n. 1), pp. 417–34.

22. *A Policy Framework for Commissioning Cancer Services: A Report by the Expert Advisory Group on Cancer to the Chief Medical Officers of England and Wales* (known as the Calman Hine report), Department of Health, London, 1995.

France in the use of radium. This was a project for "scientific medicine," drawing on tuberculosis services, but ultrascientific in its elaboration. The real developments in France took a different path, however—not (just) because plans of that scale and professional complexity commonly tend to be reduced and compromised in practice, but because there was a popular magic about radium that outran both the laboratories and the planners. In France as in Britain, public charities to provide radium cures had appeared in small towns as well as large cities. If local surgeons and radiologists were given free rein and local support, the resultant services would be dispersed beyond the control of the would-be specialist radiotherapists and such surgeons as took radium seriously; it would therefore be better to limit the geographic spread, to allow most cancer surgery to continue locally, and to centralize for radiotherapy (and for closely associated surgery). As Pinell showed, this new logic, now focused on a therapeutic modality rather than "cancer," was strengthened by the shift to teleradiotherapy, which used huge amounts of radium at a distance from the patient. The cost and dangers here were so high that such treatments had to be centralized.[23]

Where the French were planning a network, the Swedes already had the Radiumhemmet, a more or less national institution established in Stockholm in 1910 by a radiologist working with a surgeon, and with access to private funds. By 1939 the Radiumhemmet had a worldwide reputation for radiation physics, cancer staging, and statistics, as well as for radium treatments. Similar clinics were established in Lund and Gothenburg, and state and local government funding took over from the Swedish Cancer Society. Stockholm was especially famous for its work on gynecological cancers, for which a separate department had been established before World War I. Gynecological oncology appears to have remained a uniquely Swedish specialism, where radiotherapy and surgery are used together, often by the same specialist, but in the context of a radiotherapy center rather than the gynecological wards of a general hospital.[24]

The French and Swedish systems initially benefited from charitable funds, but both had elite political backing and they soon gained substantial state funding. They came to epitomize the public face of cancer, well beyond the nations directly concerned. In 1926 an international conference on cancer held at Lake Mohonk under the auspices of the American Society for the Control of Cancer had called for more public education

23. Pinell, *Fight against Cancer* (n. 6), pp. 106–42.

24. Lars-Gunnar Larsson, "Organisation of Radiotherapy and Clinical Oncology in Sweden: A Historical Review," *Acta Oncologica*, 1995, *34:* 1011–15.

and had heard Claudius Regaud extol the French system of centralized care.[25] In the United States, some state governments invested in radium as part of their public health programs, and interest was also strong in Britain, among public health doctors and the national Medical Research Council (MRC). How, then, did this governmental interest affect cancer services in the two countries that are most central to this paper?

British Varieties

Britain's first Radium Institute had been prompted by King Edward VII, who was cured of a rodent ulcer by methods deriving from Paris. Opened in 1911, it was restricted to radium therapy. Patients were referred by doctors or other hospitals, as outpatients; the London Radium Institute radiotherapist decided on the form of the treatment, but the diagnosis and further care of the patient were not his responsibility, and there was little opportunity for follow-up. Essentially, this was philanthropic provision of an expensive treatment in a way that did not disrupt the normal patterns of private and charity medicine; it fitted the liberal model. By contrast, the special cancer hospital in London (the Marsden) developed a famous radiotherapy department, and some of the London teaching hospitals—especially St. Bartholomew's (Bart's), the Middlesex, and the Westminster—were noted for both cancer surgery and radiotherapy. In some other teaching hospitals, radiotherapy was marginal to diagnostics and to surgery, and the long-standing rivalries between the charity teaching hospitals meant that effort in London was dispersed.[26] It was in the dense industrial region of Manchester that the idea of a centralized service came to be most fully realized.

The Manchester Radium Institute started in a similar way to the London Institute, except that its originator was a surgeon on the staff of the teaching hospital and its chief patron was a local brewer rather than a monarch. Money was raised, partly by (novel) newspaper campaigns, and used to provide a service available to most of the hospitals in the Manchester district. The Institute was located in the basement of the new teaching hospital, alongside the diagnostic radiology and medical electricity services; but it was separately staffed, and eventually the radiotherapist gained a few beds so he could have patients of his own. He also served

---

25. The conference is discussed in Charles Hayter, *An Element of Hope: Radium and the Response to Cancer in Canada* (Montreal: McGill-Queens University Press, 2005), pp. 81–84.

26. Murphy, "Cancer and Radiotherapy" (n. 15), chaps. 4–5.

the cancer hospital on the same site—de facto another department of the teaching hospital.[27]

After much contention at the end of the 1920s, both the Radium Institute and the Christie cancer hospital moved off the main site to cohabit in a fine new building in a southern suburb. At about the same time they jointly appointed a new director: Ralston Paterson, a Scottish-trained radiologist who had worked in North America, including a spell at the Mayo Clinic (which already employed a research-minded radiotherapist in addition to a diagnostic radiologist).[28] At the new hospital-cum-radium-institute, in a region more populous than Sweden, Paterson was able to develop a service more like Stockholm's than that in London. The hospital was directly responsible for the patients, all radiotherapists followed the same regimes, statistics were built up, a research laboratory was developed, there was a mold workshop, and surgeons visited the hospital for complex mixed treatments (or to repair the effects thereof). Paterson worked with a physicist to develop dose regimes that attained international recognition, especially in the British Empire.

By the late 1930s, the Christie was a world center along with Paris and Stockholm. It was also exemplary as a regional service. Some local towns had bought their own radium, but this was brought under Christie control. In all the local towns, clinics were held by specialists from the Christie, and patients requiring radiotherapy were referred to the regional center. There was fund-raising for the Christie throughout the region, and most local authorities also contributed. In effect it was a regional service that monopolized radium treatment, and it was seen as *the* center for cancer treatment.[29]

The Cancer Act of 1939, which (because of the war) never came into effect, sought to extend similar arrangements to other regions. Some big-city regions with independent cancer hospitals, such as Glasgow, already had arrangements approaching those of the Christie—though there was often friction with elite surgeons in the regional teaching hospital. In some other provincial cities, the service was provided through the main teaching hospital.

The patterns varied, but centralization was gaining by the 1930s, partly because of the power of central government over radium. The Medical Research Council had become responsible for the "war-surplus" radium

27. Magnello, *Centenary History* (n. 17), pp. 23–34.
28. Biography of Paterson in del Regato, *Radiation Oncologists* (n. 10), pp. 155–66.
29. Magnello, *Centenary History* (n. 17), pp. 49–70.

after World War I, and initially used it for a radium bomb (teleradiotherapy) at the Middlesex Hospital in London. The MRC was then persuaded to distribute the radium to several centers that had technical expertise but not enough radium of their own. A National Radium Trust and a National Radium Commission were set up by the government in 1929 for the purchase and controlled distribution of radium. They encouraged specialist cancer centers and the differentiation of radiotherapy from radiology.[30] By the late 1930s in Britain, the subprofession of radiotherapy was well recognized; that its separate development was supported by the leading diagnostic radiologists seems to have contrasted with attitudes in the United States and also in France.[31]

Where radiotherapists controlled beds they could try new treatments, systematize record keeping and follow-up, and extend the uses of radiotherapy. They could include brachytherapy, especially if they had some surgical training. Thus for some conditions radiotherapy became an alternative to surgery, and for these conditions, whether a patient received surgery, radiotherapy, or some combination could depend heavily on the accidents of referral and consultation; at limit, the day on which you attended the hospital might determine whether you saw a surgeon or a radiotherapist, and hence the treatment. Thus, as noted earlier, some surgeons and most radiotherapists came to stress *teamwork*, and some ran joint clinics. For example, the Westminster Hospital was known for its Wednesday clinics where the (Russian-born, European-educated) surgeon Stanford Cade led discussions with other surgeons, radiotherapists, pathologists, physicists, and others. He himself was a national expert in radiotherapy and histopathology as well as surgery; his juniors were more specialized.[32] At the Christie in Manchester there were daily lunchtime clinics, with the same range of expertise but for different cancer sites each day, depending on which surgical clinics were held on that day.

30. David Cantor, "The MRC's Support for Experimental Radiology during the Interwar Years," in *Historical Perspectives: Essays on the Role of the MRC*, ed. Joan Austoker and Linda Bryder (Oxford: Oxford University Press, 1989), pp. 181–204.

31. R. Paterson, "Radiotherapy 1925–59," *Brit. J. Radiol.*, 1973, *46:* 168–70; Murphy, "Cancer and Radiotherapy" (n. 15), p. 7.41.

32. Obituary of Stanford Cade, *Lancet*, 1973, *302*: 745–46. The Wellcome Contemporary Medical Archives Collection, London, includes a useful transcript of its interview with some of Cade's younger colleagues (from 13 October 1993).

The United States and Socialized Radium

In the United States, by contrast, radiotherapy was rarely separated from diagnosis before the 1960s.[33] As we have noted for the late 1920s, there were key sites of international importance for radium work, including the Memorial Hospital under James Ewing. The Mayo Clinic had separated radiotherapy from diagnostic radiology, and indeed X-ray therapy from radium therapy;[34] but this differentiation was not much followed, especially after World War II. From the late 1930s, the Memorial had turned to surgery and biochemistry, a shift that seems to have been very influential.[35] The few would-be radiotherapists, many of whom were European in origin or education, were limited by the professional associations of general radiology on the one hand, and by the dominance of surgeons on the other; they tended to be isolated, for safety, in the basements of hospitals.

In the United States, as mentioned, radium was not regulated, but it was sometimes supplied by governments—and could have been more so, had the politics of organized medicine been less resistant. The radium used at the Memorial in New York, the Huntingdon in Boston, and the Johns Hopkins in Baltimore was supplied through an agreement with the U.S. Bureau of Mines, brokered by Ewing and Howard Kelly. In 1934, Congress was pressed to accept repayment of ten million dollars of Belgian war debt in the form of radium; the American Radium Society, dominated by surgeons, lobbied *against* the proposal, and "the spectre of a government controlled medical specialty was not raised again until after WWII."[36]

In the 2001 Stetten lecture, David Cantor has described the radium scheme operated by the National Cancer Institute (NCI) from its foundation in 1937. He sees it as a New Deal public health program, extending the cancer-treatment schemes that had been established in some states and that provided radium treatment for the indigent poor (we

33. See the X-ray Centenary History volumes of the American Radiological Society; and esp. three chapters in *Radiation Oncology*, ed. Gagliardi and Watson (n. 20): James D. Cox, "Clinical Practice," pp. 21–41; Nancy Knight, "Training and Education," pp. 165–84; and Bogardus, "Intersociety" (n. 20).

34. See del Regato, *Radiation Oncologists* (n. 10), for the collection of biographies, esp. those of Ewing (Memorial Hospital), Paterson (Christie/Holt, Manchester), and Fletcher (MDA); and the biographical notes on Desjardins of the Mayo.

35. See "Report of a Visit to Canada and the United States by a Delegation from the British Empire Cancer Campaign, July 1948," pp. 5 and 36, in the F. P. Spears Papers, ser. E, box 14, Wellcome Contemporary Medical Archives, London.

36. Bogardus, "Intersociety" (n. 20), p. 218.

have already noted the Missouri state cancer hospital).[37] Public provision (and centralization) was advocated by some of the leaders of the vocal American Cancer Society, but it was opposed by the AMA and by American radiologists who saw it as a threat to private practice. In the words of an officer of the American College of Radiology: "Private medical practice has everything to offer that could be offered by a bureaucratic government in a war on cancer."[38] In 1940, the doctors lobbied (successfully) against a bill to provide federal health insurance that would have covered "medical services and facilities which had become standardized in their nature but which, because of high cost, were seldom used."[39] Concerning radium, as with "socialized medicine" more widely, the doctors had their way—though not without contestation. In Canada, the social democratic government of the province of Saskatchewan led other provinces into a radium scheme, as it did later for provincial health insurance.[40]

Generally, the NCI focused on research rather than treatment; but its radium fund was low-profile after the initial purchase, and the radium was not used to support clinical research or to reorganize existing services.[41] Indeed, by the time the NCI got under way (and here it contrasts with the MRC earlier in the United Kingdom), cyclotrons were attracting attention as a possible means for treatment, and the United States, through the University of California at Berkeley, was a pioneer in that technology.[42] But for the most part, American radiotherapy remained an appendage of diagnostic radiology, and American cancer hospitals remained dominated by surgeons.

The British government's research agency, the MRC, had invested in radiotherapeutics from the 1920s, and it was not much influenced by surgeons or the clinical elites more generally.[43] In the United States, the

37. David Cantor, "Radium and the Origins of the National Cancer Institute," The DeWitt Stetten Jr. Lecture given at the National Institutes of Health, Bethesda, Maryland, 28 June 2001.

38. Mac Cahal, executive secretary, to the ARC Board of Chancellors, 19 August 1937, quoted in Bogardus, "Intersociety" (n. 20), p. 215.

39. Ibid.

40. For Canada, see Hayter, *Element of Hope* (n. 25); Antonia Maioni, *Parting at the Crossroads: The Emergence of Health Insurance in the United States and Canada* (Princeton: Princeton University Press, 1998).

41. Cantor, "Radium" (n. 37).

42. For example, see the Minutes of the National Advisory Cancer Council for its initial meetings on 9 and 27 November and 13 December 1937, U.S. National Archives, Washington, D.C., RG G443, box 6; and the biography of Albert Soiland in del Regato, *Radiation Oncologists* (n. 10), pp. 77–86.

43. Joan Austoker, *A History of the Imperial Cancer Research Fund 1902–1986* (Oxford: Oxford University Press, 1988), pp. 69–90.

main government investments came *after* World War II, and it was a new form of cancer treatment, chemotherapy, that benefited most.

Post–World War II Cancer Services in the United Kingdom and United States

The wartime atomic program helped produce isotopes and large-scale generators, both of which were soon adapted to medical uses (partly to demonstrate the peacetime potential of nuclear physics). In the United Kingdom these new tools, plus a higher level of funding for research and the provision of more salaried posts under the new National Health Service (NHS), all boosted radiotherapy—though inasmuch as the NHS generalized such benefits across most of specialist medicine, it reduced radiotherapy's uniqueness as a scientific and salaried service. The National Radium Commission was abolished, but the radiotherapists remained close to the MRC, and in the 1950s when "chemotherapy" was high-profile for several diseases and clinical trials became the preferred mode of assessment of treatments, the MRC also supported some trials of radiotherapy and surgery.

All teaching hospitals now had salaried professorships of medicine, surgery, and obstetrics and gynecology; these departments were expected to do clinical research, to which the MRC was now more friendly than it had been in the 1920s.[44] But trials of surgery and radiotherapy generally proved harder to manage than trials of new drugs, in part because they had to build on existing treatments. Lung cancer was then conspicuous, because of its increasing incidence and the emergent interest in smoking as a cause, but systematic trials of radiotherapy on nonoperable cases laboriously confirmed the poor expectations.[45]

The case was different for breast cancer, and that radical mastectomy continued to be questioned in Britain after World War II owed much to the strength of the radiotherapists—especially Robert McWhirter of Edinburgh, who challenged the surgeons in territory they regarded as their own. By introducing the statistical methods that were the mainstay of their own modality, radiotherapists increased the sophistication of surgical case-assessment and results appraisal. (As Lerner notes, Britons and other Europeans were also important for the growth of surgical skepticism

44. *Clinical Research in Britain, 1950–1980*, vol. 7 of *Wellcome Witnesses to Twentieth Century Medicine* (London: Wellcome Centre for the History of Medicine, 2000).

45. See Carsten Timmermann, "As Depressing As It Was Predictable? Lung Cancer, Clinical Trials, and the Medical Research Council in Postwar Britain," in this issue.

in the United States in the 1950s.)[46] The British debates between surgeons and radiotherapists were heated, but the latter were better placed than their American counterparts; the MRC trials were "interdisciplinary" and well supplied with independent statistical expertise. Such were the conditions for the postwar "rationalizations" across radiotherapy and surgery, into which cancer chemotherapy was also fitted.

In the United States, by contrast, the new and massive state funding went to research rather than public medical services. New machines were developed, which might have offered a path to independence for radiotherapists, and the heavy involvement of government with physics research and the licensing of isotopes might have offered scope for a large-scale training program to man the new machines—but the radiological profession remained wary of government interference, resisting, for example, the regulation of linear accelerators and other technology. Instead, the numbers of cobalt units and high-voltage units increased rapidly, spreading well outside the main centers, while specialists relied on a handful of training programs, especially in new centers such as Stanford University, the M. D. Anderson in Houston, and the Penrose hospital in Colorado (to which del Regato had moved).[47]

At Stanford, very much a center of postwar technology, Henry Kaplan claimed cures of Hodgkin's disease by wide-field radiation. At the M. D. Anderson, Gilbert Fletcher, who also worked in diagnostic radiology until the 1960s, applied European methods, especially for the head and neck. Like Juan del Regato at the Penrose, Fletcher was European-trained, as were several of the rare medical physicists—another indication, perhaps, of the field's relatively low status in the United States.[48] From the 1950s there were attempts to run clinical trials that included radiotherapy—some involving the NCI, and usually led by practitioners of other modalities—but most of them failed; only after 1967 was there a standing organization for radiotherapy trials. Especially in the United States a subprofession that in prewar Europe had been built around analytical treatments and statistics was slow to adapt to the postwar pattern of experimental trials that had emerged from chemotherapeutic laboratories.[49] Not until the late 1960s were there enough American trainees to establish a subprofession substantially independent of diagnostic radiology; but from

46. Lerner, *Breast Cancer Wars* (n. 8), pp. 93–101.

47. See Knight, "Training" (n. 33), pp. 176–82; Cox, "Clinical Practice" (n. 33), pp. 28–36.

48. See the biographical notes on Kaplan, Fletcher, and del Regato himself in del Regato, *Radiation Oncologists* (n. 10), pp. 246, 237–38, and 259.

49. Cox, "Clinical Practice" (n. 33), pp. 35–36.

the 1970s it expanded rapidly, as trial programs became well established, especially for radiotherapy and chemotherapy as adjuncts to surgery, and then as facilities were established outside hospitals, in many cases owned by radiotherapists.[50]

But in some ways, the separate facilities underlined the separation of radiotherapy from the mainline clinical charge of cancer patients. American radiotherapy remained bound to its modality and did not become so formative of *cancer* services, or of the public image of cancer—in part perhaps because it achieved its limited autonomy alongside the rise of chemotherapy. Radiologists of any kind were not prominent in the general politics of medicine; they were, however, much occupied with disputes about conditions of employment, though they were among the best remunerated of American doctors.[51] In a cross-national survey of attitudes toward advanced and metastatic cases ca. 1990, American radiologists were more likely than Europeans or Canadians to "give hope," accompanied by relatively intensive radiotherapy; they were less likely to manage the terminal care themselves, and more likely to involve a medical oncologist.[52]

Post–World War II Chemotherapy

If radiotherapy was most obviously developed in European health systems that were state supported and centralized, chemotherapy was led from America, the land of liberal medicine. Indeed, as we shall see, market medicine probably accounts for its later prominence and professional form—but not for its technical origins. From the start of this new modality, government-funded institutions were central, especially the war-work (including antimalarial and chemical warfare) programs. The three strands of postwar American chemotherapy research grew from research programs on mustard gas (alkylating agents), on nutrition (aminopterin), and on antibiotics (streptomycin). One need hardly stress here the key role of the National Cancer Institute and its clinical program from 1955, the Cancer Chemotherapy National Service Center. This acted like a

50. Bogardus, "Intersociety" (n. 20), pp. 225–27; Cox, "Clinical Practice" (n. 33), pp. 30–36; Jean B. Owen et al., "Recent Patterns of Growth in Radiation Therapy Facilities in the US: A Patterns of Care Study Report," *Internat. J. Radiat. Oncol. Biol. Phys.*, 1992, *24*: 983–86.

51. Bogardus, "Intersociety" (n. 20), pp. 205–6.

52. E. J. Maher et al., "Treatment Differences in Advanced and Metastatic Cancer: Differences in Attitude between the USA, Canada and Europe," *Internat. J. Radiat. Oncol. Biol. Phys.*, 1992, *23*: 239–44.

pharmaceutical company, testing remedies on standardized mice, and organizing multicenter clinical trials in hospital units where treatments were free and doctors (several of whom were avoiding military service by serving research in Bethesda) were salaried, albeit poorly. Even the drug company most involved initially, Burroughs-Wellcome, was sometimes seen as a research charity.[53]

The cancer drug programs were models of laboratory experimentalism extended into clinical experiments; they variously drew on antibacterial research and therapies, especially those for tuberculosis. The borrowed elements included kinetic models, animal models, additive therapies, large organized programs, and clinical trials as central features of an essentially new form of clinical experimentation.[54] But the story as commonly told has a twist that is curious in historic context: the prominence of blood and lymph diseases in the new image and practice of cancer.

Leukemias, in some senses, had not been cancers before World War II. They were the preserve of general physicians and especially of hematologists. Since there was little to be done for the patients, they lacked clinical interest—but they were attractive for laboratory-based hematologists: there was a good animal model, blood was easy to handle and observe, there were lots of parameters to measure and cell types to distinguish, and hematology, in the United States, if not in Britain, already spanned laboratory and clinic. The medicines developed in the 1940s and 1950s were not considered curative: they would be given until a relapse occurred, then another would be tried, until no further therapy was possible. Here was therapeutic addition in sequence, mostly for palliation; but some long-term remissions were obtained, as well as a few "cures," especially with choriocarcinoma and some lymphomas.[55]

These medico-professional conditions were present in most advanced

53. For the cancer-screening programs, see R. Bud, "Strategy in American Cancer Research after World War II: A Case Study," *Soc. Stud. Sci.*, 1978, *8*: 425–59; C. G. Zubrod, "Origins and Development of Chemotherapy Research at the National Cancer Institute," *Cancer Treat. Rep.*, 1984, *68*: 9–19; John Laszlo, *The Cure of Childhood Leukemia: Into the Age of Miracles* (New Brunswick, N.J.: Rutgers University Press, 1996).

54. For experimentalism in biomedicine generally, see Ilana Löwy, "The Experimental Body," in Cooter and Pickstone, *Medicine* (n. 1), pp. 435–50. For clinical trials as a new form of medicine, see Peter Keating and Alberto Cambrosio, "Cancer Clinical Trials: The Emergence and Development of a New Style of Practice," in this issue.

55. For an excellent account of medical oncology in the United States, Britain, and France, see Ilana Löwy, *Between Bench and Bedside: Science, Healing, and Interleukin-2 in a Cancer Ward* (Boston: Harvard University Press, 1996), pp. 36–83. See also W. G. Jones, "Cancer Chemotherapy," in *Cancer Topics and Radiotherapy*, ed. C. A. F. Joslin (London: Pitman, 1982), pp. 31–45.

countries, but in the United States, at the NCI, leukemia was chosen as a major focus for public funding linking clinic and laboratory for cancer. The American initiative was marked by the intensity of funding, by regular experimental trials, and then by the intensification of combination treatments in search of cures rather than simply remissions. Different cytotoxic drugs seemed to have similar effects but different side effects—so using them in parallel might increase their effectiveness. The task force for acute lymphoblastic anemia managed to produce cures in children in the early 1960s, and these successes raised hopes and standards. In the 1960s, doctors who specialized in children's cancers were formed into networks for trials, and other physicians were enrolled to try various drug combinations on adult cancers. New regimes for cancer had been created outside the old limits of the disease, and by the intensive cumulation of chemicals.

Britain and France had a few key centers that featured in these stories. Jean Bernard was the French prince of hematology;[56] and in Britain from before World War II, Alexander Haddow at the Chester Beatty Institute had been making and testing chemical remedies, with collaborations in Manchester and at the Marsden Hospital in London.[57] Various single drugs were developed that increased remissions, but many physicians and most pediatricians were skeptical about the benefits of toxic treatments in extending remissions. In Britain, the American remedies seemed unduly aggressive; to some, they were an example of overprescribing.[58] But there was also a structural question: in post–World War II Britain, radiotherapists were the "keepers of cancer," and to the extent that they claimed treatment of lymphomas, say, the freedom accorded to physicians (internists) could be restricted.[59]

In countries where physicians had beds for blood diseases, they were well placed to adopt the leukemia therapies. But the fact that chemotherapy

56. Cristelle Rigal, "Contributions à l'histoire de la recherche médicale: Autour des travaux de Jean Bernard et de ses collaborateurs sur la leucémie aiguë, 1940–1970" (doctoral diss., Université Paris 7—Denis Diderot, 2003).

57. "Alexander Haddow," *Biog. Mem. Fell. Roy. Soc.*, 1977, *23*: 133–91, on pp. 153–60.

58. See J. S. Tobias et al., "Who Should Treat Cancer," *Lancet*, 1981, *1*: 884–86, on p. 885; Gareth J. G. Rees, "What Is Best for the Patient? A European View," in *Cost and Benefit in Cancer Care*, ed. Basil Stoll (Basingstoke: Macmillan, 1988), pp. 31–38, esp. pp. 34–35.

59. Tobias et al., "Who Should Treat" (n. 58); Rees, "What Is Best" (n. 58); M. J. Peckham, "Clinical Oncology: The Future of Radiotherapy and Medical Oncology," *Lancet*, 1981, *1*: 886–87. Also see the editorial in *Lancet*, 1981, *2*: 674; and David Galton's comments on a period of hostility from radiotherapists, in D. A. Christie and E. M. Tansey, eds., *Leukaemia*, vol. 15 of *Wellcome Witnesses to Twentieth Century Medicine* (London: Wellcome Centre for the History of Medicine at UCL, 2003), p. 23.

often required intensive care meant that laboratory-based hematologists were not keen to take leukemia patients; nor were radiotherapists well placed for diseases and types of management that largely fell outside their previous experience and training. Generally speaking, the lymphomas, which already involved surgeons and radiotherapists, were a bridge or boundary across which expertise in leukemias and chemotherapies could be extended to solid cancers. In the United Kingdom from about 1974, a few physicians interested in cancer chemotherapy began to seek recognition as medical oncologists, rather than clinical hematologists or general physicians. They stressed the difficulty of the treatments, but also their length and the integration with general medical care.[60] In this move, as in their therapies, they were following American examples.

The U.K. radiotherapists immediately felt threatened by this tendency to divide oncology into surgical, medical, and radiation aspects. Radiation oncology, they maintained, was an American, not a British, specialism; their U.K. discipline was "radiotherapy and oncology" (a definition that in turn worried the physicians).[61] Radiotherapists were focused on collecting statistics to incrementally improve the application of radiotherapy, whether by novel machines, or isotopes, or new routines—but they did not experiment (much) on the basis of laboratory work, nor did they expect breakthroughs. Indeed, they were inclined to see the chemotherapies simply as additions to the armamentarium. For them, trials were mainly analyses of established practices and of plausible variants and additions. Chemotherapy was but another way of interfering with the reproduction of cancer (and of all other fast-dividing cells); it was a further means of palliation, or of marginally improving some (poor) survival rates.[62] One sees here a key feature of additivity in medicine: where proven remedies exist, however imperfect, they set the conditions against which other remedies must be judged—and this can be very difficult, technically and politically, especially where different modalities are involved.[63] One of the great advantages of acute leukemias for cancer researchers was the lack of

60. Royal College of Physicians (RCP) Paper (78/8), to the Working Party on Oncology, 1978, Royal College of Physicians Archives, London (hereafter RCPA).

61. Minutes of the Joint Committee on Medical Oncology, meeting at Glasgow, 9 October 1974, RCPA.

62. For example: "Unlike radiotherapists, who do not expect exciting overnight improvements, the medical oncologists receive periodical bursts of enthusiasm by the perennial advent of any new *drug du jour*" (Juan A. del Regato, "One Hundred Years of Radiation Oncology," in *Current Radiation Oncology*, vol. 2, ed. Jeffrey S. Tobias and Patrick R. M. Thomas [London: Arnold, 1996], pp. 1–35, on p. 31).

63. See Timmermann, "Depressing" (n. 45).

previously established remedies, and the short time span of clinical trials. For the most part, leukemias were an open field, into which new chemical inventions could be launched.

For would-be chemotherapists, with a history of conquering anemias and bacterial diseases, randomized control trials epitomized a new form of clinical experimentalism. The companies were finding or producing a range of new drugs, which could be variously combined, as for example by Donald Pinkel at Memphis; and chemotherapists were becoming connoisseurs of trials.[64] And the cancer drug trials were well supported by pharmaceutical companies, which were rapidly expanding their range and their ties with clinicians. The successes with blood and lymph cancers (and choriocarcinoma), and especially with children, attracted much attention; they made central to "cancer" a group of disorders that had been marginal to that field.

In the United States, internists and radiotherapists developed rival treatments for Hodgkin's disease, but the professional situations were not symmetrical: internists had beds and could act as the doctor in charge; radiotherapists were largely confined to a service role—combined with their service role in diagnostics. The therapeutic returns for most solid cancers were marginal, but the support for the research effort, both from the U.S. government and from industry, was enough to create a new branch of internal medicine called medical oncology. The National Cancer Act of 1971 encouraged the formation of cancer centers in which medical oncologists took most of the nonsurgical cases, calling on radiotherapists as necessary. From the 1970s, multimodal trials became common, and medical oncologists were in a good position to recruit surgeons and radiotherapists. Their position was further secured in the 1980s by a massive increase in the number of drugs to be tested, and by the spread of medical treatments beyond the main centers.[65]

64. See the account of Pinkel in Laszlo, *Childhood Leukemia* (n. 53), pp. 31–32, 234–38.

65. In 1981, it was reported that the United States had 1,700 medical oncologists certified (about 6.8 per million) since the recognition of the specialty in 1974, and that most large hospitals had set up departments. In Britain, "by contrast, departments of radiotherapy (which have historically been related to diagnostic radiology) have usually provided an outpatient service without attempting to supervise more general aspects of cancer care" (Tobias et al., "Who Should Treat" [n. 58], p. 885). In 1985 the ratio of medical oncologists to the population in the United States was about thirty-five times that in Britain (Rees, "What Is Best" [n. 58], p. 34). In 1995 there were 81 British consultants in medical oncology, less than a quarter of the number per population that the United States had supported fifteen years previously. The number in Britain increased more rapidly over the 1990s (on NHS rather than academic research funding) to 163 by 2001 and to 220 by 2006 (about 4 per million population) (Derek Crowther, personal communication).

That story of research successes received much publicity, at the time and since. But as Gretchen Krueger is now showing, there is also a story of cancer chemotherapy in "ordinary practice," especially in the United States.

Chemotherapy and Liberal Practice

The initiative for the formation of a specialist society, the American Society for Clinical Oncology (ASCO), came from the margins rather than from the NCI or the academic establishments, and it did so when chemotherapy was only just beginning to claim cures.[66] To understand this, we have to shift our focus away from the state-supported medicine we have discussed for the United Kingdom and for the American NCI programs, and onto the conditions of liberal practice in the rapidly expanding American medical market of the postwar decades.

The development of medical oncology in the United States has to be understood as part of the growth of specialism within internal medicine and the concurrent replacement of family practitioners by internists.[67] But it also seems to derive from the growth of internal medicine in cancer hospitals and of cancer centers in general hospitals. In the Memorial Hospital from the 1930s, for example, and in the M. D. Anderson through the 1950s, one can follow the ways in which internists claimed places alongside surgeons and radiologists. One claim was for the use of hormone therapies, and then after World War II for the use of radioisotopes, not least for thyroid cancer. Other claims were more generic, including internists staffing the diagnostic clinics that were a key feature of American cancer centers from the 1930s, offering diagnosis for the private patients of local doctors, as well as assigning patients who had been sent to the hospital but not to particular clinicians. As clinical instruments such as the ECG became more common after World War II, they too might be used mainly by internists, often working with surgeons.[68]

---

66. Gretchen Krueger, "The Formation of the American Society of Clinical Oncology and the Development of a Medical Specialty, 1964–1973," *Perspect. Biol. & Med.*, 2004, *47*: 537–51.

67. Rosemary Stevens, "The Curious Case of Internal Medicine: Fundamental Ambivalence, Social Success,'" in *Grand Rounds: One Hundred Years of Internal Medicine*, ed. Russell C. Maulitz and Diana E. Long (Philadelphia: University of Pennsylvania Press, 1988), pp. 339–64.

68. These processes can be followed in the (Annual) Reports of the Memorial Hospital (at the Rockefeller Archive, Tarrytown, N.Y.), and in those of the M. D. Anderson Hospital (in the Hospital Archive, Houston, Tex.).

For all cancer hospital patients, internists were also on hand for such treatments as were beyond the scope or wishes of the surgeons. After World War II at the Memorial, a research fellow examined all the surgical patients and discovered that, aside from their cancers, more than 60 percent of them were ill enough to need a general medical service.[69] This may have reflected the increased readiness of surgeons to operate on vulnerable patients and/or their undertaking of more-radical operations; either way, surgical ambition in cancer hospitals probably made more work for physicians. More generally, for diagnosis and for therapy, mutual-referral patterns were part of the economy of increased medical specialization. And where cancers were too advanced for surgical treatment, the hospital internists might take them over, sometimes trying the new chemotherapies, especially when the medicines were so toxic and the patients so ill that they required a great deal of care.

From 1964, a few private physicians who saw an opportunity for specialist business were able to recruit academic leaders and the support of the NCI. They eventually gained recognition as *medical* oncologists from the American Board of Internal Medicine (ABIM)—along with several other new specialisms, but ahead of the hematologists who had strong claims over the blood and lymph cancers, and with whom the medical oncologists then negotiated joint programs. That the ASCO and its journal used the term *clinical* oncology may have reflected a distancing from research establishments, and the aspirations of some of the society's founders that it would bring together internists, surgeons, and radiotherapists who were interested in chemotherapy.

As a branch of internal medicine, clinical oncology in America proved innovative, popular, and remunerative. Research leaders found a large group of interested clinicians, who in their turn connected to a research field with unprecedented funding and visibility, especially from the early 1970s. By 1980, only seven years after registration had started, there were more than 1,700 medical oncologists registered with the ABIM.[70] Many of these medical oncologists, including some trialists, were in community practice. In the United States, unlike Britain and France, trial organization did not remain the prerogative of special cancer centers or of teaching hospitals, it permeated all levels of practice (and this is increasingly true of radiological partnerships, involved with adjuvant trials), though

69. Memorial Hospital Report, 1947–51, Section on the Department of Medicine, Rockefeller Archive, Tarrytown, N.Y.

70. R. A. V. Milsted et al., "Cancer Chemotherapy—What Have We Achieved?" *Lancet,* 1980, 2: 1343–46, on p. 1343.

it remained organized from the academic centers. Some chemo-trials are now operated through private medical corporations that supply the therapies and franchise the physicians: US Oncology now accounts for 15 percent of the chemotherapy delivered in the United States.[71] One might here see the experimentalist mode of practice as having extended from pharmaceutical companies to service companies, and from industrial laboratories to distributed clinics. Trials became part of the market, not just for the drugs, but also for medical care; they became part of the attraction of a physician or a hospital.

British Medical Oncology and Clinical Oncology in Context

In the United Kingdom, the sustained development came in London, from a few hematologists (who in Britain were pathologists and largely confined to laboratory work) and from physicians who took a particular interest in blood diseases. The Royal Marsden, Bart's, and the Postgraduate hospital at Hammersmith were the main centers. At the Hammersmith, for example, the hematological pathologist John Dacie collaborated with the physician David Galton, who also worked at the Chester Beatty as part of Haddow's team. In the sixties there was increasing interest in American therapies (and in the work of Jean Bernard in Paris), and several trials for leukemia were organized through the Medical Research Council, which around 1967 set up a Leukaemia Unit at the Hammersmith. British radiotherapists were sometimes hostile (as indeed were some physicians), but by the later 1960s radiotherapists were collaborating in trials—for example, of bisulphan versus radiotherapy for chronic myeloid leukemia.[72]

At Bart's, Sir Ronald Bodley Scott and Gordon Hamilton Fairley led the treatment of leukemias, and the extension of chemotherapies to lymphomas and other cancers. The geographic extension of the nascent specialism of medical oncology, and its characteristic trials, was funded by cancer charities and the MRC. In the early 1970s, stimulated by the American Cancer Act of 1971, the MRC and the cancer charities designed a response to complement the lavish American funding, taking advantage of the NHS structures. The Imperial Cancer Research Fund opened the first medical oncology unit, at Bart's, and four regional units were planned. Manchester in 1973 gained the first provincial chemotherapy research unit, funded by the Cancer Research Campaign at the Christie cancer hospital under the leadership of Professor Derek Crowther, who had trained and worked

71. See Keating and Cambrosio, "Cancer Clinical Trials" (n. 54).
72. Christie and Tansey, *Leukaemia* (n. 59), pp. 12–14.

at Bart's. At the Christie, Crowther had one ward (twenty-eight beds) for chemotherapy, and he concentrated initially on lymphomas before spreading outward to hematological malignancies and solid cancers. Apart from one surgical ward, the rest (three hundred beds) were manned by radiotherapists. Adult leukemias were mostly treated at the general teaching hospital, the Manchester Royal Infirmary, and childhood leukemia at the Royal Manchester Children's Hospital (Pendlebury).[73]

There are several structural points of interest here. First, the origin and growth of a subspecialism on the basis of its research—which appears to be an international characteristic of chemotherapy in rich countries. It was through research funding that consultant positions were initially supported, and NHS funding which now supports most of the posts has continued to focus on the research centers. Second, the restriction of major chemotherapy in Britain to regional centers, at least for prescription (some of the treatment could be carried out in district hospitals). And third, the association of chemotherapy with the drive to centralize the diagnosis and treatment of rare cancers, especially of children. In some provincial regions, including Manchester, the treatment of childhood leukemia was centralized from the early 1970s, and from about that date children's cancers were largely the preserve of pediatricians.

The key here was the focus on clinical trials and on centralizing patients with relatively rare conditions. There was some published evidence that as long as new routines were followed, patients did as well in hospitals that were not pioneering—but such conservative claims were attacked: who could tolerate the "semi-routinization" of treatments when most of the patients still died? And if new regimes were to be developed with due urgency, then trials must not take too long; this meant that more patients must enter trials, so fewer could be left to "ordinary hospitals." This logic, plus arguments about the fine balance between overdoses and ineffectual underdoses, ensured the centralization of treatments, even when they did not require expensive apparatus.

The same logic might be seen as preventing the chemotherapeutic regimes' being administered by "oncologists" whose main training was in radiotherapy. If drugs are always "in development" and trials are expensive and time-consuming, and if the drugs are first used in blood diseases where existing specialists have the laboratory background, then

73. See n. 65. For comparisons of medical oncology in France, Britain, and the United States, see Löwy, *Bench and Bedside* (n. 55), esp. pp. 65–71. For British policy I am indebted to Helen Valier, who is investigating the international politics; Lord Zuckerman, *Cancer Research* (London: HMSO, 1972); and, re the Manchester scene, Derek Crowther, personal communication.

one has the makings of a new specialism of medical oncology—growing beyond the claims of clinical hematology as the drugs are applied in other conditions. But of course, this nascent specialism had to negotiate its position in a complex medical field where general physicians, hematologists, radiotherapists, as well as some pediatricians and surgeons, also had interests.

In Britain, as in the United States, there were experts who saw cancer treatment as a field in which doctors from surgery, internal medicine, and radiology could come together for common training. In Britain, some wanted to create a common specialism, and the title "clinical oncology" was often used to cover all three modalities, or perhaps as an eclectic alternative to medical oncology as a branch of internal medicine.[74] During the late 1980s and early 1990s, some eminent chemotherapists and radiotherapists tried very hard to establish a joint Faculty of Clinical Oncology, responsible to both the Royal College of Physicians and the Royal College of Radiologists, but they met opposition—including some of the leaders of their respective colleges.[75] In the United Kingdom, as in the United States, the convergent option proved a weak position; it was easier to specialize *within* each of the three institutionalized main fields. There is a logic of continued divergence here which proved powerful; in a world divided into medicine and surgery (and radiology), it proved hard to maintain that cancer (or any other focus) might become a field of convergence.

Thus in both countries, chemotherapy became largely identified with medical oncology as a branch of internal medicine, and British radiotherapists struggled to maintain chemotherapy as part of their range (and to resist the possible conversion of empty radiotherapy posts to medical oncology). In the United States, the term "clinical oncology" was appropriated early by specialists in chemotherapy; in the United Kingdom, it was unilaterally appropriated by the radiotherapists in 1990, instead of "radiotherapy and oncology," which had served as their banner from the 1970s.[76] Both American chemotherapists and British radiotherapists used "clinical oncology" in the titles of their journals, both of which claimed to represent all clinical approaches to cancer.

74. The term was used generically in the interdisciplinary Working Party on Medical Oncology in 1978–79 (see Minutes, RCPA); and as an alternative to developing medical oncology: see Minutes of the Joint Committee on Medical Oncology (n. 61).

75. See Minutes of the College Committee on Medical Oncology, 1986–94, RCPA.

76. Ibid., 15 June 1990.

Comparisons, Prospects, and the Uses of History

In Sweden, it seems, the specialization in oncology, historically based on radiotherapy, *has* been able to incorporate chemotherapy, though there are also physicians who specialize in medical treatments of cancer.[77] By contrast, in the United States, medical oncology has boomed as a very remunerative branch of internal medicine; the drugs are prescribed more readily than in Europe, and medical oncologists seem to be the lead doctors for many kinds of cancer.[78] Radiotherapists remain treatment-based specialists, their considerable incomes now exceeded by some medical oncologists; around 1990, in Florida, they had to fight to prevent medical oncologists from setting up freestanding facilities that included radiotherapy.[79]

In Britain, medical oncologists have spread out from the teaching hospitals and children's hospitals, and as chemotherapy becomes more common, especially as an "adjuvant" therapy, more drugs are given by doctors who are not specifically trained in medical oncology. But, as we have seen, the policy remains to restrict major chemotherapy to the regional cancer centers. There the medical oncologists work alongside the "clinical oncologists," who give chemotherapy in addition to radiotherapy.

These patterns are not static. In France in the 1980s, the special cancer centers that had been developed in the interwar period found themselves marginalized by the growth of specialist medicine and surgery in the regional teaching hospitals; their counteraction was led by medical oncologists who had trained in the United States, who stressed the common focus on cancer (rather than particular organs), along with multidisciplinary teams, national coordination of research, and clinical trials for the production of protocols. Their prominence in the elaboration of evidence-based medicine in France resecured their roles at the apices of regional hierarchies and as points of reference for difficult cases.[80]

Even in Sweden, the dominance of the oncology tradition was threatened by proposals to divide up cancer treatment in teaching hospitals that were departmentalized according to body sites (so, for example, physicians and surgeons would collaborate over kidney cancer as they do

77. Larsson, "Organisation" (n. 24).

78. Löwy, *Bench and Bedside* (n. 55), pp. 65–71; Tobias et al., "Who Should Treat" (n. 58); Gareth Rees, "What Is Best" (n. 58), p. 34.

79. Bogardus, "Intersociety" (n. 20), pp. 225–27.

80. Patrick Castel and Erhart Friedberg, "Institutional Change as an Interactive Process: The Modernization of the French Cancer Centers" (Paper delivered at Institutions Conference, Stanford University, 26–27 March 2004).

over kidney failure, and would call in radiotherapy as needed). A national commission in the early 1970s preserved cancer centers, but they were now to include specialists in internal medicine as well as oncologists; and both general oncologists and gynecological oncologists were to have training in internal medicine as well as radiotherapy.[81]

In Britain, there have been moves to reorganize responsibilities and training in "cancer centers" so that all trainees will learn some radiotherapy and some chemotherapy—to create a single group of oncologists whose further specialization would be primarily by anatomical site (though allowing some specialization in practice between modalities). This would be related to the Swedish model, and it would seem to have a certain economic logic; but the proposal has been on hold since the late 1990s.[82] Cancer protocols are now required for all major hospitals, under national directions that allow limited local discretion. These are intended to equalize treatment across hospital districts by linking all of them with their regional cancer centers. For most cancers, the protocols require the collaboration of specialists in all three modalities.

Whether and how the British subprofessions reorganize may depend on factors both internal and external to clinical medicine—on the continuations of the structural dynamics of which this whole paper is a preliminary exploration. If, as some British *clinical* oncologists claim, the combinatorial possibilities of intensive chemotherapy are becoming exhausted and "routine treatments" are increasingly detached from research, then the case for a partial merger of the two nonsurgical subprofessions will be strengthened. Chemotherapy trials might come to look more like radiotherapy trials, and combined trials would be the rule—ways of making incremental improvements across the range of available modalities. Experimentalism, one might say, would merge back into extended analysis and rationalization. Indeed, in all leading countries, much of the incremental advance of treatments now depends on the testing of the many possible permutations and varieties of the three main modalities. The ever-shifting variables in these complex configurations of care ensure that the combinations tried are but a fraction of the total possible—so even at this level, judgments must still enter; the rationalization is always imperfect, even before we consider the peculiarities of individual patients.

81. Larsson, "Organisation" (n. 24).
82. For the United Kingdom, see the Royal College of Physicians and the Royal College of Radiologists, Joint Council for Clinical Oncology, *Report of the Working Party on Training and Education in a New Specialty of Clinical Oncology*, April 1998, RCPA.

Other models of the future are also in play. New waves of drugs, biological as well as chemical, could maintain the dynamism of medical oncology and of its experimental outlook. British clinical oncologists might do more with medicines and less with radiation, and perhaps cancer will come to look more like other areas of medicine, and more like the United States—divided between surgery and internal medicine, with radiotherapy as an add-on (though here one notes that since World War II, repeated predictions of the decline of radiotherapy have accompanied the steady increase of its practice).

But for the continued dynamics of clinical and medical oncologists in Britain, new contextual political factors may be important, including the increased managerialism of governments and the impact of the European Union. The new readiness of the British government to manage issues that would once have been strictly professional is striking. Clinical appraisals, the need to demonstrate competence for new procedures, and new regulations about medical training programs are all well under way. Managerial logic may come to be applied to the historical professional divisions that we have discussed here. These new political contexts, and the subspecialization of all modalities according to the cancer-site, could reinvigorate claims that, as in Sweden, cancer doctors should be expert in all nonsurgical modalities, though perhaps more specialized for research.

Here too, the interactions with Europe may be significant. Both medical oncology and clinical oncology are organized partly through European collaborations and associations, notably the European Society for Medical Oncology. If you check the ESMO website, you will find data on which countries recognize medical oncology: Britain has long recognized it, but Sweden appears to have failed to do so. There is a logic of implied deprivation here that may prove persuasive in attempts to regularize professional roles across the European Union, especially if American models are regarded as helpful. But for Europe, as for Britain, there could be other possibilities based on the integration of competences and new forms of training.

Whatever the developments peculiar to particular nations, we can be fairly sure that the treatments in leading hospitals in all of the richer countries will increasingly be carried out according to protocols for "normal" treatments. In the production of trials and protocols, if not necessarily their execution, specialists from all the modalities will take part, and most patients are likely to receive at least two of the modalities. It remains to be investigated how much the recommendations and the practices continue to differ between and within countries, and how these correlate with the differences in professional structure and dynamics that I have here submitted to historical analysis, albeit in a preliminary manner.

For the present, I hope I have at least raised some key questions about the cognitive and practical relations between modalities in medicine, about the conditions under which they developed differently, and hence about the path dependency of their interactions. Medical history as a discipline is rarely called on now by medical planners and policy analysts: they prefer economic analyses that are much simpler because they are more exclusive. But it is not these unhistorical forms of economics that explain why American cancer patients now need to see so many cancer specialists concurrently, or why the patterns are different elsewhere. Such explanations require history, albeit of a wider and more comparative form than most historians now produce.

One might reply that what really matters is that treatments be based on the best possible international evidence. Yet here too, as I have argued, full rationalization is impossible because of the incredible complexity of possible combinations of remedies. And even if the recommendations were the same the world over, they would still be "historical" for a reason that even medical historians have rarely explored. In laboratories using animals, possible treatments can be tried in any combinations, but inasmuch as all ethical human trials are constrained not to damage the chances of patients—when compared to presently effective treatments—so clinical trials must depend on the order in which treatments were devised. Even in principle, this most logical form of medical evidence is "path-dependent"—if I may again refer to the minimal tribute that analysts of the present, whether trialists or economists, must pay to history.

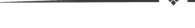

JOHN PICKSTONE founded the Centre for the History of Science, Technology and Medicine at the University of Manchester, where he is now Wellcome Research Professor and directs the project on "Constructing Cancers." He is also interested in the history of the total hip replacement, and the contemporary history of the British NHS. He has written on the history of physiology (mostly for France) and still writes on the social history of medicine (mostly for NW England). He continues to develop the ideas in his *Ways of Knowing: A New History of Science, Technology and Medicine* (Manchester/Chicago, 2000/2001). His address is: Centre for the History of Science, Technology and Medicine, Simon Building, University of Manchester, Oxford Road, Manchester M13 9PL, U.K. (e-mail: john.pickstone@manchester.ac.uk).

Cancer Clinical Trials:
The Emergence and Development
of a New Style of Practice

PETER KEATING AND ALBERTO CAMBROSIO

SUMMARY: Clinical trials are the principal vector for the development of chemotherapy, and they have become such a pervasive element of clinical cancer research that modern oncologists tend to take them for granted. Yet the system of cancer clinical trials amounts to a relatively recent (post–World War II) innovation. Its development has proceeded through ad hoc adjustments, and has produced a self-vindicating, yet open-ended, style of practice. This paper examines the historical development and articulation of the components of this new style of practice (protocols, oncologists, statistics, patients, and diseases), and of the new kind of objectivity they engender, by drawing on selected examples from American and European cancer clinical trial systems.

KEYWORDS: cancer, clinical trials, medical oncology, cooperative oncology groups, cancer patients, medical statistics

Introduction

In this paper we propose that cancer clinical trials be conceived of as a new style of biomedical practice. We explain how such a claim should be understood, and develop a preliminary analysis. Contemporary medical oncology is built around the performance of clinical trials, the principal vector for the development of chemotherapy. Clinical trials also pervade the practice of the two other anticancer therapies, radiotherapy and surgical therapy, and combinations of these referred to as multimodal

We would like to thank David Cantor for inviting us to participate in the Workshop on "Cancer in the Twentieth Century" held at the National Institutes of Health in November 2004, the participants for thoughtful comments, and Dr. Françoise Meunier and Dr. James F. Holland for their suggestions on subsequent versions of the paper. Research for this paper was supported by grants from CIHR (MOP-64372), FQRSC (ER-95786), and SSHRC (410-2002-1453), and by a CIHR/INSERM 2004–2005 International Exchange Award.

therapies. In addition, clinical trials function as an autonomous platform for the investigation of the biology and pathogenesis of cancer. Modern oncologists tend to take them for granted. Yet, from a historical and sociological point of view, the system of cancer clinical trials amounts to a relatively recent (post–World War II) innovation. Its development has proceeded through tinkering and ad hoc adjustments, and has produced what, adapting a term coined by Ian Hacking,[1] we would describe as a self-vindicating, yet open-ended, style of practice that can be clearly differentiated from, say, the laboratory style of practice and the statistical style of practice, even though it embodies elements of both.

Before outlining our thesis and presenting examples of selected components of our argument, we should clarify a possible misunderstanding. Clinical trials (in any field) can be understood as a technology. Central to this technology is a tool called a "protocol," which will be discussed in detail below. Such is the role played by protocols in clinical trials that the latter are often equated with the former; trialists, for instance, refer to a given clinical trial as "Protocol XY." From this point of view, the history of the emergence and development of clinical trials could be broadened to include the history of "protocols" as a particular way of organizing and managing biomedical activities. In turn, such a history could be understood as the history of a powerful undercurrent of twentieth-century medicine aiming at the rationalization of medical practices and leading to present-day "evidence-based medicine," in which randomized clinical trials play the role of a gold standard.[2] While there is no denying the existence and import of the rationalization trend, our goal in this paper is to provide a different (but not necessarily "alternative") view of cancer clinical trials—one that, as already mentioned, examines them as a new style of practice, viewing them as platforms, rather than "mere" technology.[3] While protocols are central to clinical trials, they are but an element of the new style of practice and do not subsume it in its entirety. The new style cannot, moreover, be explained solely in terms of the expression of a (largely external) trend toward rationalization: to understand the style, we must examine the content and the emergent properties of the com-

1. Ian Hacking, "The Self-Vindication of the Laboratory Sciences," in *Science as Practice and Culture*, ed. Andrew Pickering (Chicago: University of Chicago Press, 1992), pp. 29–64.

2. See Marc Berg, *Rationalizing Medical Work: Decision Support Techniques and Medical Practices* (Cambridge: MIT Press, 1997); Harry M. Marks, *The Progress of Experiments: Science and Therapeutic Reform in the United States, 1900–1990* (Cambridge: Cambridge University Press, 1997).

3. Peter Keating and Alberto Cambrosio, *Biomedical Platforms: Realigning the Normal and the Pathological in Late-Twentieth-Century Medicine* (Cambridge: MIT Press, 2003).

ponents of clinical trials. And, in so doing, we must be attentive to the temporal, institutional, and sociotechnical specificities of the domain (in the present case: cancer) in which clinical trials have been deployed. This is why our focus is on the post-1950 period, during which cancer clinical trials emerged and developed their distinctive style.

A New Style of Practice: The Cancer Clinical Trial System

A *style of practice* calls upon a distinctive configuration of institutions, scientific practices, and materials that generates specific ways of identifying and investigating research questions, of producing and assessing results, and of regulating these activities. We speak of a style of practice and not of a style of reasoning, as Hacking does,[4] in order to emphasize the heterogeneous nature of an arrangement that articulates tools, skills, and organizations to produce a unique form of collective endeavor. A quick description of the cancer clinical trial system in the United States and Europe illustrates the complexity of the institutional relations that underwrite the system.

In the United States more than 10,000 investigators at 3,000 individual institutions are presently registered with the largest sponsor of clinical trials, the U.S. National Cancer Institute (NCI). Each year, approximately 160 phase III protocols are actively pursued, with an average of one hundred sites participating in each trial.[5] Clinical trials, thus, are not single events, or even a series of related events: they are carried out within the context of a national (or, in the case of Europe, transnational) clinical trial and biomedical research system. As previously suggested, this institution was not designed in a single stroke; it evolved over the years in a process punctuated by numerous debates and reforms.

The NCI organized the first randomized clinical cancer trial (in acute lymphocytic leukemia) in 1954 at its Medical Center and, in the context of its cancer-drug screening program, went on to create two cooperative oncology groups known as the Acute Leukemia Group A and the Acute Leukemia Group B, later renamed the Children's Cancer Study Group and the Cancer and Leukemia Group B (CALGB). The following year, the NCI organized the first solid-cancer cooperative group, the Eastern Solid Tumor Group, which became the largest cooperative group (4,000

4. Ian Hacking, "Inaugural Lecture: Chair of Philosophy and History of Scientific Concepts at the Collège de France, 16 January 2001," *Econ. & Soc.*, 2004, *31*: 1–14.

5. M. C. Christian, J. L. Goldberg, J. Killen, et al., "A Central Institutional Review Board for Multi-Institutional Trials," *New England J. Med.*, 2002, *346*: 1405–8.

members) in the United States, the Eastern Cooperative Oncology Group (ECOG). By the 1960s, most phase II and phase III clinical cancer trial protocols in North America were devised and administered by the clinical trials network of the NCI. Not only were the groups new, but, more importantly, they constituted a new kind of *collective* (and *distributed*) biomedical actant.[6]

Initially devoted to testing chemical compounds provided by the NCI's screening program, the NCI Cooperative Group system has evolved significantly since the mid-1950s. Originally located in research organizations like the NCI or the Roswell Park Institute, in the 1970s the cooperative groups spread to community hospitals through programs designed to increase accrual to clinical trials. As a consequence, clinical investigators—"trialists" and their advanced research protocols—came into direct contact with community oncologists (most of whom had initially trained with the trialists). At the same time, as distributed research organizations, by the mid-1960s the cooperative groups no longer simply tested drugs: they tested hypotheses concerning therapy, examined pathophysiological mechanisms, and sought means for the prevention of cancer. These types of studies were integrated into the clinical trial protocols and became such a significant part of clinical cancer research that by the 1990s half of all Phase III clinical trials conducted by the groups incorporated ancillary laboratory and correlative studies.

Therapeutic modalities have likewise evolved. Initially restricted to chemotherapy, in the 1970s they became multimodal, testing therapies across the diagnostic and prognostic stages of specific tumors.[7] Moreover, following the initial successes in the mid-1960s and early 1970s with the leukemias and the lymphomas, clinical trials moved from relatively short-termed studies, using single agents and patients in advanced-stage disease, to much longer-term, Phase III studies involving the treatment of earlier phases of disease. The 1980s also saw the first wave of immunotherapies produce relatively disappointing results. In turn, the 1990s saw the emergence of a panoply of biologicals often referred to as cytostatic (as contrasted with traditional cytotoxic) agents.

Although developments within continental Europe were often derivative from American initiatives, they present significant differences and several useful comparisons. In 1962, a group of seventeen researchers from six European countries (Belgium, France, Germany, The Netherlands,

6. Peter Keating and Alberto Cambrosio, "From Screening to Clinical Research: The Cure of Leukemia and the Early Development of the Cooperative Oncology Groups, 1955–1966," *Bull. Hist. Med.*, 2002, 76: 299–334.

7. Stuart J. Pocock, *Clinical Trials: A Practical Approach* (New York: Wiley, 1983), p. 22.

Italy, and Switzerland) created the "Groupe Européen de Chimiothérapie Anticancéreuse" (GECA). As its name suggests, GECA focused on chemotherapy and consequently on a gamut of activities, running from the screening of potential chemotherapeutic agents to their testing in clinical trials. The group was established principally because this kind of work went beyond the capacities of individual European countries that lacked both the funds for purchasing research equipment and animals, and the collaborations among pharmacists, biochemists, cytologists, geneticists, immunologists, radiobiologists, virologists, clinicians, and statisticians necessary to undertake clinical cancer research. Moreover, clinical cancer trials frequently called upon a large number of patients—larger, at any rate, than those available in a single hospital and, sometimes, within a single country.[8]

The founding of the GECA was not greeted with universal applause. The group had to confront those who held that chemotherapy did not qualify as a true scientific endeavor and who considered it, at best, an empirical undertaking tinged by the commercial interests of pharmaceutical companies. GECA countered this claim by arguing not only that chemotherapy achieved positive results in cases where surgery and radiotherapy (the dominant modalities in cancer therapy)[9] failed, but also that the discovery of chemotherapeutic agents was increasingly based on the mobilization of fundamental research in biochemistry, organic chemistry, and molecular biology, and, in turn, contributed to the development of these sciences.

In 1968 GECA became the EORTC (European Organization for Research and Treatment of Cancer) and, as in the United States, it progressively expanded its activities to include multimodal therapies. The EORTC developed through trial and error in a process that shows how the status of its various subdivisions was renegotiated concomitantly with the ongoing definition of the "rules" of the new style of practice. For instance, as in the United States, clinical trials were performed by (transnational) cooperative groups specializing in a given type of cancer (but also sometimes in a given type of trial or task), and many discussions focused on the distinctive features of a cooperative group as opposed to other possible arrangements, such as working parties or task forces, and on how an

8. "Le Groupe Européen de Chimiothérapie Anticancéreuse (G.E.C.A.)," typed MS (ca. 1962–63), GECA-EORTC Proceedings of the Council, 1962–69, EORTC Archives, EORTC Headquarters, Brussels, Belgium.

9. Patrice Pinell, *Naissance d'un fléau: Histoire de la lutte contre le cancer en France (1890–1940)* (Paris: Métailié, 1992); T. Van Helvoort, "Scalpel or Rays? Radiotherapy and the Struggle for the Cancer Patient in Pre–Second World War Germany," *Med. Hist.*, 2001, *45*: 33–60.

EORTC cooperative group should perform and assess its activities. An important institutional milestone, in this respect, was the establishment of the Data Center in Brussels in 1974, in the wake of similar centralizing moves made by U.S. groups such as ECOG. The creation of a central institution staffed with statisticians and charged with the statistical design and analysis of clinical trial protocols—and, subsequently, the formation of a series of committees such as the Protocol Review Committee and the Scientific Audit Committee—coincided with the definition of common statistical approaches and procedural guidelines that came to regulate the performance of clinical trials. The institution of the Data Center thus went hand in hand with the certification of clinical cancer trials as bona fide products of the new style of practice. By 2002, about three hundred hospitals and more than twenty-five hundred scientists and clinicians from thirty-two countries participated in EORTC activities.[10]

In what follows, before describing the new style of practice instantiated by the NCI and EORTC cooperative oncology groups, we examine an institution that cuts across and draws together the various components of the cooperative groups and related organizations, running from research laboratories to patient activist groups. This institution is the clinical trial protocol, and in many respects it lies at the center of the new style of practice insofar as it articulates the style's components, such as medical oncologists, statistics, patients, and anticancer substances. We note, moreover, in passing, that protocol-type practices have engendered a new kind of objectivity that has come to characterize biomedical activities in fields other than oncology, which we have described elsewhere.[11]

The Protocol

Marc Berg has described a multi-institutional research protocol in the field of cancer chemotherapy and, using this example, has attempted to develop a synthetic view of protocols in general.[12] Whereas many

10. Françoise Meunier and A. T. van Oosterom, "Forty Years of the EORTC: The Evolution Towards a Unique Network to Develop New Standards of Cancer Care," *Eur. J. Cancer,* 2002, *38* (Suppl. 4): S3–S13. European cancer clinical trials continued, of course, to be performed outside the EORTC by national institutions.

11. Alberto Cambrosio, Peter Keating, Thomas Schlich, and George Weisz, "Regulatory Objectivity and the Generation and Management of Evidence in Medicine," *Soc. Sci. & Med.,* 2006, *63*: 189–99.

12. Marc Berg, "Order(s) and Disorder(s): Of Protocols and Medical Practices," in *Differences in Medicine: Unraveling Practices, Techniques, and Bodies,* ed. Marc Berg and Annemarie Mol (Durham, N.C.: Duke University Press, 1998), pp. 226–49.

medical authors suggest that the point of a clinical trial protocol is to impose order on some previous disorder, Berg's analysis concludes that the relevant division is not between order and disorder, but between an old order and a new order, both of which contain intrinsic elements of disorder. He nonetheless agrees that, despite its negotiated nature, some degree of imposition follows from the acceptance of a protocol by actors in biomedicine. The imposition arises from the rule-bound nature of the operation. According to Berg, "a protocol is a formalism: it operates using a collection of specific, explicit rules, which turn input data into output."[13] In virtue of the rules that they express, protocols align and articulate activities in different times and places. In the case of clinical medicine, as a device for the normalization of practices, "the protocol makes the administration of highly complex treatment schedules *possible* in the first place."[14] Aligning practices and getting others (both persons and things) to follow rules clearly requires a good deal of work and negotiation, and Berg rightly observes that the process of setting up and successfully running a clinical trial protocol is a highly political process.

While we agree with Berg on many specific aspects of his description, we find his definition and his approach somewhat restrictive in a number of ways:

> First, Berg tends to see the protocol as an organizational device or tool, and he consequently downplays the creative nature of the process. Instituting a protocol entails more than just the imposition of a new order (although we do not deny that this may often be the case): the new order implies the creation of new things or entities (DNA profiles, markers, disease categories, patient categories, etc.) and new ways of acting; it is not just the reorganization of already existing entities.

> Second, Berg's definition of a protocol tends to reduce it to one of its parts, namely, the schema—a highly stylized diagram that accompanies protocols and that shows which substances will be given to which patients on what schedule and under what conditions. As we will see shortly, rather than being simply a plan, a protocol comprises a number of other components that link it both to the past and to the future and that articulate it with other, ongoing scientific practices. To focus exclusively on the schema is to frame the protocol as a mere tool and not as a program of situated action.

13. Ibid., p. 233.
14. Ibid., p. 232 (emphasis in original).

Third, while we agree that protocols do not necessarily transform disorder into order, but create a new order out of an older order, the older order is not, in the case of oncology, "a nonprotocolized situation" where "medical personnel can allow a myriad of more or less precise laboratory tests, historical data, psychosocial circumstances, and so forth to shape the course of action undertaken."[15] We contend that prior to the imposition of any given protocol, the situation is *already* highly "protocolized"—in the sense that an archaeology of medical judgments would show that much of common practice flows from deeply embedded protocols whose "rules," so to speak, have sunk out of sight. In medical oncology, it is not so much the case, in other words, that "protocols discipline practices," as that the constitution and administration of protocols is itself a practice.

To illustrate our enlarged notion of a protocol, which is broadly consistent with the picture that emerged from Ilana Löwy's study of an experimental protocol in oncology,[16] let us now consider an example of how protocols are generated in clinical cancer trials.

In the mid-1960s, administrators of the NCI's chemotherapy program described their activities as a series of decision-making events in a process that regulated the flow of drugs (and, subsequently, of drugs combined with the two other anticancer therapies, surgery and radiation) and disease concepts through rodent models; then into phase I, II, and III clinical trials; and finally, into the hands of practicing oncologists. Although this is to some extent a simplification of a process that is considerably more complex and interactive, the image has the merit of isolating the initial components of cancer treatment research and the pervasive nature of protocol development. While the definition of phase I, II, and III trials differed somewhat in Europe, the EORTC adopted a very similar approach.

As previously mentioned, in both the United States and Europe, cooperative oncology groups are the principal vehicles of protocol development and administration. Figure 1 is a flow chart showing how an American protocol arises in a group and travels through it and the NCI (which manages the groups). As can be seen, the making of a protocol is almost as complex as the protocol itself. The tortuous nature of the process reflects, in part, a long series of administrative maneuvers undertaken by the NCI and the office that manages the groups, the Cancer Therapy

---

15. Ibid., p. 241.
16. Ilana Löwy, "La standardization de l'inconnu: Les protocols thérapeutiques en cancérologie," *Techniques & culture*, 1995, *25/26*: 73–108.

Evaluation Program (CTEP), to overcome a number of problems such as patient recruitment and the timely introduction of novel techniques that have structured protocol development in ways that are not immediately obvious. For example, all group protocols must be submitted to CTEP for final approval. CTEP sets priorities with regard to which protocols may be deemed significant (as opposed to trivial) and thus be funded—but its view of what counts as important depends in part on its constant negotiations and interactions with the groups as well as its contacts with outside experts and policymakers. Practitioners sometimes refer to this process of priority setting as "onco-politics,"[17] a term adopted by the *Journal of Clinical Oncology* as a keyword to classify domains of expertise in the cancer field.

Let us return to the process laid out in the flow chart, keeping in mind that this is merely the tip of an iceberg of corridor conversations and telephone calls, telexes, faxes, and, more recently, e-mails. More than a collection of rules, protocols embody what the U.S. trialists call "concepts" (and European trialists "rationale")—by which they refer to the therapeutic hypothesis (based on empirical or theoretical considerations) to be tested by a given protocol as well as the information to be provided by the ancillary studies included in the protocol. Concepts, in other words, concern the new information that a successful protocol produces: novelty, not routine. In practice, concepts and protocols are clearly separated. As the flow chart shows, concepts precede protocols in the sense that during the protocol development process, the initial starting point is the "idea." Ideas are communicated verbally by somebody, usually a principal investigator, to the Disease Committee chairperson, who then communicates the idea to the study chairperson. The latter, in collaboration with other investigators, produces a "concept sheet" that serves as the basis for further discussions with biostatisticians, members of the Disease Committee, the Modality Committee, and the Executive Committee. The entire process takes several weeks, and once everybody agrees, an "approved concept" can start the process of becoming an "approved protocol." In this sense it can be said that concepts drive protocols.

But since one protocol leads to another, concepts also follow protocols. This is quite obvious when we look at the development of a concept. Following their first—verbal—formulation, ideas must be reduced to a concept sheet that in turn must be submitted to a checklist that specifies what counts as a concept and how it should be presented. The "concept sheet checklist" tells us, for example, that a concept answers the question

17. Peter Keating, interview with James Holland, 24 July 2003, New York, N.Y.

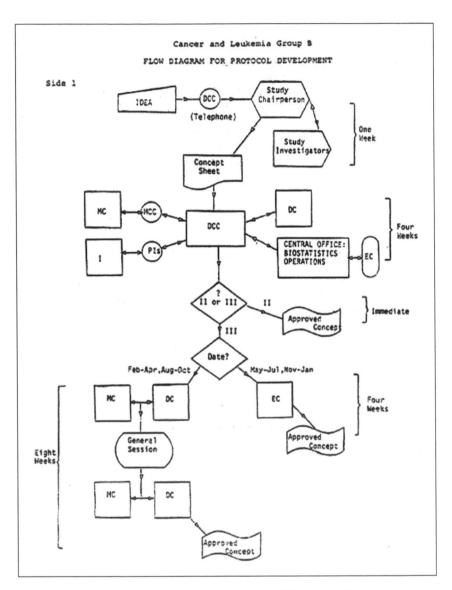

Fig. 1. Flow diagram of a CALGB protocol (ca. 1977), James Holland personal papers, New York, N.Y. *MC* = Modality Committee, *MCC* = Modality Committee Chairperson, *DC* = Disease Committee, *DCC* = Disease Committee Chairperson, *SC* = Study Committee, *EC* = Executive Chairperson, *NCI* = National Cancer Institute, *PI* = Principal Investigator(s), and *I* = Investigators.

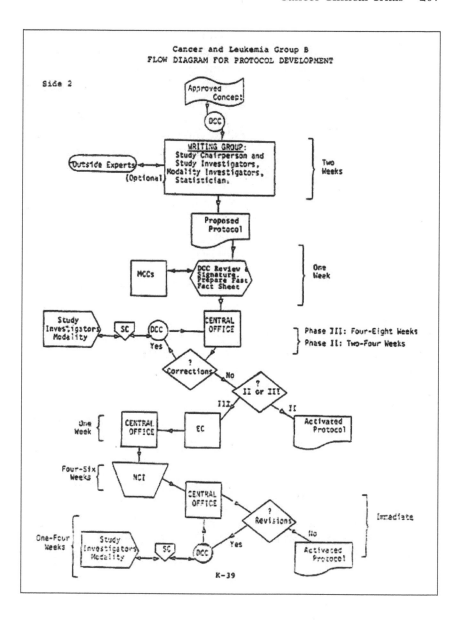

Cancer and Leukemia Group B
FLOW DIAGRAM FOR PROTOCOL DEVELOPMENT

Side 2

Approved Concept

DCC

WRITING GROUP:
Study Chairperson and
Study Investigators,
Modality Investigators,
Statistician.

Outside Experts (Optional)

Two Weeks

Proposed Protocol

MCCs

DCC Review &
Signature,
Prepare Past
Fact Sheet

One Week

Study Investigators Modality   SC   DCC

CENTRAL OFFICE

Phase III: Four-Eight Weeks
Phase II: Two-Four Weeks

Yes

? Corrections   No

? II or III

III   II

One Week   CENTRAL OFFICE   EC

Activated Protocol

Four-Six Weeks   NCI

CENTRAL OFFICE

? Revisions   No

Immediate

One-Four Weeks   Study Investigators Modality   SC   DCC   Yes

Activated Protocol

K-39

"What needs to be done and why?"[18] Thus, like a research proposal, the concept describes the history and the nature of the problem and what is new about the present solution. The concept thus becomes the introduction to the protocol and must be distinguished from previous protocols. In therapeutic cancer research, then, concepts are also proto-protocols.

Once a concept is approved, a "Writing Group" composed of the study chairperson, the study investigators, the modality investigators, and the statisticians takes about two weeks to transform the concept into a protocol. The proposed protocol then moves back through the Disease Committee, the Modality Committee, and the Executive Committee before (if Phase III) going off to the NCI for final approval. Members of CTEP often participate in these discussions; not only do they relate CTEP priorities to group members (who, in turn, relate group priorities to CTEP), but they also keep group members abreast of developments in other groups so as to reduce redundancies.[19]

Finally, in clinical cancer trials protocols themselves have protocols—in the sense that CALGB, for example, maintains a model protocol developed in the early 1980s for Phase III trials. Since Phase III trials in this period were generally different forms of combination therapy, it was possible to model protocols because of their repetitious and iterative nature; practitioners sometimes described protocols as "highly empirical complex studies."[20]

Let us now turn to an analysis of the components of the new style of practice that protocols articulate. For lack of space, we will focus on four of them.

Medical Oncologists

Conventional wisdom would hold that cancer clinical trials are the by-product of medical oncologists. We argue, however, that it is the other way around: medical oncologists are a by-product of the emergence of clinical cancer trials and cancer treatment research as a new style of practice,

18. An example of a "concept sheet checklist" can be found in CALGB, Minutes of Group Meeting, Biltmore Hotel, New York, 8–11 October 1980, p. 37, James Holland personal papers, New York, N.Y.

19. For an example of the complex interactions between CTEP and the cooperative groups, see David M. Dilts, Alan B. Sandler, Matthew Baker, et al., "Processes to Activate Phase III Clinical Trials in a Cooperative Oncology Group: The Case of Cancer and Leukemia Group B," *J. Clin. Oncol.*, 2006, *24*: 4553–57.

20. Emil Frei III, "Scientific Direction" (General Session Talk), CALGB, Fall Meeting Minutes, 31 October–3 November 1984, pp. 24–27, on p. 26, James Holland personal papers.

and the establishment and regulation of medical oncology was an explicit goal of the institutions committed to the development of the new style. In Europe, for example, the EORTC was involved from the outset in defining the new specialty: in the mid-1970s, in addition to organizing a symposium on training in medical oncology, it offered fellowships to provide training in the conduct of cancer clinical trials, organized courses for an EORTC certificate in general oncology, and formed a committee to establish the requirements for EORTC certification in oncology.[21] Although the EORTC subsequently decided that, due to different national regulatory frameworks, it was in no position to offer oncology certificates within Europe, it nonetheless deemed it useful and necessary to distinguish between three main oncology subspecialties—surgical, medical, and radiological oncology (pediatric oncology was later added)—and to prepare recommendations regarding training and expertise in these domains.[22] In the early 1980s, concomitant with the establishment of a European Society for Medical Oncology along the lines of the American Society for Clinical Oncology,[23] the EORTC articulated the official EORTC view on the requirements for establishing medical oncology as a specialty:[24] Medical oncologists had to show "a total commitment to the specialty," as opposed to part-time interest in the subject, and take into account "the importance of new developments in systemic therapy" (i.e., the new style of practice grounded in chemotherapy).[25] In addition to the emphasis on chemotherapy, training should include the relevant basic sciences (including not only tumor biology, but also medical statistics); training in research, moreover, was "highly desirable."[26]

In the United States, cooperative oncology groups trained most of the original cohort of medical oncologists. As practicing physicians, part of their work consisted of translating successful research protocols into routine treatment protocols to be adapted to individual patients.

21. Proceedings of the Council meeting, 10 November 1973, EORTC Archives; *EORTC Newsl.*, no. 35, July 1974; ibid., no. 42, October 1975; Proceedings of Administrative Board meeting, 27 February 1976, EORTC Archives.

22. Proceedings of the Council meeting, 20 June 1980, EORTC Archives; Proceedings of the Board meeting, 29 March 1980, ibid.

23. Proceedings of Board Meeting, 26 June 1981, EORTC Archives. On ASCO, see Gretchen Krueger, "The Formation of the American Society of Clinical Oncology and the Development of a Medical Specialty, 1964–1973," *Perspect. Biol. & Med.*, 2004, *47*: 537–51.

24. Proceedings of the Board Meeting, 31 October 1980, EORTC Archives; Minutes of Meeting of the Board and of the Annual Assembly, 27 February 1981, ibid.

25. "Criteria and Definition of Medical Oncology as a Subspecialty within Clinical Oncology," *EORTC Newsl.*, no. 92, March 1981, p. 1.

26. Ibid.

In this sense, even when outside a research protocol they did not act in an "unprotocolized situation." Following the expansion of the groups in the 1960s, the 1971 National Cancer Act significantly accelerated training in medical oncology, which subsequently gained recognition as a subspecialty in 1973 and went on to become one of the fastest-growing subspecialties in internal medicine in the late 1970s. Between 1973 and 1985, the American Board of Internal Medicine certified an estimated 3,500 medical oncologists.[27]

Different kinds of oncologists became associated with different kinds of protocols in the United States. In the 1970s, as more and more oncology residents rotated through hospitals and academic centers that housed cooperative oncology groups and then went out to work in community hospitals, practitioners treated an increasing number of U.S. cancer patients in the community hospitals themselves. By the end of the 1970s, according to some estimates, community hospitals treated around 80 percent of cancer patients who were thus, in practice, unavailable for research protocols, in part because of the general reluctance of community-based oncologists to put patients on the protocols.[28] As research-protocol recruitment numbers dwindled, and as community oncologists took control of the protocols that they had learned as residents, clinical cancer researchers came to the realization that through their extensive training programs they might be in the process of becoming the architects of their own demise.[29]

With patient recruitment flagging and research protocols remaining open far longer than had been programmed, clinical researchers created institutions to recruit patients in community hospitals. The NCI, for example, set up the Community Clinical Oncology Program (CCOP) in order to fund clinical trials managed by the cooperative groups but

27. Philip S. Schein, "Presidential Address: The Plight of Clinical Cancer Research," *J. Clin. Oncol.*, 1984, 2: 1433–39, on p. 1434.

28. Virginia J. Suppers and Stephen A. Sherwin, "The Organization of a National Cancer Institute Clinical Research Unit in a Community Setting," *Maryland State Med. J.*, December 1982, pp. 38–40, on p. 39. The "patient famine" and the attendant problems of recruitment were not restricted to the field of cancer. A review of the literature produced between 1986 and 1995 turned up more than 4,000 articles: see Laura C. Lovato, Kristin Hill, Stephanie Hertert, Donald B. Hunninghake, and Jeffrey L. Probstfield, "Recruitment for Controlled Clinical Trials: Literature Summary and Annotated Bibliography," *Controlled Clin. Trials,* 1997, *18*: 328–57. See also D. B. Hunninghake, C. A. Darby, and J. L. Probstfield, "Recruitment Experience in Clinical Trials: Literature Summary and Annotated Bibliography," ibid., 1987, *8*: 6S–30S.

29. Peter Keating, interview with Vincent DeVita, 23 July 2003, New Haven, Conn.; Holland interview (n. 17).

carried out within community hospitals and administered by community oncologists. The movement was not, however, simply top-down: oncologists practicing at the community level had already recognized how easily one could fall behind protocol development and how quickly protocols became dated. The establishment of clinical trials at the community level offered a means to stay abreast of the latest developments.[30]

The emergence of a third kind of medical oncologist—the "entrepreneur" oncologist—dates back to the early 1980s when the U.S. Health Care Financing Administration (HCFA) created Diagnosis Related Groups that it financed at preset levels. The groups relating to cancer chemotherapy were funded at a level that made it impossible for American hospitals to continue offering chemotherapy to patients on an in-patient basis. Since cancer patients had henceforth to be treated as out-patients, the HCFA had opened the door for oncologists to act as private practitioners and to begin treating cancer patients in their offices. These facilities operated as small enterprises, with the oncologists buying, storing, and mixing their own chemotherapeutic agents.[31]

These "mom and pop" oncology operations were, however, a relatively short-lived phenomenon. Alienated in many respects from protocol development, in the early 1990s more and more oncologists were drawn into nationwide treatment and research networks such as that developed by US Oncology. *Fortune Magazine*'s most admired company in 2004, US Oncology had absorbed the Houston-based Oncology Resources and the Dallas-based Physicians Reliance Network in 1999, to become the largest for-profit provider of cancer treatment in the United States. Presently composed of a network of 850 physicians, US Oncology treats about 15 percent of all newly diagnosed cancer patients. Given the magnitude of the enterprise, US Oncology is also, unsurprisingly, the single largest consumer of therapeutic oncology drugs in the United States.[32] More than a consumer, however, it also claims to be an important developer of protocols. Indeed, the company puts approximately 1,600 patients a year on protocols, often financed by pharmaceutical companies. Using a single, "standardized Institutional Review Board approval process," US

30. James R. Murphy, "Conducting Clinical Trials with Practicing Community Oncologists," *Controlled Clin. Trials,* 1981, *2:* 115–22, on p. 115; Robert E. Enck, "Interrelationship of Cancer Control and Clinical Research in the Community," *CA—Cancer J. Clin.,* 1984, *34:* 340–44.

31. Lee Mortenson, "Cancer Coalitions and Cancer Politics," *Semin. Oncol. Nursing,* 2002, *18:* 297–304, on p. 301.

32. Lou Fintor, "For-Profit Treatment Centers: Trailblazing a New Model of Care?" *J. Nat. Cancer Inst.,* 1999, *91:* 1272–74, on p. 1273.

Oncology boasts that "through this highly efficient organization, drugs are sped from the research lab into the real world [through clinical trial protocols], reaching patients as quickly as possible."[33]

To be sure, not all medical oncologists belong to public or private research networks, and relatively few patients are treated within a *research* protocol. Institutions have emerged, therefore, that constantly articulate research protocols and research findings with routine or standard protocols. The ideal-typical standard protocol, both in Europe and in the United States, is that described in a practice guideline. On the European side, consider the French practice guidelines. Set by the National Federation of Anticancer Hospitals, French guidelines are referred to as SORs (the acronym stands for Standards-Options-Recommendations).[34] Their establishment has been analyzed in detail by Patrick Castel and Ivanne Merle, who have shown how practice guidelines have created regulatory interfaces both between surgeons, chemotherapists, and radiotherapists within the twenty specialized anticancer hospitals, and between these institutions and community hospitals, so that "routine" cancer patients can, in principle, be treated by the latter according to the protocols (and quality standards) established by the former, which, in turn, focus on the most difficult cases.[35]

In the United States, a group of thirteen Cancer Centers—the most prestigious in the country (Sloan-Kettering, M. D. Anderson, etc.)—has developed a series of "normal protocols" for almost all cancers through consensus meetings; these practice guidelines are constantly revised. Calling themselves the National Comprehensive Cancer Network Inc. (NCCN), the Cancer Centers incorporated themselves into a private network in 1995 in order to compete in the "oncology market" and with the de facto standard protocols that were slowly being imposed by managed-care organizations.[36] The NCCN presented the consensus results at an

33. US Oncology Web site. One might easily surmise that what we have here is the privatization of public protocols. This is only partly true, however, as the lines between public and private have become increasingly blurred in the United States and the "networks" established by corporations such as US Oncology have made possible the interpenetration of nonprofit and for-profit institutions in indirect ways.

34. "Opération 'Standards, options et recommandations' (I) Fédération Nationale des Centres de Lutte Contre le Cancer," *Bulletin du cancer*, 1995, *82*: 747–890.

35. Patrick Castel and Ivanne Merle, "Quand les normes de pratiques deviennent une ressource pour les médecins," *Sociologie du travail*, 2002, *44*: 337–55. See also Patrick Castel, "Normaliser les pratiques, organiser les médecins: La qualité comme stratégie de changement. Le cas des Centres de Lutte Contre le Cancer" (doctoral diss., Institut d'Études Politiques de Paris, 2002).

36. "Cancer Centers Form Network to Compete for Managed Care, Develop Standards," *Cancer Lett.*, 1995, *21* (4): 1–4.

open meeting in March 1996 and then published them in the September issue of the journal *Oncology*.[37] In 2002, the NCCN launched its own Clinical Trials Network (CTN). Having grown to nineteen associated Centers, the Network drew together 1,600 investigators, plus an additional 400 investigators based in associated community hospitals. Like the NCI and US Oncology, the CTN preached speed and streamlined access to patients in an effort to attract private sponsors.

Statistics and Statisticians

As components of the protocols they simultaneously develop, approve, and manage, statisticians constitute a meta-element of the cancer clinical-trial configuration. Indeed, the EORTC assumed its present form with the establishment of its statistical Data Center, which, as previously mentioned, centralized the approval of protocols though the EORTC Protocol Review Committee and became the obligatory passage point for publishing trial results under the EORTC name.[38] Initially, some doubt surrounded the role of the Data Center: was it a central service available to all cooperative groups (yes); should protocols be centrally approved (yes), or was the "go ahead" of local statistic teams enough (no); should each cooperative group have a representative on the EORTC Protocol Review Committee (no); and so on. Some EORTC members initially resisted the idea that data collection should henceforth fall under "the leadership of the head of the EORTC Data Center in order to standardize the approaches to handle data generated within the EORTC groups."[39] For dissidents, the Data Center should have simply provided an interface for ensuring "smooth coordination" between the statistical centers available within participating EORTC institutions (Brussels, Ulm, Villejuif).[40] In the event, centralization trumped coordination, and subsequent EORTC guidelines mandated the submission of protocols to the EORTC Protocol Review Committee for approval, and the assignment of a statistician to every protocol.[41]

When creating the Data Center and the related statistical framework, the EORTC profited from the expertise of its U.S. counterpart. Within

37. The guidelines are published by disease. For an overview, see R. J. Winn, W. Botnick, and N. Dozier, "The NCCN Guidelines Development Program," *Oncology (Huntington)*, 1996, *11* (Suppl.): 23–28.

38. *EORTC Newsl.*, no. 32, February 1974.

39. Proceedings of the EORTC Council meeting, 30 June 1974, EORTC Archives.

40. Proceedings of the EORTC Council meeting, 9 March 1974, EORTC Archives.

41. *EORTC Newsl.*, no. 100, March 1982; ibid., no. 149, August 1986. See also M. Staquet, R. Sylvester, and C. Jasmin, "Guidelines for the Preparation of EORTC Cancer Clinical Trials," *Eur. J. Cancer*, 1980, *16*: 871–75.

U.S. cooperative oncology groups, statisticians had already gained special status. As guarantors of the validity of clinical trial protocols, they often represented a form of mechanical or a-perspectival objectivity and were thus sometimes pitted against the individual and collective expertise of clinicians.[42] In spite of this dichotomy, however, cooperative groups regularly incorporated the clinician's expertise into protocols and invariably reflected the expert understanding of the specific nature of the treated cancer patient and the cancer-treatment protocol.

The evolving role of statistics and statisticians within cancer clinical trials deserves closer scrutiny than can possibly be provided in this paper. As discussed in more detail elsewhere, this role, initially devoted to assuring the statistical validity of study design and results, has been enlarged to include more complex matters, such as interim data analysis and related issues concerning risks for both a trial's subjects and the trial itself.[43] Indeed, despite considerable interaction between clinicians and statisticians, statisticians must also guard against the production of undue risk and the corruption of data by hasty clinicians. The relationship between the two dangers depends upon how one views the application of a clinical cancer protocol: as the application of a tool, and thus a rule-bound exercise; or as a scientific experiment, for which the rules are not entirely known in advance. In this context, the definition of the role of statisticians in relation to protocols has evolved significantly, from that of "policemen,"[44] seen with some hostility by clinicians,[45] to their present ambiguous status as either technical consultants or full-fledged coinvestigators.

Patients

According to Berg, the "unequivocality" needed in order for protocols to work limits patients' expression of their views to a simple yes or no.[46] In

42. Lorraine Daston, "Objectivity and the Escape from Perspective," *Soc. Stud. Sci.*, 1992, *22*: 597–618; Marks, *Progress of Experiments* (n. 2).

43. Peter Keating and Alberto Cambrosio, "Risk on Trial: The Interaction of Innovation and Risk Factors in Clinical Trials," in *The Risks of Medical Innovation: Risk Perception and Assessment in Historical Context*, ed. Thomas Schlich and Ulrich Tröhler (London: Routledge, 2005), pp. 225–41; Alberto Cambrosio and Peter Keating, "Cancer Clinical Trials: New Style of Research, New Forms of Risk," in *Les cultures du risque (XVIᵉ–XXIᵉ siècle)*, ed. François Walter, Bernardino Fantini, and Pascal Delvaux (Geneva: Presses d'Histoire Suisse, 2006), pp. 169–86.

44. Donald Mainland, "The Clinical Trial: Some Difficulties and Suggestions," *J. Chron. Dis.*, 1960, *11*: 484–96.

45. Bernard G. Greenberg and James E. Grizzle, "Effective Statistical Consultation for Clinical Study Groups," *Cancer Chemother. Rep.*, 1969, *53*: 1–2.

46. Berg, "Order(s) and Disorder(s)" (n. 12), pp. 240–41.

this respect, his claim echoes the older medical literature that sometimes referred to patients as (mute) research material. Over the past fifty years, however, cancer patients have evolved as a collective entity along a number of interdependent lines that have delineated new images and practices for persons suffering from or surviving cancer. Presently, even though few adult cancer patients actually participate in clinical trials, virtually all of them are diagnosed, treated, and advised according to a protocol, be it a routine or an experimental protocol. The epistemic, political, and economic status of the cancer patient within protocols and the protocol-production process has been a recurring theme for both patients and practitioners, especially when the time comes to choose which road to take—which path to follow or decision to make—in that embedded series of protocols commonly referred to as the therapeutic process. Patient pathways, in other words, are oriented around protocols, and participation in protocol formulation and management has consequently become a routine (and highly politicized) activity for research scientists, practicing oncologists, and patient activists.

Cancer patients have served not only as the "raw material" and primary purpose of clinical cancer research, but also as the subject of a network of evolving rules, norms, restrictions, and ethical and epistemological dilemmas. Within this latter problematic, cancer patients have recently come to be represented, and to represent themselves, as activists.[47] Formerly concerned primarily with raising money and "awareness," patient groups have come to reject the notion that they are the silent objects of therapy, charity, and research, and have consequently demanded and received a place as participants at the clinical research table. In other words, patient activists and advocates understand that clinical trials and the protocols they generate are an obligatory point of passage for cancer patients, and that all patient pathways converge sooner or later on a protocol.

We cannot provide here a detailed history of the evolution of cancer patients as collective entities,[48] but it is clear that the emergence of new patient configurations is partly the product of medical oncology and of the advent of clinical trials: "protocol patients," initially conceived of as

47. For a sophisticated analysis of the development of patient advocate groups, see Vololona Rabeharisoa, "The Struggle against Neuromuscular Diseases in France and the Emergence of the 'Partnership Model' of Patient Organization," *Soc. Sci. & Med.*, 2003, 57: 2127–36.

48. See Peter Keating and Alberto Cambrosio, "Patients and Protocols" (Paper delivered at conference, Patients and Pathways: Cancer Therapies in Historical and Sociological Perspective, Centre for the History of Science, Technology & Medicine, University of Manchester, 7–8 October 2005).

"last chance patients," became "scarce resources" when the rise of "community oncology patients" and "private oncology patients" threatened to turn them away from the protocols coordinated by the cooperative groups. More recently, increasingly vocal "activist patients" in both the United States and Europe (albeit to a different degree, and according to different modalities) have come to play a role in protocol design, and this transformation of the rules of oncopolitics has resulted in, for instance, the mandatory presence of "minority patients" within protocols (see "Interfaces and Overlaps," below).

In many respects, the last ten years have seen the breakdown of the distinction between protocol and nonprotocol patients. This does not mean that therapy in oncology is now entirely experimental, or that all patients willingly participate in some kind of clinical trial. At best, no more than 3 percent of newly diagnosed cancer patients participate in a clinical trial in any given year.[49] In fact, the actual number of protocol patients is difficult to assess, and this is a reflection of the fact that the notion of a protocol and of related protocol practices has expanded in meaning and application. Indeed, as we have seen, the distinction between a research protocol and a standard protocol is pinchingly fine; this year's research protocol may easily become, through a single consensus meeting, next year's standard. One might even assert that, in a trivial sense, all cancer patients are now protocol patients, insofar as all present-day chemotherapeutic substances and schedules of administration have passed muster in a research protocol.

Two interesting repercussions of the protocol/nonprotocol distinction bear mention. The first concerns the financing of oncology practices. By the end of the 1980s, both clinical researchers and practicing oncologists in the United States began to observe a rise in the number of anecdotal reports concerning refusal by third-party payers to assume the clinical costs associated with clinical cancer trials, and the problem persisted throughout the following decade. When the issue first emerged at the end of the 1980s, the NCI's Cancer Therapy Evaluation Program (CTEP) organized meetings with researchers, pharmaceutical manufacturers, and "lay communities" in order to develop a consensus statement in an attempt to save clinical research from overzealous accountants.[50] An evaluation by a

49. Robert E. Wittes and Michael A. Friedman, "Accrual to Clinical Trials," *J. Nat. Cancer Inst.*, 1988, *80*: 884–85. The situation is markedly different for pediatric oncology patients, a large proportion of whom are enrolled in clinical trials.

50. Associate Director for Cancer Therapy Evaluation (Michael Friedman), "Summary Report," *Division of Cancer Treatment Annual Report*, 1 October 1988–30 September 1989, *2*: 611–15, on p. 613. See also M. McCabe and M. A. Friedman, "The Impact of 3rd Party

panel of experts appointed by CTEP of the work carried out by the cooperative groups in 1986 had detected problems in patient accrual in 35 to 80 percent of protocols, depending upon the disease category reviewed.[51] The specter of insurance companies introducing a distinction between protocol and nonprotocol patients threatened to make things worse. Clinical researchers and clinicians countered that all patients were protocol patients, for insofar as today's treatment protocol is yesterday's research protocol, the separation was purely logical; in other words, the only difference was that some protocols were new and some were old. Moreover, outside the rarefied atmosphere of insurance claims, access to the latest protocols was increasingly becoming a right, not a choice. In addition to community oncologists, clinical researchers, insurance companies, oncology corporations, and drug companies, an increasing number of "patient groups" organized along disease lines entered the mix.

In the United States, the most important of the cancer-patient advocate groups, the National Breast Cancer Coalition (formed in 1991), now comprises more than six hundred member organizations and more than 70,000 members. Unlike previous patient groups that had been content to raise money and awareness, the NBCC had a plan and a research orientation that they believed should form a part of the national agenda. Patient-driven advocacy groups reached a new plateau in 1993 with the formation of the Cancer Leadership Council, which brought together eight different patient groups in an attempt to reach a consensus on health-care reform. In 1996, prostate-cancer activists met to form the National Prostate Cancer Coalition (NPCC), and a coalition of advocacy groups came together under the name of the Intercultural Cancer Council in early 1995, calling for, among other things, greater participation of minority physicians and patients in clinical trials. Although Europeans lag somewhat in this respect, equivalent groups, such as Europa Donna (breast cancer) and Europa Uomo (prostate cancer) have been established in recent years and have come together under the umbrella of the European Cancer Patient Coalition.

The protocol/nonprotocol distinction can also become the object of controversy within the field. The recourse to harmonized protocols has recently been denounced as a "one-size-fits-all" approach to treatment and contrasted with "individualized medicine," in a recent debate

---

Reimbursement on Cancer Clinical Investigation: A Consensus Statement Coordinated by the National Cancer Institute," *J. Nat. Cancer Inst.*, 1989, *81*: 1585–86.

51. "Clinical Investigations Branch," *Annual Report, Division of Cancer Treatment*, 1 October 1985–30 September 1986, 1: 384.

pitting the French Society of Pediatric Oncology and the head of the major French cancer hospital against a medical oncologist supported by an organization of activist parents of pediatric cancer patients.[52] While this controversy appears to set patient advocates against the clinical trial system and suggests that patient groups operate outside the system, appearances are deceptive. Indeed, some patient advocate organizations insist that not only should all patients become advocates as part of the healing process, but as many patients as possible should enter clinical trials. Some patient advocates also entertain close relations with oncology companies. US Oncology, for example, sponsors approximately forty participants (most of them current and former US Oncology customers) to attend the annual Patient Advocate Foundation Patient Conference, a nonprofit patient-advocacy group founded by a breast cancer patient that "seeks to empower patients to take control of their health care."[53] By the beginning of the twenty-first century, patient advocates had gained positions at many levels of protocol production and maintenance: study design, steering committees, institutional review boards, and data and safety monitoring committees.

Diseases

Clinical cancer trials and the protocols they embody do not treat diseases as off-the-shelf entities. In keeping with the view of clinical cancer research as an autonomous enterprise, it is important to understand how clinical cancer protocols divide up diseases in new ways and create classifications that, while intended mainly for internal use, also develop careers of their own. An example of this "macroscopic" situation can be found in the development of U.K. clinical trials for leukemia.[54] The initial trials did not distinguish between adults and children, nor did they consequently distinguish between what are today considered distinct forms of leukemia, acute lymphocytic leukemia (ALL), affecting mainly children, and acute myelogenous leukemia (AML), affecting mainly adults. By conflating within the same trial "different" diseases (or categories thereof), early trials were unable to show the differential efficacy of a given substance against a given pathology. The differential reaction of patients to the substance or regimen, however, was used to produce new categories of

52. Patrick Castel and Sébastien Dalgalarrondo, "Les dimensions politiques de la rationalisation des pratiques médicales," *Sciences sociales et santé*, 2005, *23* (4): 5–40.

53. http://www.patientadvocate.org/resources.php (accessed May 2006).

54. David Galton and Humphrey Kay, *UK Leukaemia Clinical Trials for Children and Adults* (London: Leukemia Research Fund, 1977).

diseases, which then entered into general use because of their use in these trials. The design of subsequent trials built on the novel categorization. One can easily see here how trials can generate new disease categories and how, in turn, new disease categories generate new trials.

A more subtle dynamic operates for internal or "microscopic" (in the sense that they do not affect major nosological distinctions) purposes. One of the earliest protocols in the treatment of leukemia was the Protocol No. 3 of Acute Leukemia Group B, developed in the early 1960s.[55] Trialists would subsequently celebrate it as the first demonstration that an anticancer treatment had an anticancer effect in the absence of a recognizable cancer. Part of its success rested on its novel construal of a well-known disease. The innovation consisted of treating different phases of the disease, which were the direct creation of the protocol itself, as separate *kinds* of disease. For instance, remission and relapse were treated as independent events occurring in the same person with ostensibly the same disease. This shifted the focus of medical interventions from the patient to the disease process as it developed within the protocol: a division into "remission" and "relapse" created an altered natural history. Consequently, a single patient could be the site of more than one intervention within a single trial. Although heavily indebted to previous clinical knowledge and know-how, this protocol constituted a significant innovation within the field of clinical research. From Protocol No. 3 onward, the very idea of a clinical trial became something more than a test of the efficacy of a drug, as had been the case until then. The therapy—drug, dose size, dose schedule—and the disease had become intertwined; *the test had become an inquiry.*[56] Knowledge of one led directly to knowledge of the other. The phenomena of induction and remission pointed research in the direction of resistance and mutation, and showed how therapy intervened in the biology of the disease.

Oncologists do not simply diagnose and treat cancer: together with surgeons and pathologists, they also "stage" tumors according to anatomic spread,[57] and "grade" cancers according to appearance. In addition to connecting individual patients to larger biological and pathological categories, clinical protocols that stage or grade tumors determine therapeutic

55. Emil J. Freireich, Edmund Gehan, E. Frei III, et al. (Acute Leukemia Group B), "The Effect of 6-Mercaptopurine on the Duration of Steroid Induced Remissions in Acute Leukemia: A Model for Evaluation of Other Potentially Useful Therapies," *Blood*, 1963, *21*: 699–716, on p. 699.

56. Keating and Cambrosio, "From Screening to Clinical Research" (n. 6).

57. Marie Ménoret, "The Genesis of the Notion of Stages in Oncology: The French Permanent Cancer Survey (1943–1952)," *Soc. Hist. Med.*, 2002, *15*: 291–302.

choices. In this sense, clinical classifications and the trials and protocols that incorporate them clearly go beyond the mere subordination of the "art" of therapy to the more fundamental "scientific" categories of pathology and biology. The problem, in practice, is how to articulate the two. An efficient and useful staging system, for example, is not necessarily very enlightening with regard to the pathological mechanisms underlying the emergence and development of the disease in question. Similarly, the classification of diseases according to their histopathology may not be the most adequate reflection of the molecular-biological entities at play in the process. Finally, ordering pathological entities according to their biological substratum or constituents may contribute little to their immediate clinical management. In short, there are a number of problems attendant upon the articulation and confrontation of the various kinds of classification. Deciding how to frame a disease for a particular protocol or series of protocols is thus of central importance to clinical researchers.

Interfaces and Overlaps: An Example

The components of the new style of practice we have so far discussed do not exist in isolation: they obviously interact and overlap. For the present purpose, let us confine ourselves to a single example, concerning patients, patient advocates, and statisticians.

For a variety of reasons that we will not discuss here, issues of race and gender and access to clinical trials loomed large in the 1980s.[58] In the early 1990s, prodded to a large extent by patient advocate groups, the U.S. federal government decided to force all clinical trial protocols to include significant numbers of women and minorities; thus in 1993, with the passage of the NIH Revitalization Act, "minorities" and women (the two would later become absorbed into a larger group referred to as "special populations") suddenly became statutory components of clinical trial protocols.

The law was clearly going to have a direct impact on clinical cancer trials, and consequently NCI statisticians figured prominently in the NIH group of clinical trialists that was convened to write the guidelines for the

---

58. R. McCarthy, "Historical Background of Clinical Trials Involving Women and Minorities," *Acad. Med.*, 1994, *69*: 695–98; R. Merkatz and S. Junod, "Historical Background of Changes in FDA Policy on the Study and Evaluation of Drugs in Women," ibid., pp. 703–7. For a sociological analysis, see Steven Epstein, "Bodily Differences and Collective Identities: The Politics of Gender and Race in Biomedical Research in the United States," *Body & Soc.*, 2004, *10*: 183–203.

law's enactment. The resulting guidelines elicited comments that were favorable, unfavorable, and mixed: "The writers of the Guidelines are to be praised for trying to rationalize the irrational."[59] And as the previous comment cynically recognized, in writing the guidelines, the statisticians were obliged to make a number of interpretations that rendered the application of the law less disruptive than commentators had originally feared. Indeed, the statisticians had to find a way to "save the data"—and in the case of the clinical cancer trialists it was literally a matter of saving the practice, for if they had applied the letter of the law, according to statistical calculations of the required sample size, the conduct of clinical trials would have been seriously hampered.[60]

The most important among these interpretations concerned the notions of "appropriate" and "valid." Specifically, when significant gender or ethnic differences might be expected to turn up in a Phase III clinical trial, the Act stipulated that "appropriate numbers" of the target subgroup should be included in the trial so that a "valid analysis" of the difference or lack thereof could be carried out. With regard to the notion of "valid analysis," the trialists opted for a nonstatistical interpretation and concluded that "valid" simply meant "unbiased." To obtain an "unbiased" analysis, the "appropriate numbers" were considerably less than those required to conduct statistically valid tests on racial and gendered subgroups in any given trial—indeed, on the statisticians' interpretation, those numbers amounted to little more than "the usual sample sizes." The trialists also recommended that trials where differences were expected based on prior evidence also include "adequate representation" of the groups; that would allow for statistically weak (though "valid") subgroup analyses to be conducted that would then open the door for protocols specially targeting the effect.[61]

Even if any given trial managed to put together adequate representation for a valid analysis, the latter still remained more ideal than real, for the entire issue of subgroup analysis confronted the following quandary:

59. Curtis L. Meinert, "Comments on NIH Clinical Trials Valid Analysis Requirement," *Controlled Clin. Trials*, 1995, *16*: 304–6, on p. 304. For the Guidelines, see National Institutes of Health, "NIH Guidelines on the Inclusion of Women and Minorities as Subjects in Clinical Research," *Fed. Reg.*, 1994, *59*: 14508–13.

60. Laurence S. Freedman, Richard Simon, Mary A. Foulkes, et al., "Inclusion of Women and Minorities in Clinical Trials and the NIH Revitalization Act of 1993—The Perspective of NIH Clinical Trialists," *Controlled Clin. Trials*, 1995, *16*: 277–85, on p. 284. See also Curtis L. Meinert, Adele Kaplan Gilpin, Aynur Uenalp, and Christopher Dawson, "Gender Representation in Trials," ibid., 2000, *21*: 462–75.

61. Freedman et al., "Inclusion of Women" (n. 60), p. 282.

Since the 1990s, institutions had been created to ensure that clinical trials are not unduly prolonged if significant benefits or dangers are observed prior to the programmed end of the trial. Now, the problem with subgroup analysis within this framework was that, since the demonstration of benefit or harm would usually be made for the group of subjects as a whole long before it would be shown for any subgroup, unless there were a strong scientific basis for believing that the results would differ based on gender or racial/ethnic group the continuation of the trial would become unethical.[62]

As commentators pointed out at the time, the writers of the Guidelines left the definition of "appropriate" significantly vague so as to allow themselves and others considerable "interpretive" flexibility.[63] A decade later, the interpretive process continues.[64]

Conclusion

In attempting to characterize this new style of practice, we have outlined some of the components and their interconnections. One of the themes that surfaced rather consistently in this paper is the extent to which clinical cancer research counts as "true" research, or the extent to which it can be reduced to the routine testing of substances for therapeutic effects. We have seen that both perspectives are possible, and while this is perhaps a theme (or charge) that confronts all clinical research to some extent, in our case the charge and the responses take on specific contours. Clinical cancer research, despite almost fifty years of criticism and reform, has nonetheless emerged as an autonomous enterprise that typifies modern biomedicine. Viewed from a distance, and only from the perspective of Phase III clinical trials that compare well-known procedures, clinical cancer research and its incremental improvements in cancer therapy may appear to be somewhat mundane, trivial, and, occasionally, "useless." But this perspective misses two important things: first, it severs the connection between the Phase III endpoint, so to speak, and all the research that has led up to this point and that, ultimately, leads away; and second, it overlooks all the work—inventive and mundane, laboratory and institu-

---

62. Ibid., p. 283.

63. A. Sonia Buist and Merwyn R. Greenlick, "Response to 'Inclusion of Women and Minorities in Clinical Trials and the NIH Revitalization Act of 1993—The Perspective of NIH Clinical Trialists,'" *Controlled Clin. Trials*, 1995, *16*: 296–98, on p. 296.

64. Giselle Corbie-Smith, Willam C. Miller, and David F. Ransohoff, "Interpretations of 'Appropriate' Minority Inclusion in Clinical Research," *Amer. J. Med.*, 2004, *116*: 246–52.

tional—that goes into the production of even negative results. While we have here simply outlined the components of the style, in later work we hope to be able to describe in detail the forms of work and the accomplishments of this unique style of practice.

❖

PETER KEATING is a Professor in the Department of History, University of Quebec at Montreal, Montreal, Quebec, Canada H3C 3P8 (e-mail: keating. peter@uqam.ca). He specializes in the history of contemporary biomedical sciences. Previous publications include two books coauthored with Alberto Cambrosio: *Exquisite Specificity: The Monoclonal Antibody Revolution* (Oxford University Press, 1995), and *Biomedical Platforms: Realigning the Normal and the Pathological in Late-Twentieth-Century Medicine* (MIT Press, 2003).

ALBERTO CAMBROSIO is a Professor in the Department of Social Studies of Medicine, McGill University, 3647 Peel, Montreal, Quebec, Canada H3A 1X1 (e-mail: alberto.cambrosio@mcgill.ca). His work focuses on the sociology of biomedical practices and innovations, in particular on the relation between laboratory and clinical activities. Previous publications include the above-mentioned two books coauthored with Peter Keating.

Ill Patient, Public Activist:
Rose Kushner's Attack on
Breast Cancer Chemotherapy

BARRON H. LERNER

SUMMARY: In 1984 the noted breast cancer activist Rose Kushner published a controversial article, "Is Aggressive Adjuvant Chemotherapy the Halsted Radical of the '80s?" In it, she argued that chemotherapy was being used as indiscriminately as the radical mastectomy had been, before she and others had successfully discredited the disfiguring operation. As with all of Kushner's writings, this article raised valid points in an informed and provocative style, but her attack on chemotherapy was more one-sided than was typical. This may have been due to the highly personal nature of the topic: when she was diagnosed with recurrent breast cancer, she had declined chemotherapy in favor of a hormonal agent, tamoxifen. She also developed a close working and financial relationship with the manufacturers of tamoxifen. Although not seen as a problem at the time, Kushner's dual roles as patient and advocate for a particular treatment foreshadowed conflict-of-interest issues that would take center stage in medicine in subsequent decades.

KEYWORDS: breast neoplasms/therapy; drug therapy; patient advocacy; conflict of interest; medical ethics; history of medicine, 20th century; famous persons

Rose Kushner is best known for her successful campaign against the one-step Halsted radical mastectomy, which surgeons finally abandoned in the late 1970s. But she took on another foe in the 1980s: the routine use of chemotherapy for postmenopausal women with breast cancer. Kushner's efforts peaked with a polemical article, "Is Aggressive Adjuvant Chemotherapy the Halsted Radical of the '80s?" published in an American Cancer Society (ACS) journal in 1984. Using previously unpublished correspondence, I explore this article, her motivations for writing it, and

Funding for this project came from the Greenwall Foundation, the National Library of Medicine G13 grant program, the Women at Risk organization at Columbia University Medical Center, and the Schlesinger Library. Research assistance was provided by Alison Bateman-House. Special thanks go to Harvey Kushner for his support of this research.

the responses of physicians and breast cancer patients. As with all of her publications, Kushner's piece is well written and well argued, effectively merging her knowledge of science with her personal story. She identified what she believed were the limitations and toxicities of chemotherapy and also criticized the practice of oncology in the United States.

Yet Kushner's attack on chemotherapy was more problematic than her earlier crusade against radical breast surgery. In order to make her points, she painted with a broad brush stroke, giving a one-sided view. This was likely due in part to the intensely personal nature of the topic: Kushner, who had first been diagnosed with breast cancer in 1974, had experienced a recurrence of her disease in 1982. At that time, she rejected the advice of certain oncologists to undergo chemotherapy, instead opting for treatment with a less toxic hormonal agent, tamoxifen.

Rose Kushner's sophisticated brand of advocacy meant that she was hardly a representative patient. Still, her struggle to balance the available scientific data on chemotherapy with a personal risk–benefit calculus presaged what a new generation of breast cancer patients would routinely come to do. And by actively warning women about the potential downsides of routine chemotherapy, Kushner would further expand the consumerist model of medical care that she had earlier helped to pioneer. But her interactions with manufacturers of and advocates for various chemotherapeutic and hormonal agents would raise a series of challenging ethical issues that she had not previously encountered.

Kushner was born Rose Rehert in Baltimore on 22 June 1929 to a middle-class Jewish couple: Israel Rehert, a Latvian-born tailor, and the former Fannie Gravitz, a housewife originally from Lithuania. The fourth of four children, Rose was extremely bright, graduating from P.S. 49 in 1946 and then matriculating at Johns Hopkins University as a premedical student. As did many women of her generation, she did not complete her education but instead married Harvey Kushner, who later became a business executive, on 18 March 1951. The couple had three children and settled in the Maryland suburbs of Washington, D.C.[1]

Throughout these years, Kushner maintained an avid interest in medical subjects, but her B.S., earned from the University of Maryland in 1972 when she was in her early forties, was in journalism. Like many journalists of the 1970s, she was eager to challenge the status quo, and her brash (and at times abrasive) temperament helped. Among the early topics she covered was the Vietnam War, which she staunchly opposed. Kushner liked

---

1. Barron H. Lerner, "Rose Kushner," in *Notable American Women*, ed. Susan D. Ware (Cambridge: Harvard University Press, 2004), pp. 360, 361.

to recount an interview with General William Westmoreland, in which she "told him off" to his face.[2]

Kushner felt a lump in her left breast in June 1974. She was forty-four years old. Rather than first consulting a physician, she went to the nearby National Library of Medicine to do independent research on breast cancer, which she feared she had. What she learned stunned her: American surgeons, who were almost invariably men, continued to perform the disfiguring Halsted radical mastectomy, a nearly century-old operation that removed the breast, underarm lymph glands, and the chest-wall muscles on the side of the cancer. In addition, these doctors continued to perform one-step surgery, making the decision to proceed with the radical mastectomy when women were under anesthesia; that is, if the results of an intraoperative breast biopsy showed cancer, the surgeon simply completed the operation. As a result, women awoke from surgery without knowing whether they had lost a breast. Finally, Kushner discovered that doctors in Canada and Europe had replaced the Halsted procedure with less-radical operations, which they said gave equivalent results. A handful of American surgeons had followed suit.[3]

In an era promoting equal rights for women, Kushner's feminist antennae went up. She decided that she would insist on having only a biopsy of her breast lump. Not surprisingly, she had great difficulty finding a surgeon who would agree. When the biopsy was performed and the diagnosis was cancer, she had an equally hard time finding a surgeon who would perform a modified radical mastectomy, which would leave her chest-wall muscles in place. Eventually, Thomas L. Dao of the Roswell Park Cancer Institute, who had begun to question radical surgery, agreed. All of Kushner's lymph nodes were negative for cancer, suggesting there was a good chance that the operation had cured her.[4]

As she recovered from surgery, Kushner began writing furiously. She had stumbled into the story of her journalistic career. "Vietnam will have to wait," she announced in typical fashion, "while I finish a crusade to tell American women—and through them their doctors—what I have learned."[5] As described in the papers by David Cantor and Gretchen Krueger elsewhere in this volume, there was a long history of efforts to educate the public about breast and other cancers, but such propaganda

2. Barron H. Lerner, *The Breast Cancer Wars: Hope, Fear, and the Pursuit of a Cure in Twentieth-Century America* (New York: Oxford University Press, 2001), p. 175.

3. Rose Kushner, *Breast Cancer: A Personal and an Investigative Report* (New York: Harcourt Brace Jovanovich, 1975), pp. 185–205.

4. Ibid., pp. 26–27.

5. Lerner, *Breast Cancer Wars* (n. 2), p. 177.

had largely been generated by the American Cancer Society and other mainstream cancer organizations. Kushner's projects explicitly confronted "business as usual." By 1975 she had established the Breast Cancer Advisory Center, a counseling center initially run out of her home. Although she primarily served as a referral service for concerned women, she at times provided more direct advice and guidance. That same year, she published *Breast Cancer: A Personal History and an Investigative Report.* In an era before such illness narratives were common, Kushner frankly described being diagnosed with cancer and losing her breast. Yet, more importantly, she herself discussed and evaluated the medical literature. Too many physicians, she argued, had the science all wrong.

In her early years as a breast cancer activist, Kushner was highly confrontational. Gaining access to medical meetings as a journalist, she routinely gave her opinions, even interrupting physicians. To say the least, this was highly irregular behavior for a layperson, especially a woman. Many doctors responded in a hostile manner, such as the one who termed her book "a piece of garbage."[6] But Kushner was a force to be reckoned with. First, she eventually came to know the scientific literature better than most doctors, even breast cancer specialists. Second, as time went on, it appeared more and more that she was "right." That is, the Halsted radical mastectomy was an obsolete procedure that was no better than operations that removed only the breast or, in some cases, just the cancerous lump. And the one-step procedure, which silenced women as they approached a monumental decision, was equally unnecessary.

The validity of Kushner's claims became eminently clear in 1979 when a consensus panel at the National Institutes of Health rejected both the one-step operation and the radical mastectomy. As physicians gradually acknowledged these facts, they began to view Kushner not as an annoyance but as a tremendous asset. She increasingly worked with Bernard Fisher, a University of Pittsburgh surgeon who conducted many of the earliest randomized controlled trials of breast cancer treatments. In 1980 President Jimmy Carter named Kushner as the first lay member of the prestigious National Cancer Advisory Board (NCAB), which helped to set policy for cancer screening and treatment. "I'm a full-fledged member of the Establishment," the former outsider Kushner stated.[7]

But someone with Kushner's personality—inherently skeptical of authority—could never really become a supporter of the status quo, even as a member of the NCAB. Having helped to transform breast cancer

6. Ibid., p. 180.
7. Ibid., p. 227.

surgery, Kushner next turned her attention to adjuvant chemotherapy, medications given by vein or orally that were designed to kill cancer cells not removed by surgery or destroyed by radiotherapy.

Kushner's article challenging chemotherapy appeared in the November-December 1984 issue of *CA*, a journal published for clinicians by the ACS.[8] The piece had been solicited by Arthur I. Holleb, a physician and medical director of the ACS, who had a long-standing relationship with Kushner. The ACS, founded in 1913, was the United States' oldest and largest voluntary anticancer organization. It was generally quite conservative, religiously advocating a strategy of early cancer detection followed by aggressive treatment. Kushner's initial foray into the breast- cancer debate, with her advocacy of patient choice and less-radical surgery, had rubbed many at the ACS the wrong way.[9] Yet once they realized her passion and abilities, the society's leaders—including Holleb—grew increasingly inclined to work with her. Thus, Holleb had decided to give her antiestablishment views on chemotherapy an airing in a journal unaccustomed to such fiery opinion pieces. Of course, it helped that Kushner was taking on chemotherapy this time as opposed to surgery; perhaps Holleb, a former surgeon, was glad to spread the lumps around.

Kushner began her article with a scathing accusation. Most American oncologists, she charged, did not even see their patients during routine appointments, leaving nurses to deal with the substantial side effects of chemotherapy—"baldness, nausea and vomiting, diarrhea, clogged veins, financial problems, broken marriages, disturbed children, loss of libido, loss of self- esteem, and body image." Patients, moreover, were expected to display what Kushner termed the "red-badge-of-courage" syndrome: "Glue a stylish wig on your pate, chew some Rolaids, and grin and bear it."[10] In contrast, she argued, physicians in Canada and several European countries had been much less eager to jump on the chemotherapy bandwagon.

Who were these oncologists receiving Kushner's wrath? The practice of oncology in the United States was relatively new. The first effective chemotherapeutic agents for fighting cancer dated from the 1950s; gradually, a group of physicians had emerged who were interested in researching and prescribing them. Some were surgeons who hired nursing staff to administer the new drugs to patients after their mastectomies or other cancer operations, but an increasing number were internists who had decided to subspecialize in oncology and chemotherapy. The American Society

8. Rose Kushner, "Is Aggressive Adjuvant Chemotherapy the Halsted Radical of the '80s?" *CA*, 1984, *34*: 345–51.

9. Lerner, *Breast Cancer Wars* (n. 2), p. 180.

10. Kushner, "Aggressive Adjuvant Chemotherapy" (n. 8), p. 345.

of Clinical Oncology was founded in 1964 as an umbrella organization to coordinate research and clinical practice in these areas.

To what degree was Kushner's accusation—that oncologists largely ignored their patients' symptoms—accurate? She did receive at least one letter from an oncologist who resented the implication that he and his colleagues were uncaring. "Perhaps to your surprise," wrote R. W. Brownlee of Monroe, Wisconsin, "some of us worry about patients"; he added that he regularly spoke with his patients about the side effects of chemotherapy and tried to "offer some solutions."[11]

Still, the relative silence of Kushner's correspondents regarding this issue may have spoken volumes. The truth was that as of 1984, concerns about drug toxicity and the emotional burden of cancer and its treatment were only beginning to gain attention among health professionals. Indeed, it had been a layperson, Terese Lasser, who had founded an organization, Reach to Recovery, to provide postoperative breast cancer patients with information about breast forms, physical therapy, and sexual concerns. The first textbook on the subject of cancer and emotions, Jimmie C. Holland's *Handbook of Psycho-oncology*, would not be published until 1989.[12] As in her crusade against radical breast cancer surgery, Kushner had again identified a significant problem in the treatment of cancer patients in the United States.

But what Kushner had to say in the *CA* article about the value of chemotherapy itself was more complicated. Her basic argument was that the "toxic regimens" being given to the majority of women who developed breast cancer—those who were postmenopausal—were of only "marginal benefit."[13] Meanwhile, they were causing the litany of side effects that Kushner had listed at the beginning of her article, as well as the possibility of future leukemias in breast cancer patients, a late complication of chemotherapy that some researchers feared. Adjuvant chemotherapy for such women, she argued, was still experimental and thus needed to be given only in the context of randomized controlled trials. This restriction, she was careful to note, was not meant for women before menopause, whose breast cancers tended to be more aggressive and often did respond positively to chemotherapy.

Kushner traced the overuse of cancer drugs to the publication of an article by the Italian cancer researcher Gianni Bonadonna in the

11. R. W. Brownlee to Rose Kushner, 22 January 1985 (courtesy of Harvey Kushner).

12. Jimmie C. Holland, *Handbook of Psycho-oncology: Psychological Care of the Patient with Cancer* (New York: Oxford University Press, 1989).

13. Kushner, "Aggressive Adjuvant Chemotherapy" (n. 8), p. 345.

19 February 1976 issue of the prestigious *New England Journal of Medicine*.[14] Bonadonna's patients were women with operable breast cancer that had reached their underarm lymph nodes without evidence of more distant spread. Doctors knew that such women likely had invisible "micrometastases" that would eventually become clinically apparent and lead to death; the goal of Bonadonna's three-drug "CMF" chemotherapy (which consisted of cytoxan, methotrexate, and 5-fluorouracil) was to kill these invisible cancer cells, thereby delaying recurrence of the disease, possibly lengthening survival, and maybe producing cures.

Thus, when Bonadonna reported that the chemotherapy had lowered the relapse rate from 24 to 5 percent compared to controls, it was surely good news. While these data were quite early, representing a mean of only fourteen months of follow-up, it nevertheless appeared that the CMF combination was doing exactly what it was supposed to do. But Kushner believed that the value of chemotherapy had been overstated—especially in a *New England Journal* editorial, written by cancer specialist James F. Holland, that accompanied Bonadonna's article.[15] Due to Holland's use of the words "spectacular" and "monumental" to describe Bonadonna's results, Kushner claimed, no other data "have ever had such a rapid and revolutionary impact."[16] What most infuriated her was that doctors were applying the positive results shown for premenopausal women to older women outside clinical trials, even though Bonadonna's data did not justify this. "This helter-skelter zapping by individual dox," Kushner wrote to a fellow breast cancer activist, "is really making me furious."[17] Elsewhere, recalling her feminist roots, she underscored the fact that it was men who were deciding that all women with breast cancer "needed" chemotherapy: "I object to the fact that they dream up protocols over the urinal, and then go out and try them on people."[18]

Another factor in Kushner's calculus was that many postmenopausal women had breast cancers that were strongly positive for estrogen receptors—that is, their cancers grew due to stimulation by the hormone

14. Gianni Bonadonna et al., "Combination Chemotherapy as an Adjuvant Treatment in Operable Breast Cancer," *New England J. Med.*, 1976, *294*: 405–10.

15. James F. Holland, "Major Advance in Breast Cancer Therapy," *New England J. Med.*, 1976, *294*: 440–41.

16. Rose Kushner, "Adjuvant Chemotherapy Revisited" (unpublished manuscript), 21 September 1985, Rose Kushner Papers, Schlesinger Library, Cambridge, Mass., box 3, folder 51.

17. Rose Kushner to Ruth Spear, 25 October 1984 (courtesy of Harvey Kushner).

18. Dave Silburt, "Attacking Breast Cancer," *Maclean's Magazine*, 15 October 1984, p. 12.

estrogen. Not only were such cancers slower-growing, on average, but there was a drug that appeared to effectively treat them: an antiestrogen compound called tamoxifen. Tamoxifen, a pill taken twice daily, had fewer side effects than chemotherapy. And, Kushner wrote, it was what she had decided to take when she had experienced a recurrence of her breast cancer. In late 1981 she had developed a tender, red pimple on her left chest wall, which had been treated with drainage and an antibiotic. A lump remained, however, and in June 1982 a biopsy revealed a breast cancer identical to her 1974 tumor. This meant that she had metastatic, stage IV disease.[19]

After additional visits to the library and discussions with breast cancer experts, Kushner learned that even though she had gone eight years without a recurrence and thus had a relatively slow-growing tumor, she was still a candidate for adjuvant chemotherapy outside a randomized controlled trial. Three oncologists recommended that she agree to such treatment, in order to "hit cancer cells hard when the primary tumor burden is very small"; but, lacking good data, she analogized such a choice to "hitting a mosquito with a Sherman tank."[20] She eventually decided to take tamoxifen instead, supposing that the long interval between her two bouts of cancer meant that she probably had an estrogen-receptor-positive cancer (there was not enough tissue available for actual testing). At the time that her *CA* article was published (at the end of 1984), Kushner, in good health and having experienced no side effects of treatment, was very pleased with her decision.

Kushner's piece won the American Medical Writers Association's 1985 award for the best periodical article written for a professional audience. It had also received a great deal of praise from cancer specialists, suggesting that Kushner had made the frank type of comments about chemotherapy that clinicians had themselves been unwilling to make. James A. Stewart of the Vermont Regional Cancer Center wrote Arthur Holleb that the article was "excellent reading for all oncologists."[21] Toronto cancer specialist Edward B. Fish agreed: "I see the very sad result," he told Kushner, "of those who have put up with chemotherapy and still have metastases and die from their disease."[22] "It is very gratifying," Tennessee radiologist C. W. Kinsey commented, "to see a non-physician bring the medical literature

19. Kushner, "Aggressive Adjuvant Chemotherapy" (n. 8), p. 347.

20. Rose Kushner, *Alternatives: New Developments in the War on Breast Cancer* (New York: Warner Books, 1984), p. 30.

21. James A. Stewart to Arthur I. Holleb, 24 January 1985, Kushner Papers, box 3, folder 48.

22. Edward B. Fish to Rose Kushner, 21 January 1985 (courtesy of Harvey Kushner).

in to such brilliant perspective."[23] Oncologist Edward S. Greenwald of New Rochelle, New York, "heartily" agreed with Kushner, speculating that the overuse of chemotherapy stemmed from the fact that there were too many medical oncologists.[24]

The article also provided an opportunity for iconoclasts in the world of cancer to state their case. One was Michael B. Shimkin, a biostatistician at the University of California at San Diego and one of the founding fathers of the National Cancer Institute, who had become friends with Kushner in the 1970s. "We so badly need some contrary opinions in areas where the Establishment has become fixed and immobile in their [sic] views," he wrote.[25] A big problem, according to Shimkin, were the profits that chemotherapy engendered, "keep[ing] medical oncologists busy and wealthy, not to mention pharmaceutical companies."[26]

But Kushner also earned the admiration of members of the very cancer establishment that Shimkin had criticized. For example, Detroit radiotherapist William E. Powers, a fellow member of the NCAB, sent out the article with a cover letter alleging "significant inappropriate use of toxic chemotherapy in patients who have little likelihood of benefit."[27] In September 1985 the National Institutes of Health, at Kushner's urging, held a consensus conference on the topic of adjuvant chemotherapy. The committee's conclusions mirrored her beliefs, recommending only that chemotherapy be *considered* for postmenopausal women with positive underarm lymph nodes and negative estrogen receptors. For women with positive estrogen receptors, the committee concluded, "tamoxifen is the treatment of choice."[28]

Although Kushner's article was geared toward a professional audience, word got out about her argument, in part due to her frequent media appearances. Women who wrote to her appreciated her message. An Indiana breast cancer patient who had six positive lymph nodes and positive estrogen receptors told Kushner that she had chosen tamoxifen treatment instead of chemotherapy. Without Kushner's article, she stated, "I'm not sure I would have had the courage to resist."[29] A Michigan woman wrote Kushner that she had been in remission for two years: "Tamoxifen has kept my disease in check," she said, "and I am feeling great."[30]

23. C. W. Kimsey to Rose Kushner, 28 February 1985 (courtesy of Harvey Kushner).

24. Edward S. Greenwald to Rose Kushner, 31 January 1985 (courtesy of Harvey Kushner).

25. Michael Shimkin to Rose Kushner, 2 June 1985 (courtesy of Harvey Kushner).

26. Shimkin to Kushner, 24 August 1984 (courtesy of Harvey Kushner).

27. William E. Powers to Dear Colleague, [1984] (courtesy of Harvey Kushner).

28. Rose Kushner to Ezra M. Greenspan, 21 May 1986 (courtesy of Harvey Kushner).

29. P. S. to Rose Kushner, 15 March 1985 (courtesy of Harvey Kushner).

30. M. G. to Rose Kushner, 29 February 1984 (courtesy of Harvey Kushner).

Still, the article generated considerable dissent, mostly from the oncology community. In contrast to the surgeons who had remained staunch advocates of the radical mastectomy, these physicians were not merely obstinate defenders of the status quo, but were themselves knowledgeable about the medical literature, which they believed supported the use of adjuvant chemotherapy for both premenopausal and postmenopausal women. For example, George Washington University Medical Center oncologist Robert S. Siegel reported in early 1985 that the most recent analysis of Bonadonna's data showed that, compared with untreated women, 16 percent more postmenopausal women lived five years without a recurrence if they received chemotherapy; in addition, another study by Bonadonna, which used a five-drug—as opposed to a three-drug—regimen, was even more effective.[31] Two oncologists associated with the National Cancer Institute, Marc Lippman and Bruce Chabner, agreed, citing results reported at an October 1984 meeting held in London: controlled trials involving 10,000 patients with early breast cancer, they stated, had shown a 22 percent reduction of mortality among postmenopausal women receiving CMF chemotherapy.[32]

Another critic was Ezra M. Greenspan, an oncologist at Mount Sinai Medical Center in New York City, who argued that Kushner needed to make a clearer distinction between postmenopausal women who were at high risk, with aggressive-looking cancer cells and negative estrogen receptors, and those who were at lower risk. In the former instance, he argued, the data of Bonadonna and others clearly showed improved survival. To suggest that chemotherapy did not help high-risk breast cancers, both stage II and stage I (with no positive nodes), was "unethical." To imply that chemotherapy was the Halsted radical of the 1980s, he charged, was "sheer egomania."[33] These were fighting words, but Kushner was unfazed. She considered Greenspan a friend and his comments fair game, particularly the warning about her inadvertently lumping together high- and low-risk patients in her eagerness to make an important point. In a reply to Greenspan, she relied on her formidable sense of humor in trying to reach a happy medium: "To sum up, please kiss me and make up," she entreated him. "After all, I am a woman, and I think I'm a little better looking than Bernie Fisher is."[34]

31. Robert S. Siegel, "The Case for Chemotherapy after Breast Cancer Surgery," *Washington Post*, 13 February 1985, p. H6.

32. Marc Lippman and Bruce Chabner, "Adjuvant Therapy of Breast Cancer" (unpublished manuscript), n.d., Kushner Papers, box 3, folder 50.

33. Ezra M. Greenspan to Rose Kushner, 8 July 1986 (courtesy of Harvey Kushner).

34. Kushner to Greenspan, 21 July 1986, Kushner Papers, box 8, folder 129.

The fact that Kushner, her supporters, and her detractors disagreed over what the chemotherapy data showed was of considerable significance. Although researchers such as Fisher and Bonadonna had underscored the importance of randomized controlled trials, which gave data far superior to those from other types of studies, it was possible to interpret the results of these trials, especially those with subtle findings, in different ways. This was the case because even randomized studies were far from objective. For example, researchers reviewing and then analyzing randomized results used variable statistical techniques that manipulated the data in particular ways; such calculations could then lead different researchers to draw disparate conclusions from the same data (at times influenced by preexisting opinions or interest-group politics).[35] Those debating adjuvant chemotherapy in the mid-1980s were having one of these differences of opinion, although as more data came in and treatment regimens improved, it appeared that Greenspan was correct: some high-risk menopausal women clearly benefited from adjuvant chemotherapy.

But beyond the variable interpretation of the data, the debates over adjuvant chemotherapy demonstrated another key issue: different women responded differently to the same information. Or, to put it another way, women made highly personal choices about what benefits they wished to pursue and what risks they were willing to take. Although Kushner aimed at reaching all breast cancer patients considering adjuvant chemotherapy, she herself actually represented one end of a spectrum of beliefs, one that discouraged attempts at heroic cures. In contrast to poorly informed women, susceptible to false hope, she knew what her stage IV breast cancer almost certainly signified: eventual death from the disease. "The basic difference between your thinking as an oncologist and mine as a patient," she informed chemotherapy specialist Sydney E. Salmon, "is that I'm afraid this miserable disease is always incurable." As a result, she told him, "I look for symptom-free, maximum quality-of-life . . . while you still expect a cure and believe the benefits of adjuvant chemotherapy outweigh its risks."[36] Kushner, in other words, was being a realist.

But at some point, Kushner's persistent inclination to disregard the emerging data about chemotherapy may also have made her a fatalist.

35. Harry M. Marks, *The Progress of Experiment: Science and Therapeutic Reform in the United States, 1900–1990* (Cambridge: Cambridge University Press, 1997), p. 134; David S. Jones, "Visions of a Cure: Visualization, Clinical Trials, and Controversies in Cardiac Therapeutics, 1968–1998," *Isis*, 2000, *91*: 504–41; Barron H. Lerner, "When Statistics Provide Unsatisfying Answers: Revisiting the Breast Self-Examination Controversy," *Can. Med. Assoc. J.*, 2002, *166*: 199–201.

36. Rose Kushner to Sydney E. Salmon, 22 July 1984, Kushner Papers, box 14, folder 215.

After her article in *CA* was published in 1984, she began a correspondence with C. Barber Mueller, a cancer surgeon at McMaster University in Hamilton, Ontario. Mueller had sent her a copy of an article he had published in the journal *Surgery* in 1983: "Asymptomatic Metastases—To Treat or Not to Treat?" In it, Mueller had discouraged both hunting for asymptomatic areas of metastatic cancer and treating them if they were inadvertently discovered.[37] Kushner agreed with Mueller, telling him that "metastatic disease that isn't causing a woman any pain or problems should simply be watched."[38]

In her own case, even though some oncologists sincerely believed they might be able to cure her breast cancer with aggressive chemotherapy, Kushner remained highly pleased with her choice of tamoxifen. True, she wrote to Arthur Holleb, she probably had invisible metastases, but they were not causing her any problems. "In the meantime," she told him, "I'm taking only Nolvadex [the brand name of tamoxifen], my hair is on my head, I'm not vomiting, I have no stomatitis [mouth ulcers], and my white-cells and platelets are normal. To me, this is all that matters."[39]

One of Kushner's critics, Bruce Chabner, explicitly raised this risk–benefit calculus when he argued with her about the routine treatment of postmenopausal women with adjuvant chemotherapy. Kushner had estimated that there were roughly 46,400 cases of postmenopausal breast cancer diagnosed annually in the United States that had positive nodes. If Bonadonna's latest 16 percent figure was used, this meant that roughly 7,800 of these women might benefit from the drugs. For Chabner, such a trade-off was clearly worthwhile: "I do believe," he wrote Kushner, "that delaying recurrence in 8,000 postmenopausal women is worth the risk of chemotherapy."[40] Kushner completely disagreed: "I do believe," she stated, that "it is wrong to subject 46,000 women to toxic drugs for the marginal benefit of 7,800 women or fewer."[41]

In other words, until there were more definitive data from randomized controlled trials demonstrating the virtues of adjuvant chemotherapy, Kushner remained skeptical of its value. Other women, however, appeared to prefer Chabner's calculus, something that Kushner herself grudgingly admitted; the public appeal of chemotherapy was growing, even though it

37. C. Barber Mueller, "Asymptomatic Metastases—To Treat or Not to Treat?" *Surgery*, 1983, *93*: 328–29.

38. Rose Kushner to C. Barber Mueller, 6 September 1985 (courtesy of Harvey Kushner).

39. Rose Kushner to Arthur I. Holleb, 24 June 1983, Kushner Papers, box 3, folder 48.

40. Bruce A. Chabner to Rose Kushner, 15 March 1985 (courtesy of Harvey Kushner).

41. Rose Kushner to Arthur I. Holleb, 11 March 1985, Kushner Papers, box 3, folder 48.

caused side effects and probably did not help most women who underwent treatment. "Patients nowadays," she wrote to Mueller, "have been educated by the general media to believe there is, indeed, a 'magic bullet' out there that will cure breast cancer."[42] Nor did this situation change after the 1985 consensus conference had urged caution regarding adjuvant chemotherapy: both premenopausal and postmenopausal women with positive lymph nodes, Kushner wrote in 1986, "want to take as much as they can of everything to be cured or to delay a recurrence."[43] Even oncologists who were measured in their use of chemotherapy were in a bind. As Michael Shimkin told Kushner, "they are expected professionally and publicly to give their patients poisonous agents that won't do much."[44]

Kushner might have been more willing to consider chemotherapy had there not been the alternative of tamoxifen. Given her ardent concerns about quality of life, the fact that tamoxifen appeared to have very few side effects made it quite appealing. Still, the degree to which the hormonal treatment delayed the recurrence of breast cancer or improved survival was itself a subject of debate. In her 1984 article, Kushner cited two studies published in 1981 that showed prolonged disease-free survival among postmenopausal women taking adjuvant tamoxifen.[45] As she was writing her piece, British cancer specialist Michael Baum wrote her about his ongoing tamoxifen trial, which was "producing the most unbelievably good results."[46]

Others, however, challenged these data. For example, Sydney Salmon believed that the research conducted on tamoxifen was of shorter duration than the chemotherapy data and was thus less conclusive.[47] Even Dana-Farber Cancer Institute oncologist I. Craig Henderson, a staunch supporter of Kushner, had to agree. "The use of tamoxifen in your setting," he wrote to her in September 1984, "is just as experimental as the use of aggressive chemotherapy."[48] Kushner did not deny this, and had admitted in her *CA* article that the existing tamoxifen data were too preliminary to be definitive. And she was careful never to suggest that her decision to take tamoxifen and not chemotherapy was the "right" one

42. Rose Kushner to C. Barber Mueller, 6 September 1985 (courtesy of Harvey Kushner).

43. Kushner to Greenspan, 21 July 1986 (n. 34).

44. Shimkin to Kushner, 2 June 1985 (n. 25).

45. Kushner, "Aggressive Adjuvant Chemotherapy" (n. 8), p. 346.

46. Michael Baum to Rose Kushner, 6 March 1984 (courtesy of Harvey Kushner).

47. "Community Oncologists Are Justified in Using Adjuvant Therapy for Breast Cancer: Salmon," *Clin. Cancer Lett.*, 1984, *7* (8): 1–5.

48. I. Craig Henderson to Rose Kushner, 19 September 1984, Kushner Papers, box 14, folder 215.

for other women in her situation. Kushner, after all, had been one of the earliest health activists to preach the importance of women's making their own individual decisions based on the best data available. Her approach was always less proscriptive than consumerist: "Let the buyer beware."

But Kushner's advocacy of tamoxifen was complicated. Just as in her discussions of radical breast surgery, in her writings on adjuvant therapy she interspersed her own story amid the scientific data. As a result, her personal beliefs about various treatment options became subtly conflated with her "objective" advice on the subject. And when Kushner—America's preeminent lay expert on breast cancer—chose tamoxifen, it potentially carried a powerful message for other women about what was "best."

By Kushner's own admission, she had long been "prejudiced" against chemotherapy, dating at least as far back as the highly favorable 1976 *New England Journal* article and editorial.[49] By 1979 she had begun an "anti-chemo" file, the name of which sent a clear message about her strong beliefs on the subject.[50] In May 1982 she had received a letter from her surgeon, Thomas Dao, describing a series of patients he had evaluated whose breast cancer had recurred despite treatment with CMF. Believing that these women should not have received CMF in the first place, Dao criticized "the almost indiscriminate use of adjuvant chemotherapy" among breast cancer patients. He also worried about the generation of drug-resistant cancers because of this overuse.[51] Ironically, the biopsy of Kushner's chest-wall lump took place the next month. Although the three oncologists had recommended chemotherapy, Dao had advised only tamoxifen, based on the assumption of estrogen-receptor positivity. Kushner had eventually taken the advice of Dao, the one surgeon who had been willing to give her a modified operation in 1974 and was now her trusted doctor and friend.[52] At this same time, Kushner later wrote, her anti-chemo file began to grow.[53]

This series of events, I would argue, set up a type of self-validating feedback loop. Kushner's basic mistrust of chemotherapy for postmenopausal women, coupled with that of her doctor, led her to reject this therapy for her own situation. This decision, in turn, led her to view ongoing chemotherapy studies with a skeptical eye and to write her *CA* article when Holleb had suggested it. The article, finally, led Kushner to be identified

49. Kushner, *Alternatives* (n. 20), p. 34.

50. Rose Kushner to Serena Stockwell or Michael Braun, 17 August 1984, Kushner Papers, box 3, folder 48.

51. Thomas L. Dao to Rose Kushner, 21 May 1982, Kushner Papers, box 9, folder 142.

52. Kushner, "Aggressive Adjuvant Chemotherapy" (n. 8), p. 348.

53. Kushner to Stockwell or Braun, August 17, 1984 (n. 50).

as one of the most vocal critics of routine adjuvant chemotherapy in the country, a stand she then felt obligated to maintain.

This discussion should not suggest that it was only Kushner who made decisions based on some combination of medical knowledge, doctors' advice, and personal preference. As breast cancer and other patients, following Kushner's lead, became more empowered in the 1980s, they increasingly used a model of "shared decision-making" to guide their treatment choices.[54] Physicians—even those who communicated the latest science to their patients—also potentially incorporated personal beliefs or value judgments into their discussions. Their opinions reflected a series of factors, such as reliance on anecdotal clinical experiences, excessive allegiance to familiar modalities, and information obtained from pharmaceutical companies.

The influence of the drug industry was also relevant in Kushner's case. As her opposition to chemotherapy continued, her confidence in tamoxifen as an alternative treatment grew. At some point, she purchased stock in Imperial Chemical Industries (ICI), the British company that manufactured Nolvadex, and regularly mentioned the medication in her frequent articles and lectures on breast cancer. When her book, *Alternatives: New Developments in the War on Breast Cancer*, was published in 1984, a natural alliance was formed: ICI and its American affiliate, Stuart Pharmaceuticals, were eager to help publicize the book, which was not only an excellent treatise on the disease but also spoke very favorably about their product.[55] Kushner received travel funding from the two companies, enabling her to appear at meetings and to sell her book.[56] Stuart Pharmaceuticals also bought 10,000 copies of *Alternatives*, distributing them to physicians as gifts.[57]

By 1987 ICI was also donating money to Kushner's Breast Cancer Advisory Center for general operating expenses and specific projects, such as mailings to support mammography legislation.[58] In February 1988 Kushner actually wrote the text for "Nolvadex and You," a patient-information leaflet being prepared by ICI. "This leaflet is being written," she told readers, "to help your doctor explain why you are an excellent

54. Analee E. Biesecker and Thomas D. Biesecker, "Patient Information-Seeking Behaviors when Communicating with Doctors," *Med. Care*, 1990, *28*: 19–28; Raisa Deber, Nancy Kraetschmer, and Jane Irvine, "What Role Do Patients Wish in Clinical Decision-Making?" *Arch. Internal Med.*, 1996, *156*: 1414–20.

55. Rose Kushner to John Harvey-Jones, 27 February 1984 (courtesy of Harvey Kushner).

56. Rose Kushner to Larry Thompson, 20 January 1985 (courtesy of Harvey Kushner); Susan J. Smitten to Rose Kushner, 19 November 1987, Kushner Papers, box 9, folder 142.

57. Gene H. Zaiser to Rose Kushner, 24 October 1983 (courtesy of Harvey Kushner).

58. Rose Kushner to Trisha P. Conti, 28 October 1987, Kushner Papers, box 9, folder 141.

candidate for 'adjuvant' Nolvadex hormonal therapy."[59] Her optimism about the product was palpable; at one point the text stated that the two daily pills of Nolvadex "have no side effects."[60]

By this time, tamoxifen had become a highly respected medication—one that was both effective and safe. In December 1986 the U.S. Food and Drug Administration had approved it as standard therapy for postmenopausal women with positive lymph nodes and estrogen-receptor-positive breast cancers.[61] Still, Kushner had put herself in a very difficult situation, becoming embroiled in a volatile medical and commercial controversy. "I have bet my life on Nolvadex," she admitted to ICI Chairman John Harvey-Jones in 1984.[62] Providing scientific information to the public about a drug that had such incredible personal importance to her necessarily created a conflict of interest.

Twenty years later, how should we judge Kushner's interactions with the manufacturers of tamoxifen? Today, relationships between health-related industries and their professional and lay spokespeople receive intense scrutiny. Full disclosure statements about any financial ties are expected to accompany all lectures and published articles.[63] Some critics have persuasively charged that pharmaceutical companies—including AstraZeneca, the current manufacturer of tamoxifen—have co-opted aspects of breast cancer activism.[64] But it would be unfair to hold someone even as progressive as Kushner to our modern ethical standard. The mid-1980s, when she published her article in *CA*, was a period of transition from an earlier time in which largesse from industry was tolerated and even lauded. Indeed, it was in the fall of 1984, just before Kushner's piece appeared, that the *New England Journal of Medicine* inaugurated a new policy that required all authors to disclose commercial and entrepreneurial interests.[65] As the decade proceeded, other physician organizations adopted similar policies.[66]

59. Rose Kushner, "Nolvadex and You" (draft), 15 February 1988, Kushner Papers, box 4, folder 58.

60. Ibid.

61. Rose Kushner to Arthur I. Holleb, 29 July 1986, Kushner Papers, box 4, folder 58.

62. Kushner to Harvey-Jones, 27 February 1984 (n. 55).

63. International Committee of Medical Journal Editors, "Statement on Project-Specific Industry Support for Research," *Can. Med. Assoc. J.*, 1998, *158*: 615–16.

64. Barbara A. Brenner, "From the Executive Director: Seeing Our Interests Clearly," *Breast Cancer Action Newsl.*, vol. 52, February–March 1999, at **http://www.bcaction.org/Pages/SearchablePages/1999Newsletters/Newsletter052B.html** (accessed on 7 June 2006).

65. Arnold Relman, quoted in "Dialogue: Disclosure of Conflicts of Interest," *Sci. Tech. & Hum. Val.*, 1985, *10*: 36–40, on p. 37.

66. Committee on Ethics of the American College of Obstetricians and Gynecologists (ACOG), "Guidelines for Relationships between Industry and the American College of

Kushner apparently never publicly commented on her relationship with ICI and Stuart Pharmaceuticals; nor does it seem that anyone raised the issue of her potential bias. This is unsurprising, given that she always readily discussed that she was taking the same drug that she was plugging. Intelligent consumers could have deduced the possibility that she was a biased commentator. In addition, Kushner might have argued that the money from the manufacturers of tamoxifen helped her sell books and maintain her financially strapped Breast Cancer Advisory Center, but did not require her to spout the company line.

Still, Rose Kushner's award-winning article comparing adjuvant chemotherapy to the Halsted radical mastectomy provides a cautionary tale about individuals who function simultaneously as patients and spokespeople. Over the past twenty years, celebrities—ranging from Parkinson's disease patient Michael J. Fox to cancer survivor Lance Armstrong—have become the most prominent faces of disease in America. Some, such as Magic Johnson, who has AIDS, have been hired by pharmaceutical companies to promote specific drugs.[67] If Rose Kushner, "the best informed person around,"[68] could not maintain a clear line between personal decisions and public advice, it is unlikely that any of these other individuals will be able to do so either.

❖

BARRON H. LERNER is the Angelica Berrie-Arnold P. Gold Foundation Associate Professor of Medicine and Public Health at the Columbia College of Physicians and Surgeons and the Mailman School of Public Health, Columbia University, 722 West 168th Street, Room 938, New York, NY 10032 (e-mail: BHL5@columbia.edu). He is the author, most recently, of *When Illness Goes Public: Celebrity Patients and How We Look at Medicine* (Johns Hopkins University Press, 2006). His previous book, *The Breast Cancer Wars: Hope, Fear, and the Pursuit of a Cure in Twentieth-Century America* (Oxford University Press, 2001), won the American Association for the History of Medicine's William H. Welch Award in 2006 for a book of outstanding scholarly merit.

Obstetricians and Gynecologists and Its Fellows," *ACOG Commit. Opin.*, no. 45, October 1985.

67. Alex Kuczynski, "Treating Disease with a Famous Face," *New York Times*, 15 December 2002, pp. H1, H15. See also Barron H. Lerner, *When Illness Goes Public: Celebrity Patients and How We Look at Medicine* (Baltimore: Johns Hopkins University Press, 2006).

68. This phrase came from Ann Landers, who served with Kushner on the National Cancer Advisory Board: Ann Landers to Harvey D. Kushner, 26 November 1990 (courtesy of Harvey Kushner).

Part III / Prevention and Risk

Breast Cancer and the "Materiality of Risk": The Rise of Morphological Prediction

ILANA LÖWY

SUMMARY: This paper follows the history of "morphological risk" of breast cancer. In the early twentieth century, surgeons and pathologists arrived at the conclusion that specific anatomical and cytological changes in the breast are related to a heightened risk of developing a malignancy in the future. This conclusion was directly related to a shift from macroscopic to microscopic diagnosis of malignancies, and to the integration of the frozen section into routine surgery for breast cancer. In the interwar era, conditions such as "chronic mastitis" and "cystic disease of the breast" were defined as precancerous, and women diagnosed with these conditions were advised to undergo mastectomy. In the post–World War II era, these entities were replaced by "carcinoma in situ." The recent development of tests for hereditary predisposition to breast cancer is a continuation of attempts to detect an "embodied risk" of cancer and to eliminate this risk by cutting it out.

KEYWORDS: breast cancer, surgical pathology, biopsy, frozen section, mastectomy, in situ cancer

"Molecular Lesions"

The starting point of this paper was an expression overheard during a consultation in cancer genetics. Trying to explain to a woman with a family history of breast cancer the meaning of a mutation in a BRCA gene, a clinical geneticist described such a mutation as a "molecular lesion." On one level, this term may be viewed as an oxymoron. The term "lesion" describes damage to organs and tissues. It was introduced in the early nineteenth century in the context of efforts to correlate clinical signs with morbid changes in the body, first analyzed in terms of gross pathology, and later also as changes observed in histological preparations. This term, the French philosopher of medicine Georges Canguilhem has proposed, is central to the distinction between the normal and the pathological.[1]

1. Georges Canguilhem, *The Normal and the Pathological*, trans. Carolyn R. Fawcett (1964; New York: Zone Books, 1989).

Molecules belong to a different domain: that of the chemistry of life. The term "molecular lesion" collapses a distinction between two distinct levels of functioning of the organism, and between two different levels of explanation: pathological and biochemical.

On another level, however, "molecular lesion" points to two important phenomena: the central role of pathology in the diagnosis and monitoring of cancer, and similarities between predictive tests grounded in the analysis of DNA sequences and those grounded in cytological observations. In this paper, focused on breast cancer, I trace the history of "predictive morphology"—that is, attempts to link specific changes in breast tissue to an increased danger of developing breast cancer in the future. I am also interested in the main consequence of the development of predictive morphology: the rise of preventive surgery.

Cytological diagnosis of proliferative changes in breast tissue is rarely presented as a predictive process. Typically, a woman who undergoes a biopsy—either following the discovery of a lump in the breast or, nowadays, often because of abnormal mammographic findings—is told that the pathology laboratory has found "atypia," "hyperplasia," or "in situ carcinoma," and for this reason she has a higher-than-average chance to develop breast cancer in the future. Today such a pronouncement is usually associated with a quantitative evaluation—"X times increased risk," "Y chances to develop a breast cancer in the next five years." Such a prediction is fully integrated into the usual diagnostic procedures—clinical examination, mammography, echography, and biopsy—that aim to confirm the existence of a malignancy. A routine part of screening for breast cancer or of diagnosis of a suspicious lump in the breast, "predictive morphology" has a low level of public visibility and has not become a subject of ethical debate. By contrast, "predictive genetics"—testing to reveal the presence of mutations that increase the chances to develop cancer—has a high level of visibility. Such tests were presented as an entirely new development that introduced new ethical and psychological dilemmas. Thus the development of tests for BRCA mutations was followed by an impressive production of studies dealing with the psychosocial effects of these tests. In France, the preoccupation with moral and psychological consequences of genetic prediction led to changes in legislation. According to French law, tests of "late onset genetic conditions," such as mutations in the BRCA gene, can be made only by a multidisciplinary team that includes genetic counselors (in France, always M.D.'s) and psychologists or psychiatrists.[2]

---

2. The French legal *dispositifs* are Decree (décret) no. 2000-570 of 23 June 2000, and Health Ministry order (arrêté) of 2 May 2001. See also Christine Sevilla, Pascale Bouret,

The high level of concern for the psychological well-being of people who discover that their genetic makeup puts them at increased risk to develop a malignancy contrasts with a much lower level of preoccupation with the psychological well-being of people who learn that morphological changes in their tissues greatly increases their chance of developing a cancer in the future. However, as the pathologist Elliott Foucar has noted, predictive genetics and predictive morphology pursue a very similar goal: the search for structural anomalies that allow risk assessment in "asymptomatic" (that is, clinically healthy) patients.[3] In both cases, the prediction is linked to uncertainty about whether an illness will develop, when it will develop, and how severe it will be; and in both, the stress level of those who test positive varies according to the efficacy of the proposed preventive steps and their cost to the patient: laser treatment for cervical dysplasia and preventive mastectomy are viewed as efficient preventive measures, but the first is much less traumatic than the second. Finally, in predictive morphology, as in predictive genetics, the population-based notion of risk is translated into a demonstration of the presence of physical changes in the body, using specific techniques: cytology, or molecular biology. Genetic testing may be seen as a way of making hidden aspects of the body visible, and thus as an approach that is not qualitatively different from a microscopic observation. While from a strictly logical point of view molecules cannot have lesions, the expression "molecular lesions" makes intuitive sense.

Radical Mastectomy and the Rise of Microscopic Diagnosis of Breast Cancer

Cancer is a pathologist's disease. In the early twenty-first century, pathologists still have the last word in the diagnosis of solid cancers (the diagnosis of hematological malignancies is a somewhat more complicated issue).[4] The maintaining of the pathologists' near-total control over the diagnosis and monitoring of malignancies is unusual. The decades after World War II have been seen as a period of intensive "molecularization" of biology and medicine driven by the rapid expansion of biological and

Catherine Noguès, et al., "L'offre de tests de prédisposition génétique au cancer du sein ou d'ovaire en France," *Médecine/Sciences*, 2004, *20*: 788–92.

3. Elliott Foucar, "Predictive Genetics and Predictive Morphology Have Certain Similarities," *Brit. Med. J.*, 2001, *323*: 514.

4. On the history of the diagnosis of hematological malignancies, see Peter Keating and Alberto Cambrosio, *Biomedical Platforms: Realigning the Normal and the Pathological in Late-Twentieth-Century Medicine* (Cambridge: MIT Press, 2003).

biomedical research, and accelerated by the growing automation of laboratory tests that played an increasingly important role in the diagnosis and monitoring of diseases.[5] By contrast, cancer diagnosis continues to be grounded primarily in the nontransmissible knowledge of the pathologist. Tests for biological markers linked with a given malignancy (e.g., PSA for prostate cancer, C-125 for ovarian cancer) are seen mainly as an indication to start a search for the presence of malignant cells, or, alternatively, as a means to refine a cancer diagnosis, not to establish it. In 2007 too, a patient has a cancer because a pathology report says so.

The absolute reign of the pathologist in the jurisdiction of breast cancer did not automatically follow the definition of cancer as a cell disease.[6] In the late nineteenth century, experimental studies of cancer conducted in the laboratory included detailed microscopic observations, but the knowledge generated by these studies was only slowly incorporated into the routine diagnosis of malignant growths (a process that can be compared to the slow integration of bacteriological knowledge into the routine diagnosis of transmissible diseases). Diagnosis of cancer was the exclusive domain of the surgeon. Surgeons who treated cancer were usually confident in their ability to recognize the disease either clinically, when examining the patient, or anatomically, during an exploratory surgery. The pathologist remained, in the main, the "Keeper of the Dead"; his job was to dissect cadavers, and from time to time to study surgically excised tissues in order to confirm or disprove the surgeon's diagnosis. In the late nineteenth century, Stephen Jacyna has shown, surgeons were well aware of the existence of pathological diagnosis of malignancies and occasionally asked for a pathologist's opinion before undertaking an extended breast surgery. These were, however, rare and sporadic events: in the majority of cases, surgeons relied exclusively on their clinical judgment and, at most, sent the excised tissues for analysis once the operation was completed.[7]

5. Soraya de Chadarevian and Harmke Kamminga, eds., *Molecularization of Biology and Medicine* (Amsterdam: Harwood Academic, 1998); Keating and Cambrosio, *Biomedical Platforms* (n. 4).

6. Lelland J. Rather, *The Genesis of Cancer: A Study in the History of Ideas* (Baltimore: Johns Hopkins University Press, 1978); David Cantor, "Cancer," in *Companion Encyclopedia to the History of Medicine,* ed. William F. Bynum and Roy Porter, vol. 1 (London: Routledge, 1993), pp. 537–61; Ilana Löwy, "Cancer—The Century of the Transformed Cell," in *Science in the Twentieth Century,* ed. John Krige and Dominique Pestre (Amsterdam: Harwood Academic Press, 1997), pp. 461–77.

7. L. Stephen Jacyna, "The Laboratory and the Clinic: The Impact of Pathology on Surgical Diagnosis in the Glasgow Western Infirmary, 1875–1910," *Bull. Hist. Med.,* 1988, *62:* 384–406.

The diffusion of W. S. Halsted's radical mastectomy in the late nine-teenth and early twentieth centuries reflected a growing conviction that breast cancer always starts as a local event, and becomes generalized only in a later stage.[8] The local-to-general theory was consolidated by the accep-tance of the principle that the cancer spreads through the lymphatic sys-tem and migrates from one lymph node to another, and then to adjacent tissues. This view, propagated by Sampson Handley, replaced the earlier "embolic theory" that stressed the role of blood circulation in the genesis of metastasis. In Handley's descriptions, metastatic breast cancer had a quasi-anatomical continuity with the primary tumor, and the main issue was, "how can the cancer of the breast, with all its microscopic ramifica-tions, be completely excised?"[9] The adoption of radical surgery—named "the complete operation," a term that strongly hinted that all the other forms of surgery were incomplete and therefore dangerous—consolidated in turn the local-to-general view of the natural history of breast cancer. All the remissions were attributed to a successful extirpation of malignant tissue, and were seen as confirmation of the view that breast cancer always starts as a localized disease.[10]

Unfortunately, many women succumbed to metastatic cancer in spite of having had a successful radical surgery. A follow-up published in 1927 found that 40 percent of women who underwent Halsted's mastectomy were alive five years after the initial diagnosis, as compared to 22 percent of the patients in the untreated group.[11] This disappointing result was attributed to the fact that the majority of these women were diagnosed too

8. Simple mastectomy is the removal of the breast gland alone, while radical mastectomy includes the removal of underlying muscles and regional lymph nodes and is a much more mutilating operation.

9. W. Sampson Handley, *Cancer of the Breast and Its Operative Treatement* (London: Mur-ray, 1906), pp. 1–2.

10. The majority of historians believe today that Halsted's radical surgery was unneces-sarily mutilating, and that it is difficult to assess the clinical efficacy (if any) of early uses of this technique. On the history of breast cancer surgery and of early-detection campaigns, see Jane Austoker, "'The Treatment of Choice': Breast Cancer Surgery 1860–1895," *Bull. Soc. Soc. Hist. Med.*, December 1985, *37*: 100–107; Barron Lerner, *The Breast Cancer Wars: Fear, Hope and the Pursuit of a Cure in Twentieth-Century America* (New York: Oxford University Presss, 2001); Robert Aronowitz, "Do Not Delay: Breast Cancer and Time, 1900–1970," *Mil-bank Quart.*, 2001, *79*: 355–86. For a different view of the efficacy of Halsted's mastectomy, see James Olson, *Bathsheba's Breast: Women, Cancer, and History* (Baltimore: Johns Hopkins University Press, 2000).

11. Ernest M. Dalland, "Untreated Cancer of the Breast," *Surg. Gyn. & Obstet.*, 1927, *44*: 264–68. The untreated group included many women diagnosed with inoperable, and there-fore often more advanced, cancer—a finding that may indicate that the curative efficacy of radical mastectomy was even smaller.

late, when the tumor had already spread to lymph nodes and probably to other tissues as well. When cancer was treated early, surgeons affirmed, the results were much better. For example, the British surgeon Gordon Taylor claimed that he was able to cure surgically up to 90 percent of women with early cancer.[12] Janet Lane-Claypon's pioneering statistics of the results of breast cancer surgery confirmed these claims. According to her data, nearly 80 percent of women diagnosed with early breast cancer—that is, with small, localized tumors, without lymph-node involvement—were alive five years after a radical breast surgery. However, only about one-fifth of the women operated on for breast cancer were in this category, while four-fifths had a more advanced disease.[13]

The logical next step was the call to women to see a doctor immediately when they noticed a suspicious lump in their breast.[14] The "do not delay" message, relayed by doctors and by cancer charities, incited more women with tumors of the breast to see doctors.[15] A shift in the population of women who consulted for breast pathologies complicated in turn the diagnosis of breast malignancies: in the early twentieth century, the majority of these women suffered from an advanced disease, sometimes with dramatic manifestations, such as suppurating, painful abscesses; tumors that covered all the chest wall ("cancer *en cuirasse*"); or a breast literally "eaten by the crab." Surgery textbooks from that period enumerated the clinical signs of breast cancer: the puckering of the skin and dimples, reversal of the nipple, adhesion to the skin and the chest wall, immobility of the tumor, enlarged lymph nodes.[16]

12. R. S. Handley, "Gordon Taylor, Breast Cancer and the Middlesex Hospital," *Ann. Roy. Coll. Surg. Engl.*, 1971, *49*: 151–64.

13. Janet E. Lane-Claypon, *Report on the Late Results of Operation for Cancer of the Breast* (London: HMSO, 1928).

14. American Medical Association (AMA), Prevention of Cancer Series, leaflet no. 1 (undated); J. C. Bloodgood, *What Every One Should Know about Cancer* (AMA leaflet, undated); Aronowitz, "Do Not Delay" (n. 10).

15. Aronowitz rightly points out the absence of quantitative data on the efficacy of the "do not delay" campaigns (in terms of a reduction of cancer mortality, or a shift to the diagnosis of less-advanced tumors): Aronowitz, "Do Not Delay" (n. 10). Testimonies in medical articles seem to indicate, however, an increase in the number of women who consulted for nonmalignant or "early" lumps in their breast, at least in major cancer-treatment centers.

16. E.g., Alfred Velpeau, *Traité des maladies de sein et de la région mammaire* (Paris: Masson, 1858); Samuel W. Gross, *A Practical Treatise of Tumors of the Mammary Gland, Embracing Their Histology, Pathology, Diagnosis and Treatment* (New York: Appleton, 1880); A. Marmadike Shields, *A Clinical Treatise on Diseases of the Breast* (London: Macmillan, 1898); Handley, *Cancer of the Breast* (n. 9).

Cancer experts increasingly realized, however, that their ability to diagnose breast cancer on the basis of clinical signs was, alas, inversely proportional to their chances to cure it through surgery: the cases that were the most suitable for treatment were also those in which a differential diagnosis of cancer was the most difficult.[17] The key for therapeutic success, they believed, was the treatment of truly early cases, those that could be diagnosed only by a microscopic observation. For example, experts reported in 1913 that in Johns Hopkins Hospital, 80 percent of women who could be definitively diagnosed with breast cancer only after an exploratory incision survived for five years following the radical operation; by contrast, only 25 percent of those who underwent radical mastectomy after a diagnosis made on the basis of clinical signs of cancer survived for a similar length of time.[18]

The improvement of the results of the treatment of breast cancer, some specialists accordingly proposed, would not come from the perfection of surgical techniques, but from the improvement of diagnostic ones. "It is monumental," the British surgeon Edred Corner explained in 1908, "that, as a matter of fact, of late years every improvement in treatment has been done in the way of extending our operations, while little or nothing has been done in the way of improving our powers of diagnosis"; ideally, he proposed, cancer should be diagnosed at a microscopic stage, before the development of a fully formed tumor.[19] James Ewing, one of the leading U.S. pathologists and the founder of the American Society for the Control of Cancer, shared this view. Ewing was skeptical about the curative power of radical mastectomy in a declared breast cancer, and he proposed to concentrate instead on the surgical treatment of very early and, if possible, borderline cases. Such cases, he argued in 1913, were the only ones that offered real chances of a surgical cure.[20] The injunction to focus on the early stages of malignancy, and the strong encouragement of women to see a doctor as soon as they noticed any suspicious changes in their breast, favored the rise of systematic microscopic diagnosis of breast cancer.

17. "Discussion on the Diagnosis and Treatment of Cancer of the Breast," *Brit. Med. J.,* 1908 (October 31), 2: 970–81.

18. Joseph Colt Bloodgood, *Control of Cancer,* AMA Prevention of Cancer Series, no. 7 (text of a speech delivered by Bloodgood, 17 June 1913).

19. Edred M. Corner, in "Discussion of the Diagnosis and Treatment" (n. 17), pp. 976–77.

20. James Ewing, "Precancerous Diseases and Precancerous Lesions, Especially in the Breast," *Fourth Report of the Collis P. Huntington Fund for Cancer Research and the Memorial Hospital, 1913–14* (New York: 1913–14), 4: 1–32.

Malignant and Benign Changes in the Breast: 1880–1910

The first aim of a differential diagnosis of proliferative changes in the breast (mainly, but not exclusively, suspicious lumps) was to decide whether a given lesion was dangerous; an additional goal was to decide whether such a lesion might become dangerous later. The dominant theory of carcinogenesis in the nineteenth and twentieth centuries viewed malignant tumors as distant consequences of a trauma or a chronic irritation, which induced pathological changes in the affected tissues (inflammation, involution, hyperplasia) that in some people led to the development of true malignancies. Carcinogenesis was, however, a slow process that often took many years. Breast cancer was thus linked to the blocking of milk ducts during lactation, while the disease was more often observed in women past their reproductive years.[21]

If premalignant changes in the breast always preceded the appearance of the disease "cancer," a correct identification of such changes and their appropriate treatment could prevent malignancies. This was, however, a difficult task. Surgery textbooks provided detailed descriptions of nonmalignant breast lesions—such as cystadenoma, hyperplasia, hypertrophy, papillary adenoma, periductal fibroma, periductal sarcoma, fibromata, myxomata, abnormal involution, keloid tumors, and chronic inflammation—often with estimates of their potential to become malignant in the future.[22] But authors also insisted on the fluidity of gross and microscopic definitions, and the difficulties of rigorous differential diagnosis. "In no department of surgery," the Boston surgeon Collins Warren explained in 1905, "has the classification of the diseases of an organ or the pathological nomenclature been more confusing than it is in the diseases of the mammary gland. . . . in this case national and even local systems have added again to the confusion."[23]

Confronted with a confusing diagnostic situation, some surgeons energetically promoted radical surgery for all suspicious lesions of the breast, especially in women nearing or past menopause. A practitioner who usually sees breast cancer cases, William Rodman explained, needs to

21. Shields, *Clinical Treatise* (n. 16), p. 34.

22. Ewing, "Precancerous Diseases" (n. 20); William L. Rodman, *Diseases of the Breast with Special Reference to Cancer* (Philadelphia: Blackinson, 1908).

23. J. Collins Warren, "The Surgeon and the Pathologist: A Plea for Reciprocity as Illustrated by the Consideration of Classification and Treatment of Benign Tumors of the Breast" (talk delivered at the 56th annual session of the AMA, Portland, Ore., 11–14 July 1905; reproduced in an AMA leaflet, printed in Chicago, 1905), Dept. of Rare Books, Countway Library, Harvard Medical School, Boston, Mass.

be taught that 80 percent of all the mammary neoplasms are malignant.[24] Historians of medicine like to quote the statement made in 1903 by the Johns Hopkins surgeon Joseph Bloodgood: "in regard to tumors, lynch law is by far the better procedure than 'due process.'"[25] The depicting of Bloodgood as spokesman for the most extreme branch of surgical activism may be unfair, however: other experts criticized Johns Hopkins surgeons for their excessive caution, because they were unwilling to conduct radical mastectomies without a previous attempt at a differential diagnosis of the breast tumor.[26]

The enthusiasm for radical mastectomy for doubtful tumors of the breast was grounded in the conviction that nearly all such tumors are either malignant or "premalignant" (a term that was coined in the early twentieth century).[27] Dr. Clark Stewart grounded his argument in favor of radical surgery for all women over forty with breast pathologies on the view that linked breast cancer to inflammation: "the danger of transition of chronic cystic mastitis to adenocarcinoma is sufficient to make the removal of the whole gland advisable in all except very early, slight degrees of the affection."[28] Dr. William Jepson similarly affirmed that a large number of benign growths are really benign only temporarily: a growth in at least nine out of ten "involuted" breasts must be looked on as malignant, and the right treatment for such breasts was therefore an entire extirpation.[29]

Confronted with surgeons who assumed that every single suspect lesion of the breast should be treated by a radical mastectomy, women might have had a very good reason to hesitate to consult when they discovered a lesion. Bloodgood, his "lynch" statement notwithstanding, understood that an excessive surgical activism was in direct contradiction to the goals of the "do not delay" campaign. The solution, he proposed in 1913, was the improvement of the differential diagnosis of breast lesions. More

24. Rodman, *Diseases of the Breast* (n. 22), p. 235.

25. Joseph Colt Bloodgood, "The Relation of Surgical Pathology to Surgical Diagnosis," *Detroit Med. J.*, 1903, *3*: 337–52, on p. 338. After the demise of radical mastectomy, the "quotablity" of this sentence was greatly enhaced by an implicit parallel between the brutal treatment of blacks and of women.

26. J. Clark Stewart, "What Is the Proper Surgical Treament of Suspicious Tumors of the Involuting Breast?" *JAMA*, 1904, *53*: 365–69, on p. 366.

27. George Herbert Fink, *Cancer and Precancerous Changes* (London: Lewis, 1903), pp. 93–95.

28. Stewart, "What Is the Proper Surgical Treament" (n. 26), pp. 366–67.

29. William Jepson, "A Comment on Clark Stewart's, 'What Is the Proper Surgical Treatment of Suspicious Tumors of the Involuting Breast?'" *JAMA*, 1904, *53*: 368.

precise diagnosis would reduce the number of unnecessary radical surgeries, and would encourage women to see a doctor as rapidly as possible. This would lead in turn to the prevention of malignant tumors:

> in every location that we encounter cancer, we also meet lesions that, histologically, are not cancer. When these lesions are radically removed, we never observe recurrence or death from cancer which could be attributed to the tumor removed. . . . These lesions, which histologically are not cancer, and which are curable up to 100% by radical removal, may be called precancerous. . . . The hope for almost complete eradication of cancer rests on the recognition and the complete eradication of the precancerous lesion, whatever this may be.[30]

The key word here was "recognition." Premalignant changes and early tumors did not produce distinct clinical symptoms. Many surgeons were nevertheless confident in their ability to diagnose a true breast malignancy during a surgery, especially when they linked gross anatomical findings with previous clinical observations. One of the leading British cancer experts, Sir Harold Stiles, declared in 1908 that

> a knowledge of the histological structure of a lump in the breast is of little value for the patient unless the surgeon can associate it with a correct life-history. With this knowledge at his command, it will be very rarely necessary for the surgeon to be supported in the operating theatre by an expert pathologist armed with a freezing microtome.[31]

Other surgeons, however, such as Joseph Bloodgood, maintained that in many cases macroscopic examination of the tumor was not sufficient and the only valid diagnosis was microscopical.[32] For Sampson Handley, "the future of breast surgery rests as much with the early diagnosis of doubtful swellings by means of exploratory incision and microscopic examination as with improved methods for the extirpation of fully developed, clinical carcinoma."[33] But "exploratory incision," the precondition of the microscopic diagnosis of cancer, was problematic: some surgeons feared that the removal of a suspicious lump or a part of it, without a wide excision of surrounding tissues, might lead to the rapid spread of malignancy through the bloodstream—precisely the effect they wanted to prevent through surgery.[34] The solution to this dilemma was the generalization of the frozen section.

30. Bloodgood, *Control of Cancer* (n. 18).

31. Harold J. Stiles, "The Diagnosis and Treatment of Malignant Disease of the Breast," in "Discussion on the Diagnosis and Treatment" (n. 17), p. 973.

32. Bloodgood, *Control of Cancer* (n. 18).

33. Handley, *Cancer of the Breast* (n. 9), p. 191.

34. James Wright, "The 1917 New York Biopsy Controversy: A Question of Surgical Incision and the Promotion of Metastasis," *Bull. Hist. Med.*, 1988, *62*: 546–62.

Frozen Section in Breast Surgery and the Development of Surgical Pathology

A microscopic examination of tumor cells was perceived as a reasonably safe procedure, if the suspected lesion was superficial or if it secreted cell-containing liquid. By contrast, a "two-stage procedure"—first, a biopsy (often, the excision of the whole suspicious lump) with fixation and staining of the excised tissues (a process that took several days) and examination of the slides by a competent pathologist, and then, if the tumor was found to be malignant, a radical mastectomy—was seen, especially in the United States, as extremely dangerous. A woman who has a small, highly curable tumor and who undergoes a two-stage procedure, Bloodgood affirmed in 1913, will be almost surely doomed to death.[35] This was a vicious circle: only a careful microscopic diagnosis could spare women unnecessary radical mastectomies, but such a diagnosis was seen as too dangerous if it was not followed immediately by a radical surgery.

The answer to this dilemma was the generalization of the frozen section: suspicious tissue was frozen, sliced with a chilled microtome, fixed in formaldehyde, and rapidly stained; the subsequent microscopic examination took only a few minutes, and could be done during a surgery. If the result was positive, the surgeon changed his instruments, redraped the patient, and proceeded immediately to a radical mastectomy.[36]

Frozen section was developed in the late nineteenth century. This method, like diagnostic fixed section, was occasionally used by surgeons—hence Stilles's allusion, in 1908, to the presence of a microscopist with his microtome in the operating room. It became gradually integrated into the routine surgical diagnosis of breast cancer when an increasing proportion of patients consulted for tumors that could not be diagnosed with certainty without a microscopic examination.[37] In the 1920s, even doctors who worked in small clinics might occasionally be confronted with doubtful

35. Bloodgood, *Control of Cancer* (n. 18).

36. Samuel R. Haythor, "Advantages and Disavantages of the Frozen Section Method for the Diagnosis of Malignancy," *Reports of the William H. Singer Memorial Research Laboratory, Pittsburgh*, 1931; J. Arthur B. McGraw and Frank W. Hartman, "Present Status of Biopsy," *JAMA*, 1933, *101*: 1205–9; James Wright, "The Development of the Frozen Section Technique, the Evolution of Surgical Biopsy, and the Origins of Surgical Pathology," *Bull. Hist. Med.*, 1985, *59*: 295–326; Wright, "1917 New York Biopsy Controversy" (n. 34). Some surgeons claimed, however, that they made diagnostic biopsies of breast tumors several days before radical surgeries, with no ill results for the patients: e.g., Kenneth W. Monsarrat, in "Discussion on the Diagnosis and Treatment" (n. 17), pp. 976–77.

37. Stilles, "Diagnosis and Treatment" (n. 31); Wright, "Development of the Frozen Section Technique" (n. 36).

or borderline tumors. This shift in the population of patients increased the need for arrangements for a frozen section in all operating rooms. It also increased the demand for pathologists trained in this technique.[38] The generalization of frozen section favored close interactions between surgeons and pathologists. Surgeons' initial resistance to the microscopic diagnosis of cancer may have reflected, among other things, a fear of the loss of an essential element of their authority and its transfer to distant, anonymous experts; with the development of the frozen section, the pathologist became a direct collaborator of the surgeon and worked under surgeons' orders in the operating room. This arrangement benefited pathologists, too: their presence during surgeries allowed them to take a part in surgeons' activities, and to view themselves as experts involved in the care of living patients, not only as guardians of dead flesh.

In the late 1920s, frozen section became a "state of the art" technique in the treatment of breast tumors. Frozen and fixed sections were seen as complementary: frozen sections made possible a rapid diagnosis and an appropriate intervention; in parallel, fixed sections, systematically used to confirm and refine the initial diagnosis, favored exchanges among experts, the establishment of libraries of reference slides, and the standardization of microscopic diagnoses of cancer. The status of the frozen section as an indispensable diagnostic tool was made official by standards issued in 1930 by the American College of Surgeons, whose Committee for the Treatment of Malignant Diseases stated that

> the diagnosis of cancer in its early stages is extremely difficult and it may be impossible without an exploratory operation. In order that the patient's possibility of cure will not be jeopardized, such exploratory operation should be conducted only under such conditions that the appropriate treatment, whether by surgery or by radiation, may be carried out immediately when the diagnosis is established by the pathologist by the means of frozen section.[39]

Data from the surgical ward of New York Hospital illustrate the progress of frozen section as a norm in breast cancer surgery. In the years 1914–18, in more than 90 percent of the cases surgeons were confident in their abil-

---

38. Joseph Bloodgood, "When Cancer Becomes a Microscopic Disease, There Must Be a Tissue Diagnosis in the Operating Room," *JAMA*, 1927, *88*: 1022–23; Bloodgood, "Biopsy in the Treatment of Malignancy," *J. Clin. Lab. Med.*, 1931, *16*: 632–703; McGraw and Hartman, "Present Status of Biopsy" (n. 36); Wright, "Development of the Frozen Section Technique" (n. 36).

39. Committee for the Treatment of Malignant Diseases of the American College of Surgeons (R. B. Greenough, chairman), "Organization of a Service for Diagnosis and Treatment of Cancer," *Surg. Gyn. & Obstet.*, 1930, *51*: 570–74, on p. 572.

ity to make a diagnosis of malignancy on the basis of clinical findings and the macroscopic appearance of the tumor. Where they failed to do so, they used frozen section, indicating that at least in that hospital, experts probably did not see this technique as dangerous; it was nevertheless an exceptional procedure, systematically legitimated in surgery accounts by the undecided nature of the breast growth. In the years 1925–28 frozen section became the norm, and it was introduced into the majority of surgeries for breast tumors. Where no frozen section was made (between 15 and 20 percent of the cases), surgeons felt obliged to explain its omission by stressing that the malignacy of the tumor was evident from its gross appearance.[40]

In the 1920s and 1930s, the intransmissible knowledge of the pathologist became the cornerstone of the diagnosis of cancer:

> The major responsibility of the pathologist in this field is still the very basic, practical task of differentiating cancer from nonmalignant lesions of the breast. This can be done on a strictly empirical basis with a high degree of accuracy. A cancer is a cancer, histologically, not because it fulfills certain a priori criteria but because of its resemblance to other lesions that have proved to be clinically malignant. The criteria of malignancy vary in different sites of the body and must be modified from organ to organ. The technique is essentially that of the natural historian, or if you will, of the sophisticated bird watcher.[41]

In the 1930s, the pathologist's verdict became a key element of the diagnosis of a breast malignancy. Microscopic diagnosis could nevertheless take two forms: synchronic and diachronic. A synchronic diagnosis focused on the status of breast tissue at a given moment, and classified breast lesions into two mutually exclusive categories: malignant and non-malignant ones—that is, into those that needed to be treated immediately by radical mastectomy (or, if the lesion was judged inoperable, by radiotherapy), and those that could be treated by less drastic approaches or could be left alone. A diachronic approach attempted to evaluate whether a given lesion would become dangerous in the future, and if it would, to propose an appropriate preventive therapy.

Frozen sections were expected to distinguish malignant from nonmalignant tissue. In some cases, however, they did not yield a definitive answer. Some surgeons preferred in such cases to wait for the results of fixed section rather than to proceed immediately with a radical mastectomy. The accumulation of the results of the two-stage procedure indicated that

40. Breast Cancer files, Surgical Divisions I and II, New York Hospital, Archives of New York Hospital, New York, N.Y.

41. William H. Sternberg, "The Pathology of Breast Cancer," in *Breast Cancer*, ed. Albert Segaloff (St. Louis: Mosby, 1958), pp. 46–52, on p. 52.

earlier fears concerning this procedure were exaggerated. Janet Lane-Claypon had found in 1928 that among patients with small, localized tumors, those who underwent a two-stage surgery had a slightly better five-year survival rate than those who underwent a one-stage operation, a result that she attributed to the fact that the former often had a very early cancer.[42] Bloodgood in 1935 revoked his earlier warnings about the two-stage procedure. The danger of this procedure, he explained, was much smaller than had been thought, especially when the biopsy was combined with an irradiation of the axilla and of the wound. In the case of doubtful tumors, he said, doctors should submit slides to a number of the best microscopic diagnosticians and wait for their verdict: "this statement is absolutely the reverse of what I have advocated in previous publications, but it is forced upon me by facts, just as previous statements were."[43]

The danger of biopsy was more strongly accentuated in the United Kingdom and the United States than in France. Faced with an uncertain diagnosis of a breast tumor, experts at the Curie Foundation (the first French center that specialized in cancer treatment) did not hesitate to excise the tumor, send it to the pathology laboratory, and, if the laboratory verdict (usually given after 4–7 days) was that the tumor was malignant or borderline, to recommend a radical mastectomy. A few months' delay between lumpectomy and mastectomy was seen as dangerous, but a difference of a few days, or even a few weeks, was considered acceptable. The acceptability of the two-stage procedure, combined with surgeons' confidence in their ability to diagnose a malignancy of the breast macroscopically, may account for the relative rarity of frozen sections at the Curie Foundation in the interwar era.[44]

Confronted with increased numbers of "early" tumors, pathologists and surgeons became more aware of the complex meaning of diagnosis of a small localized tumor without lymph-node involvement. They were also more attuned to the temporary dimension of such diagnosis. French authors stressed the great heterogeneity of the entity "breast cancer," and explained that it included two categories of growths: fast-growing and highly malignant tumors, and slow-growing ones with a much more favorable prognosis.[45] The Massachusetts General Hospital surgeon Rob-

42. Lane-Claypon, *Report* (n. 13).

43. Joseph Colt Bloodgood, "Biopsy in Breast Lesions, in Relation to Diagnosis, Treatment and Prognosis," Proceedings of the Round Table Conference on Cancer, Memorial Hospital, NYC, *Ann. Surg.*, 1935, *162*: 239–49, on p. 248.

44. Breast Cancer records, 1919–39, Curie Foundation; Surgery reports, 1919–39, ibid., Department of Patients' Records, Curie Insitute, Paris.

45. Amadé Baumgarten, *Les maladies de la mammelle* (Paris: Ballière, 1908), p. 275.

ert Greenough explicitly stated that the term "early" does not necessarily refer to early detection: "'early diagnosis' of breast cancer means early in the course of disease, rather than early as measured by the duration of the symptoms in point of time. . . . taken in this sense, few of us will deny that 'early diagnosis' is by far the most significant factor in prognosis of cancer of the breast."[46] Anatomical and histological data provided a spectrum of possibilities: at one extreme was a fully malignant lesion, and at the other a fully benign one—with a wide range of intermediate possibilities in between. The great difficulty of gathering reliable information on the precise meaning of those intermediary forms contributed to the popularity of preventive surgery.

Frozen Section and Preventive Surgery

The increasing role of the pathologist in cancer diagnosis had a double effect on the treatment of breast lesions. On one hand, it helped to reduce the number of unnecessary radical mastectomies: with the generalization of a systematic microscopic study of tumors during surgery, it was impossible to maintain that 90 percent of lumps found in breasts of women over forty were malignant, or that the only answer to the finding of such lumps was a highly mutilating surgery. On the other hand, the increasing numbers of women who became persuaded by the "do not delay" campaigns to consult for suspicious lumps in the breast, combined with the generalization of cytological diagnosis of such lumps, increased in all probability the number of women diagnosed with a precancerous or borderline condition, and therefore of those who underwent surgical treatment of such a condition, often a simple mastectomy.

James Ewing championed preventive mastectomy, especially in cases of inflammation of the breast, for him an important stage in carcinogenesis. "Chronic mastitis," he explained, "is a very important predisposing condition for mammary cancer. It appears also from histological evidence that many cancers arising from chronic mastitis do not represent a wholly new process but, on the contrary, the natural result of steadily increasing epithelial overgrowth. . . . 50% of the breasts excised for cystic mastitis show pronounced precancerous changes or miniature carcinomas."[47] Such

---

46. Robert B. Greenough, "Early Diagnosis of Cancer of the Breast," Proceedings of the Round Table Conference (n. 43), *Ann. Surg.*, 1935, *102*: 233–38, on p. 238.

47. James Ewing, *Neoplastic Diseases: A Treatise on Tumors* (Philadelphia: Saunders, 1922), p. 493. Chronic mastitis was initially seen as leading nearly always to the development of a malignant tumor. Later, cystic mastitis was removed from the list of precancerous conditions, and became reclassified as moderately increasing the chances of development of

a high percentage of association between cystic mastitis and carcinoma fully legitimated for Ewing a systematic preventive surgery in each case of a definitive-grade cystic mastitis. The same rule, he proposed, should be applied for other conditions of the breast known to be associated with the ulterior appearance of malignancies.[48]

Ewing argued in parallel that partial diagnostic procedures, such as the excision of a lump or of a breast lesion, might be too dangerous. It seemed to be a safe rule to remove the whole breast when an incision is required for diagnosis: "in this field too much reliance should not be placed on the examination of resected areas and nodules . . . it is usually safer to excise the whole breast, to make the diagnosis *complete*, and to remove the source of anxiety or actual danger."[49] Ewing was skeptical about the virtues of the "complete operation" (that is, Halsted's mastectomy) in an already declared breast cancer; for him, the results usually did not justify the suffering and the mutilation induced by this operation. By contrast, he supported a "complete diagnosis"—that is, the elimination of a breast that harbored changes that could lead to the development of a malignant tumor in the future. Greenough similarly argued that in some supposedly benign lesions, such as cystic disease, an adequate gross and microscopic examination cannot be conducted without the removal of the whole breast.[50]

Drs. M. C. Tod and E. K. Dawson, from the Edinburgh Royal College of Physicians, also explained that a simple mastectomy is the best treatment for the great majority of the so-called borderline conditions of the breast. They proposed a slightly different term for this procedure: "diagnostic mastectomy." Precancerous conditions of the breast are often associated with the presence of small foci of carcinoma, and only careful analysis of the entire tissue of a breast can confirm, without any doubt, that no malignancy is present and no radical surgery is needed.[51] "Diagnostic mastectomy," Tod and Dawson concluded, is an efficient means to ensure

---

malignancy (in today's language, a moderate risk factor). See S. Warren, "The Relations of Chronic Mastitis to Carcinoma of the Breast," *Surg. Gyn. & Obstet.*, 1940, *71*: 257–62; Laureen V. Ackerman and Juan A. del Regato, *Cancer: Diagnosis, Treatment, and Prognosis* (St. Louis: Mosby, 1947), pp. 924–29. A related and partly overlapping condition, "fibrocystic breast disease," was seen as a risk element until the 1980s (and for some experts, it remains one today): Susan M. Love, R. S. Gelman, and W. Silen, "Fibrocystic 'Disease' of the Breast—A Nondisease?" *New England J. Med.*, 1982, *307*: 1010–14.

48. James Ewing, "Classification of Mammary Cancer," Proceedings of the Round Table Conference (n. 43), *Ann. Surg.*, 1935, *162*: 249–52; Ewing, *Neoplastic Diseases* (n. 47), p. 493.

49. Ewing, *Neoplastic Diseases* (n. 47), p. 541 (emphasis added).

50. Greenough, "Early Diagnosis" (n. 46).

51. M. C. Tod and E. K. Dawson, "The Diagnosis and Treatment of Doubtful Mammary Tumours," *Lancet*, 1934, *2*: 1041–45.

that premalignant lesions are not intermingled with true cancer, and is a much safer approach than the resection of the suspicious area alone. Doctors who are too anxious to avoid mastectomies may put the lives of their patients at risk: "that the psychological effect of such removal might be injurious can hardly be denied, but in our view this possibility has been allowed to weigh too heavily, and it is noteworthy that the women surgeons with whom we have discussed the matter lay little stress on this factor."[52]

The double trend—a more careful diagnostic evaluation of the necessity for a radical mastectomy, and, in parallel, an enlargement of the criteria for a simple mastectomy—may be illustrated by the treatments proposed to women with pathological changes in the breast in the Huntington Hospital, attached to Harvard Medical School, in the 1930s. Changes in the population of women that consulted for breast affections at the Huntington Hospital between 1920 and 1940 reflect the shift toward early detection of breast pathologies, a possible consequence of the "do not delay" campaigns. At the beginning of this period the great majority of the women who came to Huntington were diagnosed with an invasive breast cancer; at the end of that period, about half of them were diagnosed with benign diseases of the breast.[53] The number of patients diagnosed with invasive breast cancer remained stable between 1920 and 1940, oscillating between 80 and 100 cases per year (1937/38 was the only exception, with 136 cases). By contrast, the number of diagnoses of benign conditions of the breast increased steadily: 10 to 20 cases per year between 1920 and 1926, 40 to 60 per year between 1927 and 1936, over 80 between 1937 and 1940.

Between 1920 (the first year for which there are detailed data on treatment of tumors of the breast) and 1940 (the last year such data are available), there was a sharp rise of amputations for benign conditions of the breast, a trend that started in 1931/32. Before that date there were very few breast amputations for this indication (4 for the whole period 1920–30). The number of breast amputations increased considerably in the 1930s (Table 1), when the main indications for simple mastectomy were "cystic mastitis" or "cystic breast disease," but not "fibroadenoma," "fibroma," or "mazoplasia."[54]

52. Ibid., p. 1045.

53. The following data were collected from Annual Reports of the Harvard University Cancer Commission, Dept. of Rare Books, Countway Library, Harvard Medical School, Boston, Mass.

54. The last category, defined as a "nodular mastitis," appeared in the 1930s: there were no cases of this pathology before 1933, and 31 cases in both 1936/37 and 1937/38 (among, respectively, 81 and 87 diagnoses of benign breast conditions). The sudden prominence of

Table 1. Diagnosis of non-malignant breast disease and breast amputation,
1930–1940. Data in Annual Reports of the Harvard University
Cancer Commission, Dept. of Rare Books, Countway Library,
Harvard Medical School, Boston, Mass.

Year	No. of amputations	% of women with nonmalignant disease
1931/32	10	22%
1932/33	14	27%
1933/34	18	27%
1934/35	7	17%
1935/36	13	19%
1936/37	22	27%
1937/38	13	15%
1938/39	10	12%
1939/40	7	10%

The high proportion of simple mastectomies for benign breast disease
in the Huntington Hospital is surprising. It may reflect a pattern of recruitment (the hospital may have attracted patients with uncertain diagnoses
of breast tumors) and/or a local policy of predilection for an extensive
surgery in all the doubtful cases, especially if the patient was already on
the operating table. It may also reflect technical constraints of the frozen
section technique, as it was performed at that time. The standard procedure, when biopsy was conducted as a part of the surgery, was to pack the
wound with gauze soaked with formaldehyde while waiting for the results.
If malignancy was found, the patient was redraped, the instruments were
changed, and the surgeon proceeded with Halsted's complete operation.
If no tumor was found, it was necessary to excise all formaldehyde-soaked
tissues—that is, to make a very extensive excision—and if the tumor was
large, or the breast small, a simple mastectomy could become the only
cosmetically acceptable solution.[55] The more frequent choice to do exploratory surgeries for suspicious breast conditions, coupled with a reluctance
to use the two-stage procedure (it was no longer viewed as lethal, but in
the United States it continued to be seen as less safe than one-stage sur-

---

"mazoplasia" (a mild version of chronic mastitis) may have reflected a more finely tuned
classification of the entity "cystic mastitis" or "cystic disease," the inclusion of women earlier
classified as healthy in the category "benign breast disease," or both.

    55. Richard Joseph Behan, *Cancer, with Specific Reference to Cancer of the Breast* (St. Louis:
Mosby, 1938), pp. 330–31.

gery), may have nearly automatically led to an increase in the number of simple mastectomies.[56] Technical reasons, and not only male doctors' perception of the female breast (especially in women past their reproductive years, and presumedly past concerns about their sexual attractiveness) as a useless, nonfunctional organ, may account for the high number of mastectomies for benign growths of the breast in the 1930s.

Carcinoma in Situ—From Predictive Histology to Predictive Radiological Images

In the 1920s and 1930s pathologists acquired a greater familiarity with a wide range of breast lesions, and improved the classification and the codification of such lesions.[57] The stabilization of histological classifications of borderline breast lesions was not followed, however, by a parallel stabilization of their prognostic meaning. The gray zone of precancerous or potentially cancerous changes in the breast is a domain that continued to resist pathologists' and oncologists' attempts to firmly link cytological images with "morphological prognosis."[58] A better homogenization of histological diagnoses, pathologists and surgeons hoped, would favor quantitative and comparative studies of the distant fate of "premalignant" or "doubtful" breast lesions.[59] The latter aim was hampered, however, by the great morphological and clinical variability of breast lesions. The classification of subsets of malignant transformations of the breast, the French surgeon Pierre Masson explained, is mostly a convention, generated by the pathologist's habit of examining a limited number of slides prepared from an excised lump:

> analysis of larger sections of the breast shows, however, that breast malignancies are, as a rule, polymorphic. Fundamental, glandiform, atypical, and metaplastic forms can be found in the same breast, together with numerous intermediate forms. . . . The names that we give to these various forms may be useful for classification, but one should beware of perceiving them as truly distinct entities.[60]

56. Bloodgood, "Biopsy in Breast Lesions" (n. 43), p. 248.

57. Lerner, *Breast Cancer Wars* (n. 10), pp. 197–202.

58. Eliott Foucar, "Do Pathologists Play Dice? Uncertainty and Early Histopathological Diagnosis of Common Malignancies," *Histopath.*, 1997, *6*: 495–502; Foucar, "Predictive Genetics" (n. 3).

59. Ellis McDonald and William C. Hueper, "Cancer and the Laboratory," *J. Lab. Clin. Med.*, 1931, *16*: 713–33.

60. Pierre Masson, *Diagnostic de laboratoire: Tumeurs—Diagnostic histologique* (Paris: Maloine, 1923), p. 301.

Moreover, correlation between histological and clinical data was very problematic: "the anatomical types of the disease are so numerous, the variations in clinical course so wide, the paths of dissemination so diverse, the difficulty of determining the actual conditions so complex . . . as to render impossible in the majority of cases a reasonably accurate adjustment of means to ends."[61]

Faced with the difficulty of attributing clinical meaning to their findings, some pathologists elected to focus exclusively on transformations in breast cells. The conviction that specific cytological changes—"carcinoma in situ"—were early stages of the development of breast tumors, was grounded in an analysis of microscopic images, not in clinical data. In situ carcinomas and areas of cellular atypia were first described by pathologists who analyzed tissues removed during a mastectomy and occasionally found areas that contained modified, but not fully malignant, cells. With the generalization of biopsies, proliferative changes in breast tissue such as breast hyperplasia, atypia, lobular carcinoma in situ (LCIS), and ductal carcinoma in situ (DCIS) were also observed in intact breasts. Before the era of mammography, the observation of these conditions was nearly always accidental. Typically, a woman underwent a biopsy for a suspected lump; the lump was found to be benign, but a detailed histological analysis of the biopsy sample revealed proliferative changes in the surrounding tissue.

The first description of in situ carcinoma was made in 1932 by the pathologist Albert Broders. Broders described "a condition in which malignant epithelial cells and their progeny are found in or near positions occupied by their ancestors before the ancestors underwent malignant transformation."[62] He did not attempt to correlate this condition with clinical outcomes: its morphological characteristics, and the proximity, observed in some slides, of foci of in situ carcinoma to foci of invasive cancer, were sufficient to classify carcinoma in situ as a cancer. The failure to recognize this condition, Broders explained, is fraught with a grave danger for the patient: "if it goes unrecognized, carcinoma is allowed to masquerade as a benign or no more than precarcinomatous process, with the possibility of its becoming too far advanced to be amenable to treatment."[63] He added that a malignant but noninvasive carcinoma in situ

---

61. Ewing, *Neoplastic Diseases* (n. 47), p. 541. French authors, attuned to the heterogeneity of breast tumors, had a tendency to view attempts to correlate histological diagnoses with outcomes as hopeless. See, e.g., Pierre Hermert, "La radiothérapie dans le traitement du cancer du sein," *Paris médical,* 1936, *26*: 233–46.

62. Albert C. Broders, "Carcinoma in situ Contrasted with Benign Penetrating Epithelium," *JAMA,* 1932, *99*: 1670–74, on p. 1670.

63. Ibid., p. 1673.

should be carefully distinguished from a benign but invasive penetrating epithelium, a breast pathology associated with inflammation. The difference between malignant and nonmalignant cells, Broders concluded, is grounded in the nature of cells, not in their anatomical position: "it is therefore imperative that the microscopist take into consideration the character of the epithelial cells above everything else in order to arrive at a correct diagnosis."[64]

The description of lobular carcinoma in situ (LCIS), made by F. W. Foote and F. W. Stewart in 1941, was similarly grounded in a careful analysis of histological preparations; the condition, called "a rare form of mammary carcinoma," was, like DCIS, classified as a true malignancy on the basis of the nature of the cells involved.[65] The classification of noninvasive lesions as "carcinoma" was made possible by the redefinition of cancer as a disease of the cell.[66] Not all the cancer experts agreed, however, with an identification of the disease cancer with the transformed cancer cell. Robert Greenough argued in 1935 that one should stick to the definition of cancer as the infiltration of epithelial cells beyond the basal membrane for the ducts: "it is wise to regard anaplastic morphology of single cells or cells within their normal structural confines as evidences of hyperplasia, precancerous if you will, but not as justification for the diagnosis of cancer."[67]

The definition of "carcinoma in situ" was consolidated through standardized classifications of cancer. The American Cancer Society's *Manual of Tumor Nomenclature* of 1951 proposed a binary nomenclature, inspired by traditional biological classification: a histogenicity code that indicated the tissue from which a given neoplasm originated, and a malignancy code that described the level of malignancy of a given tumor. The first two numbers indicated the tissue of origin: for example, tumors with the first two digits 00 to 09 originated from a glandular epithelium. The last number, separated by a full stop, indicated the degree of malignancy. Tumors were graded from 1 to 9: 1 and 2 were benign tumors; 3 and 4, indeterminate; and 5 and higher, malignant. According to this classification, ductal carcinoma in situ was 00.5 and infiltrating ductal carcinoma, 00.6—a terminology that stressed the close proximity of these two conditions.[68] On the

64. Ibid., p. 1674.

65. F. W. Foote and F. W. Stewart, "Lobular Carcinoma in situ: A Rare Form of Mammary Carcinoma," *Amer. J. Surg. Path.*, 1941, *19*: 74–99; Foote and Stewart, "Comparative Studies of Cancerous versus Non-Cancerous Breasts," *Ann. Surg.*, 1945, *212*: 6–39.

66. Löwy, "Cancer—The Century of the Transformed Cell" (n. 6).

67. Greenough, "Early Diagnosis" (n. 46), p. 233.

68. American Cancer Society, *Manual of Tumor Nomenclature and Coding* (New York: ACC, 1951).

other hand, some experts continued to stress the morphological complexity of breast cancer: they criticized a linear model of carcinogenesis that did not take into consideration both the inherent capacity of neoplasm of the breast epithelium to differentiate simultaneously in several directions, and the multifocal origins of many breast carcinomas.[69]

From the 1950s to the 1980s, DCIS and LCIS were systematically treated by mastectomy. Mastectomy for DCIS was usually described as a treatment of a declared cancer. Mastectomy for LCIS was often described as a prophylactic procedure, and occasionally also as a diagnostic one. LCIS is often mutifocal, and random biopsy did not always detect its presence; simple mastectomy, some specialists argued, was a "safer and more thorough biopsy technique."[70] In the 1950s and 1960s some cancer experts, observing that women who had cancer in one breast were in greater than average danger of malignancy in the other breast, advised a preventive ablation of that breast; such preventive surgery was recommended, for example, to those with a family history of the disease. It was also recommended by some experts to women diagnosed with "good prognosis" cancers: cancers in the contralateral breast, oncologists observed, were not detected earlier than the first ones, and were often of different histological type.[71] Women diagnosed with lobular, in situ, comedo, colloid, and medullar breast tumors could benefit most from the elimination of the nonaffected breast, because a bilateral mastectomy provided them a near-complete certainty of a long-term cure.[72]

Some cancer specialists argued that since *all* the women diagnosed with breast cancer had a higher than average probability of developing a malignancy in the second breast, ideally one should propose to them a preventive ablation of the nonaffected breast, either at the same time as their radical mastectomy or a year or two after the first operation. It is unfortunate, said Robert Pollack and others, that despite its advantages, preventive mastectomy is viewed with abhorrence by many patients and

69. Sternberg, "Pathology of Breast Cancer" (n. 41), pp. 46–52.

70. John R. Benfield, Aaron G. Gingerhut, and Nancy E. Warner, "Lobular Carcinoma of the Breast, 1969," *Arch. Surg.*, 1969, *99* (2): 129–31, on p. 130.

71. The observation that cancer in the contralateral breast was not detected in an earlier stage than the first one (and occasionally, was detected in a more advanced stage) may be an indirect indication of the inefficacy of the "do not delay" campaigns, and an argument in favor of the claim that the extent of spread of a tumor is mainly related to its biological traits.

72. Forum: "When Primary Cancer of the Breast Is Treated, Should the Second Breast Be Prophylactically Removed?" *Mod. Med.*, 1966, *34*: 242–60. Bilateral mastectomies for DCIS and LCIS, and preventive mastectomies for women with a family history of breast cancer, follow a similar logic.

is not performed as frequently as it should be.[73] It is rather surprising, George Pack argued, that preventive mastectomy—that is, the removal of a nonfunctional organ—is much more strongly resisted than preventive oophorectomy: "the surgeon who knowingly removes a malignant tumor of one ovary and conserves the opposite ovary and the uterus is vulnerable to authoritative criticism, yet the sexual mutilation by bilateral oophorectomy is greater and more fundamental than by double mastectomy. By a strange paradox, women tolerate the loss of both ovaries better than the removal of both breasts."[74] For Pack, "there is no valid excuse for retention of the opposite breast if one becomes cancerous. . . . the sacrifice of a useless organ such as the remaining breast does not make the patient a functional cripple, as would the complete removal of other paired organs, such as the testes."[75]

The generalization of mammography screening in the 1970s and 1980s popularized the notion of breast cancer without a palpable lump. Thanks to this technique, preclinical tumors, once a very small proportion of cases of cancer, are now about a third of all breast cancer diagnoses.[76] The presence of cancer was dissociated from the presence of a lump. As one patient put it: "it is imperative that women become aware that no tumor does not necessarily mean no cancer. Only a mammogram can reveal what cannot be felt—the presence of deadly cancer cells."[77] Or, to be more precise, mammography reveals a suspicion of a presence of such cells, to be confirmed by a pathologist. Mammography screening drastically expanded the number of breast biopsies, which led in turn to an important increase in diagnoses of in situ cancers—especially of DCIS, both deliberate (DCIS can be visible on a mammogram as a cluster of microcalcifications) and accidental, when the biopsy is made for a different reason.

Before the generalization of mammography, DCIS was a rare, accidental, diagnosis. Since the introduction of mammography, 12 to 15 percent of women treated for breast cancer are diagnosed with DCIS, and in

73. Robert S. Pollack, *Treatment of Breast Tumors* (Philadelphia: Lea & Feibiger, 1958), pp. 83–84; Walter L. Mersheimer, "The Problem of Second Primary Breast Cancer," *CA—Cancer J. Clin.*, January–February 1966, pp. 33–35; Henry Patrick Leis, "Prophylactic Removal of the Second Breast," *Hosp. Med.*, January 1968, pp. 45–49.

74. George T. Pack, "Editorial: Argument for Bilateral Mastectomy," *Surgery*, 1952, *29*: 929–31, on p. 930.

75. Ibid., p. 931.

76. Vivianne Le Doussal, "Trente ans de pratique en pathologie mammaire dans un centre anti-cancéreux," *Annales de pathologie*, 2003, *23*: 486–91.

77. Joanne Lyeck, "Breast Cancer in the Family," *Plus Magazine*, March 2004, pp. 38–39.

more than 90 percent of these women, the diagnosis is made by mammography.[78] The treatment for this condition is, as a rule, highly successful; the survival rates of DCIS patients are very high irrespective of the treatment they receive (lumpectomy or mastectomy).[79] This is not a new finding: Bloodgood had already observed that all the patients diagnosed with "borderline tumors of the breast" survived, independently of their treatment; "the surprising finding was that they lived no matter what the operation or the diagnosis was. . . . in 1915, *I gathered this group together and removed it from the group of cancers in the breast in which the glands were not (microscopically) involved.* The withdrawal of the borderline group reduced the five-year cures from 85 to 70 percent."[80]

The systematic treatment of DCIS (today mainly by lumpectomy and radiation) is compared to the systematic surgical treatment of cervical dysplasia.[81] This comparison may be inaccurate: Experts agree that the great majority of cervical tumors pass through a detectable dysplasia phase.[82] The causal relationships between DCIS and invasive breast cancer are more controversial.[83] Moreover, the important reduction in the incidence of cervical cancer is usually attributed to a systematic treatment of cervical dysplasia, while population-based data indicate that the treatment of DCIS has only a marginal effect on the overall incidence of invasive breast cancer.[84] Doubts about the contribution of DCIS therapy to the

78. David P. Winchester, Jan M. Jeske, and Robert A. Goldschmidt, "The Diagnosis and Management of Ductal Carcinoma in situ of the Breast," *CA—Cancer J. Clin.*, 2000, *50* (3): 184–200.

79. Michael D. Lagios, "DCIS: Current Concepts in Diagnosis and Management," *Breast J.*, 2003, *9* (Suppl. 1): s22–s24; Harold J. Burstein, Kornelia Polyak, Julia S. Wong, et al., "Ductal Carcinoma in situ of the Breast," *New England J. Med.*, 2004, *350*: 1430–41.

80. Bloodgood, "Biopsy in the Treatment of Malignancy" (n. 38), p. 701 (italics added). The classification of borderline tumors of the breast changed over time, and it is very difficult to determine what present-day lesions correspond to the ones described by Bloodgood.

81. Experts no longer recommend systematic mastectomy for DCIS, but this diagnosis is still more frequently considered as an absolute indication for a mastectomy than an invasive tumor: 33 percent of patients with stage 0 tumor are seen as having absolute counterindications for breast-conserving surgery, versus 10 percent of those with stage 1 cancers. See Monique Morrow, C. Bucci, and A. Rademaker, "Medical Contraindications Are Not a Major Factor in the Underutilization of Breast-Conserving Surgery," *J. Amer. Coll. Surg.*, 1998, *186*: 269–74.

82. One should remember, however, that the opposite is not true: the great majority of cervical dysplasias do not evolve to a malignancy.

83. Elliot Foucar, "Carcinoma in situ of the Breast: Have Pathologists Run Amok?" *Lancet*, 1996, *347*: 707–8.

84. S. W. Duffy, L. Tabar, B. Vitak, et al., "The Relative Contributions of Screen-Detected in situ and Invasive Breast Carcinomas in Reducing Mortality from the Disease," *Eur. J. Canc.*, 2003, *39*: 1755–60.

reduction of breast cancer mortality did not, however, affect the norm of a systematic therapy of this condition, and DCIS was presented as a "gold standard," the lesion against which all the other breast lesions need to be compared.[85] The precise correlation of observed changes in cells and tissues to clinical developments remains nevertheless problematic.[86] According to a 2004 review, advances in molecular biology confirm that DCIS is indeed a stage in the development of an invasive breast cancer, strengthening the arguments in favor of a systematic treatment of this condition. In parallel, this review states that "after 10 years of follow-up, *14 to 60 percent* of the women who underwent diagnostic biopsy alone received a diagnosis of invasive cancer in the affected breast"; it is not surprising that the authors conclude that "treatment choices are complicated by the varied clinical behavior of ductal carcinoma in situ."[87]

Recently, in situ cancers and atypia were linked with a hereditary predisposition to breast cancer. Pathologists reported unusually high levels of histological abnormalities (DCIS, LCIS, atypical ductal hyperplasia [ADH], and atypical lobular hyperplasia [ALH]) in the breast tissue of BRCA-positive women.[88] The translation of "molecular lesions" into morphological ones transformed the preventive amputation of healthy organs into an elimination of flawed, and potentially diseased, ones, and reinforced the case for preventive mastectomy for BRCA-positive women. It also constructed a solid bridge between genetic and morphological prediction. In the mid-1990s, the description of mutations that increase the susceptibility to breast cancer was accompanied by the hope of a rapid development of therapies able to neutralize the effects of mutated genes. Ten years later, this hope has not materialized (yet). In the meantime, prophylactic surgery was recognized as the most effective preventive measure

85. David L. Page, "Breast Lesions, Pathology and Cancer Risk," *Breast J.*, 2004, *10* (Suppl. 1): s3–s4.

86. Edwin R. Fisher, "Pathobiological Considerations Relating to the Treatment of Ductal Carcinoma in situ of the Breast," *CA—Cancer J. Clin.*, 1996, *47* (1): 52–64; Winchester, Jeske, and Goldschmidt, "Diagnosis and Management" (n. 78).

87. Burstein et al., "Ductal Carcinoma" (n. 79), p. 1433.

88. K. K. Khurana, A. Losmann, P. J. Numann, and S. A. Khan, "Prophylactic Mastectomy: Pathological Findings in High Risk Patients," *Arch. Path. Lab. Med.*, 2000, *124*: 378–81; N. Hoogerbrugge, P. Bult, L. M. de Widt-Levert, et al., "High Prevalence of Premalignant Lesions in Prophylactically Removed Breasts from Women at Hereditary Risk for Breast Cancer," *J. Clin. Oncol.*, 2003, *21* (1): 41–45; N. D. Kauf, E. Brogi, L. Scheurer, et al., "Epithelial Lesions in Prophylactic Mastectomy Specimens from Women with BRCA Mutations," *Cancer*, 2003, *97*: 1601–8; C. Adem, C. Reynolds, C. L. Soderberg, et al., "Pathological Characteristics of Breast Parenchyma in Patients with Hereditary Breast Carcinoma, Including BRCA1 and BRCA2 Mutation Carriers," ibid., pp. 1–11.

that can be proposed to women at high risk of breast cancer—even in countries such as France, where this approach was initially strongly resisted by oncologists.[89] In 2007, too, experts continue to believe that the most effective way to deal with uncertainty is to cut it out.

❖

ILANA LÖWY is a senior research fellow at INSERM. Her address is: CERMES, 7 rue Guy Môquet, 94801 Villejuif Cedex, France (e-mail: lowy@vjf.cnrs.fr). Her research interests include the history of bacteriology, immunology, virology, and oncology; relationships between the laboratory and the clinics; the history of tropical medicine; and intersections between gender studies and biomedicine. Her most recent book, *L'emprise de genre: Masculinité, féminité, inégalité* (Paris: La Dispute, 2006), investigates the consequences of the asymmetric construction of immanent attributes of masculinity and femininity on the maintaining of women's subordinated status. Her current research focuses on the history of "precancer" and of the efforts to prevent the development of malignant tumors.

89. Timothy Rebbeck, H. T. Lynch, S. L. Neuhasen, et al., "Prophylactic Oophorectomy in Carriers of BRCA 1 and BRCA 2 Mutations," *New England J. Med.*, 2002, *346*: 1616–22; François Eisinger, Brigitte Bressac, Damienne Castaigne, et al., "Identification et prise en charge des prédispositions héréditaires aux cancers du sein et de l'ovaire: Mise à jour, 2004," *Bulletin du cancer*, 2004, *91* (3): 219–37.

From Cancer Families to HNPCC: Henry Lynch and the Transformations of Hereditary Cancer, 1975–1999

RAUL NECOCHEA

SUMMARY: Hereditary non-polyposis colorectal cancer (HNPCC) helps us understand how medical genetics has changed over the last forty years. The concept of the "cancer family" emerged from the realization that members of some families developed cancer more frequently than members of others, which led to a series of strategies by clinicians in the 1960s to persuade others of this. By the early 1990s molecular genetics had transformed the disease, from one that a few physicians believed ran in families, to one with precise genetic components that researchers generally accepted, and that could be detected through genetic tests. Nevertheless, a diagnosis of HNPCC still requires that the mutated genes be found within a kin group that is generally accepted as a cancer family. Moreover, the "cancer family" construct was crucial in the search for the HNPCC genes. HNPCC's trajectory can be mapped onto important debates about the complex relations between clinical and molecular genetics knowledge and practice.

KEYWORDS: HNPCC, genetics, colorectal cancer, family medical pedigree

In the last forty years, hereditary non-polyposis colorectal cancer (HNPCC), also known as the Lynch syndrome, has grown from clinical nonentity to well-defined disease. The standard story of this shift, from poorly recognized or even nonexistent ailment to one whose existence and mode of transmission are clinically beyond doubt, is generally told as one of the

This research was funded in part through U.S. National Institutes of Health contract #263MQ311650. David Cantor, John Krige, Steven Vallas, Maren Klawiter, Asad Umar, Andrea Tone, and the *Bulletin*'s reviewer provided crucial insights and encouragement. Drafts have been presented at the annual meeting of the American Association for the History of Medicine, Madison, Wisc., 2 May 2004; and the American Sociological Association, San Francisco, Calif., 2004. Drs. Henry Lynch, Jukka-Pekka Mecklin, Richard Boland, Bert Vogelstein, Albert de la Chapelle, Annika Lindblom, Lauri Aaltonen, Nickolas Nicolaides, and Nicholas Papadopoulos have generously given their time to share their experiences working on cancer genetics.

triumphs of molecular genetics. In this story, the identification of particular genes associated with HNPCC transformed biomedical attitudes toward this disease, and ended years of doubt about its existence and nature. It is a tale of a transition from doubt to certainty, from statistical speculations to solid science, and from the collection of family histories to molecular genetics. It is also a story of the vindication of Henry Lynch, the man who had championed HNPCC since the 1960s, and whose claims about the disease's hereditary nature were doubted by the cancer establishment for decades. In this paper I argue that the story is more complicated. I claim that a preexisting concept, the "cancer family," drawn from research done with family histories in the 1960s, was crucial to the search for the HNPCC genes in the 1990s. Moreover, a diagnosis of HNPCC still requires that the mutated genes responsible for HNPCC be linked back to a kin group that is generally accepted as a "cancer family."

This, then, is a story of the complex interactions of molecular genetics and earlier traditions of medical genetics based on the collection of family pedigrees. In this paper I make three arguments. First, molecular genetics was crucial in the transformation of hereditary cancers, from diseases that only a few physicians believed in and that could be detected through family pedigrees, to diseases with precise genetic components that could be detected through genetic tests. Focusing on HNPCC, I will show how its acceptance as a medical entity today is inextricably bound to the discovery of a few genes, collectively known as "mismatch repair genes," in the early 1990s. During this decade it became possible to link specific genes to particular cancers for the first time, and to calculate the statistical risk of succumbing to cancer for those bearing the genes. At the same time, and this is my second argument, molecular genetics techniques were not simply applied to cancer research: in HNPCC, these techniques interacted with a longer tradition of cancer detection and prevention based on the elaboration of family medical pedigrees. The 1960s "cancer family" construct, in particular, was crucial to the search for the above-mentioned mismatch repair genes. Moreover, the family history is still key to the contemporary diagnosis of HNPCC. Finally, I also argue that the impetus for much of this research was clinical. Lynch's interest in hereditary cancers was inspired, in part, by a search for ways to improve cancer control, and this clinical interest sustained his research endeavors in this field despite considerable opposition to his methods from the cancer establishment. It was only in the early 1990s, with growing clinical interest in HNPCC and the identification of mismatch repair genes, that Lynch's efforts to improve control gained wider acceptance.

The "Cancer Family" in Nebraska

Henry Lynch's interest in cancer and heredity began in the early 1960s, shortly after his arrival in Omaha, Nebraska, where he held posts at the University of Nebraska College of Medicine and the Eppley Institute for Research in Cancer and Allied Diseases. He joined the faculty of the Creighton University School of Medicine in 1967, where he remains today. In 1962 or 1964 a gastroenterologist at the Omaha Veterans Administration Hospital requested that Lynch consult on a patient with a strong family history of colorectal cancer. The gastroenterologist suspected that familial adenomatous polyposis (FAP) would be the likely diagnosis, since FAP was the only known hereditary disorder predisposing to colorectal cancer. However, when Lynch drew a detailed pedigree, he found the strong tendency for colorectal cancer in the family to exist in the absence of multiple colonic polyps (which characterize FAP). Lynch presented his findings at a meeting of the American Society of Human Genetics in 1964. The story goes that his presentation reminded Marjorie Shaw, a medical geneticist at the University of Michigan, Ann Arbor, of another family with similar genetic and clinical traits. In 1966, Shaw, Lynch, and other colleagues published their first report on the two families—family N from Nebraska, and family M from Michigan.[1] This was the beginning of Lynch's long-standing interest in what would come to be known as "cancer family syndrome" (CFS), now "hereditary non-polyposis colorectal cancer," or "Lynch syndrome." For Lynch, the term "cancer family syndrome" referred to the particular features he observed among members of these families, which included a high occurrence of adenocarcinomas of multiple anatomical sites (most frequently in the endometrium and colon), multiple primary malignant neoplasms, an early age at onset, and autosomal dominant inheritance.[2]

As David Cantor has argued, when Lynch identified CFS in Nebraskan families he saw this as an opportunity to improve cancer control. In his view, the identification of a hereditary cancer in one family member allowed physicians to target other family members for signs of the disease, and so to identify cancers at an earlier stage than was hitherto possible.[3] Early detection and treatment was the dominant approach to cancer

---

1. Henry Lynch, Marjorie Shaw, Charles Magnuson, Arthur Larsen, and Anne Krush, "Hereditary Factors in Cancer," *Arch. Internal Med.*, 1966, *117*: 206–12.

2. Henry Lynch, "Heredity and Cancer," *Nebraska State Med. J.*, 1969, *54*: 298–99.

3. David Cantor, "The Frustrations of Families: Henry Lynch, Heredity and Cancer Control, 1962–1975," *Med. Hist.*, 2006, *50*: 279–302.

control in the 1960s,[4] but Lynch's efforts to improve early detection and treatment were not greeted with the enthusiasm he might have hoped for. First, many physicians and scientists doubted his claim to have identified a new form of hereditary cancer, arguing that he had not taken adequate account of environmental or viral factors in his studies of cancer families, and that his results could be accounted for by chance clusters of cancer or by bias. Second, for years cancer experts had sought to discredit popular beliefs that cancer was a hereditary disease, fearing that they promoted complacency about or paralytic fear of cancer, and encouraged individuals to delay seeking qualified medical help until the best opportunities for effective treatment were no longer viable. To his critics, Lynch's focus on hereditary cancers threatened to perpetuate these problems, and consequently to undercut the very programs of control that he sought to improve. During the 1960s and 1970s, therefore, his efforts to promote CFS as a hereditary disease were not very successful.

From Cancer Family Syndrome to HNPCC

Despite his initial failure to ignite medical and scientific enthusiasm, Lynch's research on the cancer family syndrome continued through the mid-1970s and 1980s and focused on finding a reliable genetic marker for the disease before it struck. His work was that of a clinician treating patients on a day-to-day basis. The immediate concern was to make the CFS a distinct entity—separate, especially, from the classic type of hereditary colorectal cancer known as familial adenomatous polyposis.[5] FAP was characterized by the presence of hundreds of polyps blanketing the rectal and sigmoid areas of the colon—that is, the areas closest to the anus. Cancer developed from these polyps years after they first appeared. Moreover, the polyps themselves were easy to spot with a sigmoidoscopy, and easy to remove as well. Thanks to the lengthy clinical experience with FAP, the polyp-covered rectal and sigmoid areas had become such reliable biological markers of a future colorectal cancer that other physicians were very skeptical about hereditary cancer emerging when there was no polyposis. Therefore, much of Lynch's subsequent work on colorectal cancer went both into documenting more cases of the disease that emerged from a paucity of polyps and into looking for a biological marker that was as reliable as the polyp-covered rectum.

4. Robert Aronowitz, "Do Not Delay: Breast Cancer and Time," *Milbank Quart.*, 2001, 79: 355–86.
5. Paolo Palladino, "Between Knowledge and Practice: On Medical Professionals, Patients, and the Making of the Genetics of Cancer," *Soc. Stud. Sci.*, 2002, 32: 137–65.

By the late 1970s, a few other physicians had become interested in this intriguing type of cancer. One of them was Richard Boland, then completing his studies at the Yale School of Medicine; another was Jukka-Pekka Mecklin, then working on his dissertation at the Medical Faculty of the University of Helsinki. Upon independently contacting Lynch, each received a warm welcome to work on the subject, and also access to the cancer family data that Lynch had been collecting for years. In 1984, Boland suggested renaming CFS the "Lynch syndrome" in honor of Henry Lynch,[6] a term still used. The name "HNPCC" also began to be used in the mid-1980s.[7]

From the 1960s to the 1980s the number of reported CFS families increased in Europe and the United States. Without including Henry Lynch's numerous publications, three articles on this subject were published between 1967 and 1969, eleven in the 1970s, and twenty-one in the 1980s.[8] In 1983, the Johns Hopkins Hospital alone had a registry of eighty CFS families.[9] Moreover, by the mid-1980s a small cohort of physicians—including gastroenterologists Giuseppe Cristofaro in Brindisi, Italy, and Paul Rozen in Tel Aviv, Israel, in addition to Boland and Mecklin—was convinced of the greater number of non-polyposis colorectal-cancer cases relative to the polyposis cases in the family data they had collected.[10] Their autonomous efforts meant that more "cancer families" were being identified, now in different parts of the world. The slow but steady pattern of growth in interest in CFS indicates that, despite facing considerable opposition, Lynch's propositions did not always meet antagonism and hostility from the cancer establishment. Although not mainstream, these ideas were not entirely marginalized, and over time they began to reach a sympathetic audience, composed mainly of clinicians who, like Lynch, were committed to improving interventions in cancer control.

6. C. Richard Boland and Frank J. Troncale, "Familial Colonic Cancer Without Antecedent Polyposis," *Ann. Internal Med.*, 1984, *100*: 700–701.

7. Asad Umar, Richard Boland, Jonathan Terdiman, et al., "Revised Bethesda Guidelines for Hereditary Nonpolyposis Colorectal Cancer (Lynch Syndrome) and Microsatellite Instability," *J. Natl. Cancer Inst.*, 2004, *96*: 261–68.

8. See Fig. 1 and Jukka-Pekka Mecklin, "Cancer Family Syndrome: Studies on the Hereditary Nonpolypous Colorectal Carcinoma Syndrome" (medical diss., University of Helsinki, 1987). I gratefully acknowledge Dr. Mecklin's generous sharing of his dissertation.

9. Anne Krush, "Research Efforts in Hereditary Intestinal Polyposes and Cancer of the Gastrointestinal Tract," *Dis. Colon & Rectum*, 1983, *26*: 399–400.

10. Henry Lynch, "Frequency of Hereditary Nonpolyposis Colorectal Carcinoma (Lynch Syndromes I and II)," *Gastroenterology*, 1986, *90*: 486–89; Henry Lynch, Thomas Smyrk, and Jane Lynch, "Molecular Genetics and Clinical-Pathology Features of Hereditary Nonpolyposis Colorectal Carcinoma (Lynch Syndrome)," *Oncology*, 1998, *55*: 103–8.

In addition to documenting more cases of the disease that emerged from a paucity of polyps, CFS researchers in the late 1970s had a parallel task: locating a biological marker for CFS that was as reliable as the polyp-covered rectum was for FAP. This task was considerably more difficult, and success dodged them for another decade.[11] Researchers tested carcinoembryonic antigen, skin fibroblast tetraploidies, mucosal proliferation indexes, lectin from *Amaranthus caudatus*, and other assays in hopes that one of these could work as a marker that might some day single out specific people for cancer surveillance. Their search for markers, again, indicates strongly that their main concern was clinical: treating patients whom they knew personally, not necessarily finding an ultimate cause of cancer at the molecular level. In fact, for people like Lynch, Boland, and Mecklin one of the most valuable outcomes of finding a reliable marker would have been to develop more-sensitive and less-invasive screening technologies (as opposed to the dreaded and expensive colonoscopy) in order to minimize the discomfort and pain of patients who were under surveillance, to assess risk more accurately within a cancer family so that not all its members would have to submit to the harsh surveillance regime, and to make the risk-assessment tools themselves less expensive to use. Even as the researchers delved more deeply into the territory of molecular genetics to identify markers, they had not stopped relying on the collection of patient histories and the construction of cancer family pedigrees. Yet as the early CFS researchers became more conversant in the language of recombinant DNA, and as they developed research alliances with molecular geneticists, the field increasingly focused on the search for genes "responsible" for CFS.

By the mid-1980s there were quite a few researchers trying to characterize CFS at the molecular level. However, further work was difficult because of the lack of a uniform definition of the disease. The fact that many used the terms "cancer family syndrome," "hereditary non-polyposis colorectal cancer," and "Lynch syndrome" interchangeably was symptomatic of this. The 1989 International Conference on Gastrointestinal Cancer in Jerusalem provided a venue for Drs. Paul Rozen and Henry Lynch to address the lack of a standard definition. The next year, in August 1990, thirty researchers met in Amsterdam for that purpose. This group was the basis of the International Collaborative Group on Hereditary Non-Polyposis

11. Henry Lynch, Claude Organ, Jr., Randall Harris, Hoda Guirgis, Patrick Lynch, and Jane Lynch, "Familial Cancer: Implications for Surgical Management of High-Risk Patients," *Surgery*, 1978, *83*: 104–13; Henry Lynch, Paul Rozen, and Guy Schuelke, "Hereditary Colon Cancer: Polyposis and Nonpolyposis Variants," *CA—Cancer J. Clin.*, 1985, *35*: 95–114.

Colorectal Cancer (ICG-HNPCC). The researchers reached a consensus about the defining features of HNPCC, which came to be known as the Amsterdam Criteria: (1) at least two relatives of a person with cancer should also have laboratory-confirmed colorectal cancer; (2) one of the relatives had to be a first-degree relative of the primary patient; (3) at least two successive generations in the family should be affected; (4) one of the relatives should be diagnosed before age fifty; and (5) the diagnosis must rule out the possibility of familial adenomatous polyposis. The ICG also emphasized that early detection was crucial: members of families in which hereditary cancer was suspected should have colonoscopies or sigmoidoscopies combined with a barium enema every two years, starting at age twenty-five. Just as significantly, the term "cancer family syndrome" was less and less used from then on, and the term "hereditary non-polyposis colorectal cancer" gained more purchase because of the specificity of the pathology it described.[12]

But the Amsterdam Criteria did not go unchallenged. Early on, a group of Italian researchers from Rome and Modena considered the criteria too strict to be helpful in determining which families should be considered for studies and for clinical surveillance. For one thing, some families that the Italian researchers thought of as candidates for further study were too small to have three or more relatives at all, let alone three that had cancer. More importantly, the critics argued that the Amsterdam Criteria unfairly excluded tumors outside the colon as part of the expression of HNPCC. Instead, they suggested that colorectal, endometrial, stomach, laryngeal, kidney, or urinary tract cancers in two consecutive generations could work as a set of alternative criteria.[13] The mounting criticism led to a modification of the Amsterdam Criteria in 1999, and their renaming as the "Amsterdam II Criteria." Accordingly, certain hereditary cancers were considered "HNPCC-related extracolonic cancers," such as those occurring in the endometrium, small bowel, ureter, and renal pelvis. The remaining criteria remained unchanged.[14]

12. Henry Lynch, Giuseppe Cristofaro, Paul Rozen, et al., "History of the International Collaborative Group on Hereditary Nonpolyposis Colorectal Cancer," *Fam. Cancer*, 2003, 2: 1–3; Hans Vasen, Jukka-Pekka Mecklin, P. Meehra Khan, and Henry Lynch, "The International Collaborative Group on Hereditary Non-Polyposis Colorectal Cancer (ICG-HNPCC)," *Dis. Colon & Rectum*, 1991, *34*: 424–25.

13. Maurizio Ponz de Leon, "Prevalence of Hereditary Nonpolyposis Colorectal Carcinoma (HNPCC)," *Ann. Med.*, 1994, *26*: 209–14.

14. C. Eng, H. Hampel, and A. de la Chapelle, "Genetic Testing for Cancer Predisposition," *Ann. Rev. Med.*, 2001, *52*: 371–400.

Another criticism of the 1991 Amsterdam Criteria was that they did not offer much guidance on how clinicians could incorporate the knowledge of HNPCC genes into diagnosis when they began to be discovered after 1993, a process I discuss in detail in the next section. This was why some researchers—led by Miguel Rodriguez-Bigas, a surgeon at Roswell Park Cancer Institute in Buffalo, New York—with support from the National Cancer Institute, the American Joint Commission on Cancer, and the ICG-HNPCC, met in Rockville, Maryland, in 1996 to produce more "genetically oriented" criteria to diagnose HNPCC. What came to be known as the "Bethesda Criteria" took the Amsterdam Criteria as their departure point; should they be met, physicians must then test the tumor for "genetic instability," a trait I describe below. Although genetic instability occurred in some sporadic colon cancers, most HNPCC tumors were deemed genetically unstable. If the tumor were deemed genetically unstable, this would justify a full test for mutations in one of the HNPCC genes.[15] However, a negative genetic instability test did not rule out the possibility of HNPCC. Conversely, a positive instability test did not imply a positive diagnosis of HNPCC, but rather called for additional forms of genetic testing that were more expensive and difficult than instability tests.[16]

The Mismatch Repair Genes

Between 1991 and 1999—that is, between the development of the two Amsterdam consensus definitions of HNPCC—two groups of researchers, at Johns Hopkins University and at the University of Helsinki, reported finding the first gene locus strongly linked to the expression of HNPCC. Shortly after, a group of Swedish researchers at the Karolinska Institute reported a second locus also linked to HNPCC. These discoveries led to the subsequent characterization of the genes and the development of tests to find them. It is now widely believed that these two genes account for most cases of HNPCC.[17]

The collaboration that led to the discovery of the first gene involved in HNPCC started when Bert Vogelstein of Johns Hopkins and Albert de la Chapelle of the University of Helsinki joined forces after a meeting in

15. Bob Kuska, "New Diagnostic Criteria for HNPCC Are on the Way," *J. Nat. Cancer Inst.*, 1997, *89*: 11–12.

16. Eng, Hampel, and de la Chapelle, "Genetic Testing" (n. 14).

17. See Minna Nystrom-Lahti, Ramon Parsons, Pertti Sistonen, et al., "Mismatch Repair Genes on Chromosomes 2p and 3p Account for a Major Share of Hereditary Nonpolyposis Colorectal Cancer Families Evaluable by Linkage," *Amer. J. Hum. Genet.*, 1994, *55*: 659–65.

the early 1990s in Kobe, Japan, between Vogelstein and a colleague of de la Chapelle's. The data for these researchers' experiments came from cancer family pedigrees and tissue samples that the collaborators gathered in Canada, New Zealand, and Finland. Because of the rarity of cancer families, the researchers had to rely, in turn, on clinical and epidemiological data collected by others: Jane Green for the Canadian family, Jeremy Jass for the New Zealand family, and Jukka-Pekka Mecklin for the Finnish family. The first genetic linkage analyses did not indicate any evidence of linkage between HNPCC and any part of the genome the researchers focused on. Was colorectal cancer a common enough disease that familial aggregations such as those revealed by the cancer family pedigrees could happen by chance alone?[18] The collaborators shifted their strategy and decided to look more thoroughly at genetic regions not well covered in the initial linkage analyses, and found an association between HNPCC and a region on chromosome 2. That genetic locus would eventually be named MSH2.[19]

Meanwhile, a team of Swedish researchers led by Annika Lindblom of the Karolinska Institute performed genetic analyses on genomic regions of blood samples from three Swedish cancer families that they had collected for this purpose. Lindblom had been studying familial colorectal cancers approximately since 1980 and, fittingly, she had amassed a significant data set.[20] By the early 1990s, she was convinced that different families could have different HNPCC genes and that, therefore, it was better to perform linkage analyses using genetic materials from single large families than to combine samples from many families.[21] Her strategy paid off: shortly after Vogelstein and de la Chapelle reported the locus on chromosome 2, the Swedish researchers reported that a second locus was linked to HNPCC, on chromosome 3. That locus would eventually be dubbed MLH1.[22]

The loci for MSH2 and MLH1 had two features in common. First, they had been found in the analysis of tumors extracted from people who belonged to a "cancer family," as defined by the 1991 Amsterdam Criteria. Second, the effect of a mutation in either of the loci was the failure to repair mismatches in a sequence of nucleotides during normal cell

18. Telephone interview with Bert Vogelstein, 12 August 2005.

19. Päivi Peltomäki, Lauri Aaltonen, Pertti Sistonen, et al., "Genetic Mapping of a Locus Predisposing to Human Colorectal Cancer," *Science*, 1993, *260*: 810–12.

20. Annika Lindblom, correspondence with author, 8–12 July 2005.

21. Ibid., 18 August 2006.

22. Annika Lindblom, Pia Tannergård, Barbro Werelius, and Magnus Nordenskjöld, "Genetic Mapping of a Second Locus Predisposing to Hereditary Non-Polyposis Colon Cancer," *Nature Genet.*, 1993, *5*: 279–82.

reproduction; this is why the genes would later be collectively referred to as "mismatch repair genes." HNPCC researchers had considered mismatch repair an area of interest for familial colorectal cancer since at least 1993.[23] However, when the loci were found, their discoverers were not yet completely aware of the function of either. In fact, the very names "MSH2" and "MLH1" were derived from a crucial clue from other geneticists who focused on yeast, and who had shown that a similar kind of genetic mismatch in those organisms was caused by the mutated yeast mismatch repair genes called MSH2 and MLH1. Normally, the yeast mismatch repair enzyme corrected replication errors that could otherwise pile up on the DNA molecule, just as the typos in an essay could add up to an unreadable text. Genetic mismatches in some human colorectal cancers, the yeast geneticists suggested, could be the result of a mutation in a human homologue of the yeast mismatch repair enzyme—that is, in the human DNA's ability to correct its own replication mistakes during each cell cycle.[24] At the time, the main working assumption among cancer geneticists was that certain genes acted as tumor suppressors; the discovery of a different mechanism for human cancer development, that of mismatch repairs, was so radical that Daniel Koshland, editor of *Science*, called the mismatch repair enzyme the "molecule of the year."[25]

Once the location of the genes on chromosomes 2 and 3 was generally accepted, and once a specific function for these genes was proposed, a short and intense race to characterize and clone the genes began. At this point, new players joined too: a group of geneticists who had substantial expertise not only in cancer biochemistry, but also in the process of mismatch repair in general. This group included scientists like Manuel Perucho, Richard Kolodner, Stephen Thibodeau, Paul Modrich, Tom Petes, and Michael Liskay.[26] Numerous collaborations took place between these and more HNPCC-seasoned researchers. At the same time, the competition was intense, particularly for understanding the effects of genetic

23. Lauri Aaltonen, Päivi Peltomäki, Fredrick Leach, et al., "Clues to the Pathogenesis of Familial Colorectal Cancer," *Science*, 1993, *260*: 812–16.

24. Micheline Strand, Tomas Prolla, Michael Liskay, and Thomas Petes, "Destabilization of Tracts of Simple Repetitive DNA in Yeast by Mutations Affecting DNA Mismatch Repair," *Nature*, 1993, *365*: 274–76.

25. Daniel Koshland, "Molecule of the Year: The DNA Repair Enzyme," *Science*, 1994, *266*: 1925.

26. See C. Richard Boland, Stephen Thibodeau, Stanley Hamilton, et al., "A National Cancer Institute Workshop on Microsatellite Instability for Cancer Detection and Familial Predisposition: Development of International Criteria for the Determination of Microsatellite Instability in Colorectal Cancer," *Cancer Res.*, 1998, *58*: 5248–57.

mismatch. Within the next few months, the human mismatch repair genes MSH2 and MLH1 had been located, described, and cloned, and reports about similar findings made their way to top scientific journals, often within a few weeks of one another.[27]

Several other gene loci related to HNPCC were discovered within a few years after 1993, which were later dubbed PMS1, PMS2, MSH3, MLH3, and MSH6.[28] Unlike MSH2 and MLH1, however, these other gene loci were not found through linkage analyses. Rather, after MLH1 and MSH2 were shown to have a mismatch repair function, researchers probed other loci with similar functions. When mutations were found in them, they were associated with HNPCC, but this did not necessarily prove a strong causative relation. Thus, it has been more difficult to specify their connection to the disease.

By 1994, the number of articles dealing with HNPCC had increased exponentially (see Fig. 1), but some key issues were still being sorted out. Nomenclature was problematic, for the effect of the mismatch repair genes received different names: "microsatellite instability," "the RER phenotype," "ubiquitous somatic mutations," and "microsatellite mutator phenotype."[29] But nomenclature was only the tip of the iceberg. As had been the case when the ICG-HNPCC promoted the standardization of HNPCC via the Amsterdam Criteria, researchers now believed that a uniform definition was crucial to determining the underlying molecular basis of genetic mismatches and their clinical and pathological associations.

This time it was the U.S. National Cancer Institute that took the initiative to standardize the meaning of the phenomenon. In late 1997, a group of approximately 120 investigators from North America, Europe, Asia, and Australia convened in Bethesda, Maryland, to establish a consensus definition of "microsatellite instability," and to discuss its implications for therapy as well as the issue of microsatellite instability in non-HNPCC

---

27. John Maddox, "Competition and the Death of Science," *Nature*, 1993, *363*: 667; Manuel Perucho, "Correspondence re: Boland et al., 'A National Cancer Institute Workshop on Microsatellite Instability for Cancer Detection and Familial Predisposition,'" *Cancer Res.*, 1999, *59*: 249–56.

28. Henry Lynch, Stephen Lemon, Beth Karr, et al., "Etiology, Natural History, Management and Molecular Genetics of Hereditary Nonpolyposis Colorectal Cancer (Lynch Syndromes): Genetic Counseling Implications," *Cancer Epidemiol. Biomark. & Prevent.*, 1997, *6*: 987–91.

29. S. N. Thibodeau, G. Bren, and D. Schaid, "Microsatellite Instability in Cancer of the Proximal Colon," *Science*, 1993, *260*: 816–19; Peltomäki et al., "Genetic Mapping" (n. 19); Yurij Ionov, Miguel Peinado, Sergei Malkhosyan, Darryl Shibata, and Manuel Perucho, "Ubiquitous Somatic Mutations in Simple Repeated Sequences Reveal a New Mechanism for Colorectal Carcinogenesis," *Nature*, 1993, *363*: 558–61.

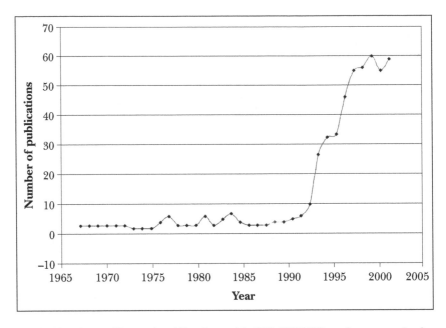

Fig. 1. Numbers of journal publications with CFS, HNPCC, and cognates in the title, excluding Henry Lynch's publications—the purpose being to show how *other* researchers began to take notice of HNPCC in the 1980s, and how the publications explode in number after the "mismatch repair genes" are found and characterized by 1994. *Sources*: PubMed; Jukka-Pekka Mecklin, "Cancer Family Syndrome: Studies on the Hereditary Nonpolypous Colorectal Carcinoma Syndrome" (medical diss., University of Helsinki, 1987).

cases. Microsatellites in genes are sequences of two to four nucleotide base pairs that are repeated. Normally, nucleotide bases are arranged in pairs in the DNA molecule, with the base adenine facing thymine, and the base cytosine facing guanine. The NCI consensus panel agreed that a change in the length of microsatellites due to the insertion or deletion of repeating units is what gives a microsatellite the trait of "instability." Hence, the panel reached a consensus: HNPCC tumors differ from non-HNPCC ones because the former have a higher level of microsatellite instability. This was important for clinical surveillance because it implied that, should the Amsterdam Criteria for identifying "cancer families" be met, the next step should be to test tumors from individuals within these families for microsatellite instability (MSI). MSI testing was both easier and less expensive than performing a full genetic test to find any of the mismatch repair genes involved in HNPCC. Only if MSI was found should genetic tests for mismatch repair genes be recommended for individuals and their families.

The 1997 NCI consensus panel reaffirmed the 1996 position, stating that "MSI testing has one clinical purpose: to identify patients with HNPCC."[30] In addition, the panel encouraged the development of high-risk clinics and cancer registries. Lastly, they suggested that HNPCC be given a new name, in light of the increasing knowledge about the link between tumors and mismatch repair. One suggestion was "hereditary mismatch repair deficiency syndrome," to underscore the connection between a peculiar genetic function and a complex pathology. However, the panel did not arrive at a consensus on this matter.

Recent studies of tumors taken from people in cancer families indicated that carriers of mismatch repair mutations had a 60–80 percent chance of developing colorectal cancer sometime in their lifetimes.[31] This kind of precision is significant: it leads to the prescription of strict surveillance through yearly colonoscopies for mutated gene-carriers; in some of the most extreme cases, it leads to the recommendation to surgically remove part of the healthy colon as a preventive measure. It has been suggested that "no group of researchers has benefited more from the recent boom in genetics and biotechnology than those who study the rare hereditary non-polyposis colon cancer."[32] Bert Vogelstein even reflected years later on how HNPCC has "gone from a total black box to pretty well worked out."[33]

Evidently, this is not the end of research on HNPCC. Although the lack of mismatch repair is commonly accepted as the underlying genetic cause of HNPCC, and although microsatellite instability has been accepted as the biological marker of the disease, questions remain or have been made possible. Among them is why microsatellite instability occurs, for not all MSI is due to HNPCC—in fact, most occurrences of MSI are not inherited at all, but acquired. To further complicate matters, HNPCC leads to cancer in various organs, not just the colon and rectum, but does not lead to cancer in other organs, like the lungs; the reason why this happens is an open area of research.[34] The future of HNPCC research also

30. Boland et al., "National Cancer Institute Workshop" (n. 26), p. 5255.

31. Bo Liu, Ramon Parsons, Nickolas Papadopoulos, et al., "Analysis of Mismatch Repair Genes in Hereditary Non-Polyposis Colorectal Cancer Patients," *Nature Med.*, 1996, 2: 169–74.

32. Kuska, "New Diagnostic Criteria" (n. 15), p. 11.

33. Telephone interview with Bert Vogelstein, 11 August 2003.

34. Telephone interview with Albert de la Chapelle, 18 August 2005.

raises challenges like the development of more sensitive genetic tests, ambitious population-screening programs, and chemopreventive pharmaceuticals.[35] These issues, however, are part of another story, to be told in the near future.

Discussion

The study of HNPCC is part of a broader story of changes in medical genetics in Europe and the United States. Has molecular genetics taken over medical genetics research, replacing disease definitions and interventions based on the collection of family histories with others derived from molecular genetics? The case of HNPCC suggests that this is not so. Rather, medical genetics has been transformed by the influx of molecular genetics, so that the latter has become interwoven with earlier traditions of medical genetics based on the collection of family histories. This is a complex blend of knowledge and practice happening on at least four levels: (1) the use of family histories to seek out cancer genes in the early 1990s; (2) the present influence of hereditary cancer registries on current molecular genetics research; (3) the potential for certain families to become consumers of new medical interventions derived from molecular genetics; and (4) the importance of "cancer families" in the formulation of standardized medical concepts, like the Amsterdam Criteria.

First, molecular genetics transformed HNPCC from a disease that ran in families, if physicians recognized it at all, to one with precise genetic components that could be detected and characterized. The acceptance of HNPCC as a medical entity today is tied to the discovery of the mismatch repair genes in the early 1990s. Thanks to these discoveries, statistical calculations of risk for HNPCC for individuals are not only possible, but increasingly routine. In addition, the discovery of a biological marker for HNPCC, microsatellite instability, has enabled a tiered approach to cancer detection, where positive cancer family histories justify MSI detection tests, which, if positive, in turn call for genetic tests to find mutations in the mismatch repair genes. However, the cancer family history is still the starting point of cancer genetics research—a point sometimes lost on the younger molecular geneticists. Existing cancer family histories were the key to finding the MSH2 and MLH1 cancer genes in the early 1990s.

---

35. Patrick Lynch, "If Aggressive Surveillance in Hereditary Nonpolyposis Colorectal Cancer Is Now State of the Art, Are There Any Challenges Left?" *Gastroenterology*, 2000, *118*: 969–71.

Second, as Figure 1 indicates, there has been an exponential increase in the HNPCC literature since the discovery of the mismatch repair genes, most of it in the field of molecular genetics. Cancer genetics as a medical specialty is over fifty years old, and yet it has become one of the most active sites of research in medicine only since the early 1990s, with the discovery of genes involved in hereditary colorectal, breast, and ovarian cancers. The work of molecular geneticists on mismatch repair has been a turning point that significantly increased the production of medical knowledge of medical genetics. This, ironically, has meant that pioneering clinicians like Lynch and Mecklin are no longer the central figures in the field that they helped to found. Hence Cantor's assertion that "while [Lynch] came to be honoured as one of the 'fathers' of cancer genetics, his 'children' sometimes quietly questioned his paternity."[36] Jukka-Pekka Mecklin recently commented: "The first 15 years (1983–1998) I had a feeling that I was fully involved with HNPCC and in the center of the circus. Since 1998 the increase of molecular genetic research on hereditary cancer and hereditary colorectal cancer has been so enormous that you must feel more and more like an outsider and you can participate only in small parts of the debate."[37]

On the other hand, the productivity of contemporary molecular geneticists continues to be made possible by the old technology of collecting family histories. The collection methods are more comprehensive and sophisticated now than in the 1960s, but the aim is still to produce thorough cancer family histories. Hereditary cancer registries for multiple organs have sprouted throughout the world. Henry Lynch established one such registry in Nebraska in the late 1960s. The M. D. Anderson Cancer Center in Texas has maintained an HNPCC registry since 1988, and has been making strides toward establishing a hereditary cancer map of Latinos in the state. Japan established a hereditary cancer registry in 1981, Finland in 1983, Italy in 1984, Holland in 1985, and Denmark in 1993.[38] The collecting of cancer family data is ongoing, and it reflects a concern with public health, particularly that of people who have familial histories of cancer.[39] It is not driven only by the needs of molecular geneticists.

---

36. Cantor, "Frustrations of Families" (n. 3), p. 302.

37. Jukka-Pekka Mecklin, correspondence with author, 27 August 2003.

38. Torben Myrhoj, Inge Bernstein, Marie L. Bisgaard, et al., "The Establishment of an HNPCC Register," *Anticancer Res.*, 1994, *14*: 1647–50.

39. Heikki Järvinen, Markku Aarnio, Harri Mustonen, et al., "Controlled 15-Year Trial on Screening for Colorectal Cancer in Families with Hereditary Nonpolyposis Colorectal Cancer," *Gastroenterology*, 2000, *118*: 829–34; Gabriela Möslein, "Clinical Implications of

Even as scorn was poured on the "cancer family" notion in the 1960s and 1970s, the idea gained some adherents. Clinicians like Lynch and Mecklin tended to interact with patients as much as, if not more than, they worked in the laboratory; neither saw it as a priority to find the molecular basis of cancer inheritance early on. The motivation for the pioneers was to find cheaper, more accurate, and less invasive ways to figure out who was at greater risk within cancer families. This is important, because these clinical priorities do not necessarily spell "find the cancer genes" at all: quite the contrary, the wide search for biomarkers to make cancer predictions did not focus on genes until the early 1990s. In the case of HNPCC, the early elite was guided not by a will to "geneticize," but by concerns to alleviate suffering and minimize costs for patients. It is clear that this kind of humane concern is still a strong motivation for many who work in the area of cancer genetics. It is also an important component of the HNPCC pioneers' charismatic influence on their colleagues and students, at least for some for whom hereditary cancer research still must start and end with the families affected. This suggests that knowledge of medical histories, pathologies, and genetics influence one another constantly, as medical geneticists try to keep all these aspects reflexively in mind. This is a richer way for researchers to view their own work, rather than as a simple and idealized one-way application of knowledge created in a neatly bound laboratory to an equally discrete and ever-receptive clinical realm.[40]

This reminds us of the importance of clinicians' leadership in the early stages of medical genetics research, and of the endurance of their priorities. It was the persistence of clinicians that helped overcome doubts about the value of the study of heredity in cancer. We now know that HNPCC is the most prevalent form of hereditary colorectal cancer in the United States,[41] and therefore that it has an impact on public health, albeit a very small one relative to the burden of sporadic colorectal cancer. The growth of hereditary cancer registries today is explicitly linked to the clinician-driven need for better cancer control, which, for members of

---

Molecular Diagnosis in Hereditary Nonpolyposis Colorectal Cancer," *Recent Results Cancer Res.*, 2003, *162*: 73–78.

40. See Susan Lindee, *Moments of Truth in Genetic Medicine* (Baltimore: Johns Hopkins University Press, 2005); Peter Keating and Alberto Cambrosio, "The New Genetics and Cancer: The Contributions of Clinical Medicine in the Era of Biomedicine," *J. Hist. Med. & Allied Sci.*, 2001, *56*: 321–52; Keating and Cambrosio, "From Screening to Clinical Research: The Cure of Leukemia and the Early Development of the Cooperative Oncology Groups, 1955–1966," *Bull. Hist. Med.*, 2002, *76*: 299–334.

41. Eng, Hampel, and de la Chapelle, "Genetic Testing" (n. 14).

HNPCC families, means interventions ranging from aggressive surveillance to prophylactic surgery. Yet, the growth of hereditary cancer registries also ensures that familial data will continue feeding our knowledge of the molecular genetics of disease and of the risk of cancer for certain populations.[42]

Third, it is clear that the intertwining of molecular genetics and family histories not only results in improved cancer control and more knowledge about medical genetics, it is also tightly linked to the commercial potential of genetic testing, diagnosis, and therapeutics. Increasingly since 1990, scientific entrepreneurs have harnessed the knowledge gained through the Human Genome Project and, with the crucial intervention of powerful computer applications, have carved potentially profitable niches in the business of pharmacogenetics, studying the role of genetic variations in drug responses by individuals.[43] Although commercial drugs for hereditary cancers are still unavailable, commercial genetic testing for breast and ovarian cancer is available, and it is dominated in the United States by Myriad Genetics, a biopharmaceuticals firm that effectively cornered the market for commercial testing of the BRCA1 and BRCA2 genes.[44] No such monopoly exists in the case of MSH2 or MLH1, but at least one biotechnology firm was founded on the basis of the discovery of the human mismatch repair genes: Nick Papadopoulos, a postdoctoral researcher in Bert Vogelstein's laboratory in the early 1990s, founded GMP Genetics to develop a patented technology to increase the sensitivity of genetic tests, particularly those used for hereditary colorectal cancers.[45]

The Human Genome Project spin-offs, sophisticated computer applications, the precedent of Myriad Genetics, and the growth of GMP Genetics suggest that we must attend to yet another aspect of the growth in knowledge about medical genetics. The commercialization of cancer genetics knowledge was not feasible in the 1960s and 1970s, but by the early 1990s it was. The shift in the potential for profit in cancer diagnosis and therapeutics is part of the economic context of the take-off of cancer genetics

---

42. Duster assumes that genetic tests used since the 1990s have been the only technologies to assess the risk of hereditary cancer, but this ignores how cancer family pedigrees were used as risk-assessment tools since the 1960s: see Troy Duster, *Backdoor to Eugenics* (New York: Routledge, 2003).

43. Adam Hedgcoe, "Terminology and the Construction of Scientific Disciplines: The Case of Pharmacogenomics," *Sci. Technol. & Hum. Val.*, 2003, *28*: 513–37.

44. Shobita Parthasarathy, "Architectures of Genetic Medicine: Comparing Genetic Testing for Breast Cancer in the USA and the UK," *Soc. Stud. Sc.*, 2005, *35*: 5–40.

45. Nick Papadopoulos, correspondence with author, 15 September 2003.

research in the early 1990s. By then the work was not only about medical genetics puzzle-solving or helping patients, it was also about money-making opportunities.

Fourth, and finally, the formation of the International Collaborative Group on HNPCC in the early 1990s also enabled the intertwining of knowledge derived from collecting family histories with that derived from molecular genetics. The Amsterdam Criteria of 1991 were a standard based on a consensus of researchers using a sizeable collection of "cancer families" as evidence. Participants in this process were aware of the shortcomings of their definition of HNPCC, particularly because they had very few clues as to the disease's hereditary cause—yet this imperfect definition was enough to lead to the crucial discovery of the mismatch repair genes. The ICG-HNPCC was quite open to revising the Amsterdam Criteria, and actively sponsored the initiative led by the National Cancer Institute to include new knowledge about mismatch repair and genetic instability in the definition of HNPCC.

The first intervention of the ICG-HNPCC was defensive: The Amsterdam Criteria assured HNPCC a degree of international recognition, moved it away from the margins of medical research, and conferred upon it some scientific legitimacy.[46] But the consensus definition still had to be defended from challengers by claiming that critiques could be reconciled with the Amsterdam Criteria with only minor variations (as was the case with the Amsterdam II Criteria), or by claiming that the changes were necessary complements to the original definition (as was the case with the Bethesda Criteria). The standards set by the ICG-HNPCC were evolving entities that defined a pathology in need of explanation, and determined which families could be used as legitimate sources of tissues and other clinical data. Indeed, the mismatch repair genes MSH2 and MLH1 were sought and found in families that fulfilled the Amsterdam Criteria. The ICG-HNPCC's standards thus defined a part of reality for the researchers who sought these genes: that of the field of data collection.

Considering the role that "cancer families" played in the identification of cancer genes, their contemporary influence on molecular genetics through cancer registries, their potential future as consumers of new

---

46. Other diseases have also moved historically away from the periphery and closer to the center of medical attention. See Elizabeth Armstrong, "Diagnosing Moral Disorder: The Discovery and Evolution of Fetal Alcohol Syndrome," *Soc. Sci. & Med.*, 1998, *47*: 2025–42; Stella Capek, "Reframing Endometriosis: From 'Career Woman's Disease' to Environment/Body Connections," in *Illness and the Environment: A Reader in Contested Medicine*, ed. Steve Kroll-Smith, Phil Brown, and Valerie Gunter (New York: New York University Press, 2000).

medical therapies, and their dynamic presence in the standardization of medical terminology, it is hard not to dwell on their remarkable endurance. Put another way, the cancer family is not part of the past of medical genetics research, but very much a part of its multifaceted, molecular, familial, commercial, present.

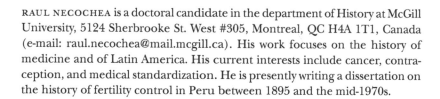

RAUL NECOCHEA is a doctoral candidate in the department of History at McGill University, 5124 Sherbrooke St. West #305, Montreal, QC H4A 1T1, Canada (e-mail: raul.necochea@mail.mcgill.ca). His work focuses on the history of medicine and of Latin America. His current interests include cancer, contraception, and medical standardization. He is presently writing a dissertation on the history of fertility control in Peru between 1895 and the mid-1970s.

Medicine and the Public:
The 1962 Report of the Royal College
of Physicians and the New Public Health

VIRGINIA BERRIDGE

SUMMARY: The 1962 report of the Royal College of Physicians on smoking was a significant event in the history of smoking. Its significance was, however, more than smoking-specific: the RCP committee's appointment, its membership, its work, and the manner of its publication signified the changes within social medicine, and within the medical profession more generally, in postwar Britain. Doctors assumed the right to speak to the public and to government on matters of individual health, and a new risk-based public health was in the process of formation. A public health "policy community" formed, and governments began to assume responsibility for advising the public on health matters. The use of research in the report, and of social research in response to it, was important in the emergence of evidence-based medicine within public health. The paper argues for greater attention to the change in public health epitomized by the report in current debates on the concept of the 1960s "permissive society." It was the harbinger of a new style of "coercive permissiveness" in health.

KEYWORDS: smoking, public health, media, evidence-based medicine, social medicine, permissive society, consumerism

This research began life in a Wellcome Trust–funded project and has since been enriched by the Wellcome-funded "Science Speaks to Policy" program that I led at the London School of Hygiene and Tropical Medicine, by the work of the Centre for History in Public Health, and by interactions with public health researchers at the School. A previous version was given at a conference on cancer organized by David Cantor at the National Library of Medicine in Bethesda, Maryland, in 2004. I am grateful to David Cantor and to an anonymous referee for their comments on drafts of the paper. My thanks are also due to the National Archives, the Royal College of Physicians, and the Wellcome Library for the History and Understanding of Medicine, whose archive deposits have been used in the course of my research.

In April 1963, D. Kelly wrote to the British Ministry of Health about an idea he had had in his head for quite a while about antismoking publicity. After discussion with a German doctor friend, he suggested: "A rhyming poster might work. . . . 'THE MODERN BLOKE—DOESN'T SMOKE'. . . . The ladies are less of a problem—but a growing one. What about 'CONTEMPORARY HAGS ABHOR FAGS' with a similar illustration of modern witches refusing temptation."[1] Another correspondent, K. Norman Reynolds, had written in the previous month. He enclosed a poster he had originally designed for a competition, but was, "alas," "too late in entering it": "The word 'Cancer' is spelt in cork tipped cigarettes, which gets across a point as well as adding to the eye appeal. This unfortunately hasn't come out in this print."[2] In the early 1960s, the Ministry was also the recipient of "puffing poems" and drawings, the results of a National Society of Non Smokers essay competition for children. Antismoking ideas poured in from members of the public.

These suggestions, now yellowing in their folders in the National Archives, are testimony to the change that occurred in the 1960s and 1970s in public health, and, indeed, in the relationship between medicine and society more generally. For the talk of posters and homemade publicity efforts represented the last gasp of an older tradition of public health and of public education, but also looked toward new developments. A new era of mass-media education and health consciousness of individual risk was dawning. Both David Armstrong and Mark Harrison have seen the war years as important for the rise of health education—either as Armstrong's "medicine of the social"[3] promoted by the wartime need to know, or Harrison's argument that wartime health education in the army promoted a new mood of citizenship and responsibility.[4] The late 1950s and early 1960s saw a reorientation of that wartime stance on the part of government: citizens who would act responsibly if given "the facts" were replaced by consumers of harmful goods or substances who needed to be persuaded about risk. In the early 1960s, medicine began to modernize itself, repositioning itself in relation to government, and to society and "the public." I argue here that the report on smoking published by the Royal College of Physicians in 1962, *Smoking and Health*, was a key stage

1. "Smoking and Lung Cancer: Publicity Suggestions," Ministry of Health files, MH 151/23, National Archives, Kew (hereafter NA).

2. Ibid.

3. David Armstrong, *A New History of Identity: A Sociology of Medical Knowledge* (Basingstoke: Palgrave, 2002), p. 51.

4. Mark Harrison, *Medicine and Victory: British Military Medicine in the Second World War* (Oxford: Oxford University Press, 2004), p. 4.

on the road to the new modernized and mediatized medicine and public health.

The repositioning and its implications are central to two areas of historical debate—to reassessments of "the permissive society" of the 1960s, and to the historiography of public health. For the former, commentators such as the health-policy analyst Howard Glennerster have noted that a new social-policy agenda was emergent in Britain in the 1960s and 1970s, which removed criminal sanctions in regard to abortion and sexuality and was hostile to state intervention in such matters.[5] But others have noted that criminal forms of regulation were replaced by medical ones, and that "permissiveness" in sexuality was dependent on new forms of medical surveillance.[6] The "myth" of 1960s permissiveness has come under scrutiny in a wider range of more recent work.[7] The revision has not, however, discussed the changes in public health in that decade that are considered in this paper. I seek to argue that the 1962 report and the changes it helped to usher in in public health in the 1960s, and especially in the 1970s, embodied the contradictions in the concept of permissiveness: on the one hand, health became a matter of individual responsibility; but that individual responsibility lay within a new framework of governmental intervention in individual behavior—what is termed here "coercive permissiveness."

The historiography of British public health is beginning to take account of the postwar changes in the ideology and outlook of public health.[8] Most attention has been focused on the organizational and professional changes that saw the Medical Officer of Health (MOH) lose his local government "empire" in the early 1970s and reemerge as the "community physician" located within the National Health Service (NHS). Medical public health professionals have been criticized in Jane Lewis's work for the failure to develop a distinctive ideology for public health, and for their tendency to define the role of public health around whatever tasks they undertook at the time.[9] Journalist doctors like James Le Fanu and Michael

5. Howard Glennerster, *British Social Policy since 1945* (Oxford: Blackwell, 1995), p. 96.

6. Jeffrey Weeks, *Sex, Politics and Society: The Regulation of Sexuality since 1800* (London: Longman, 1981), pp. 267–68.

7. See, e.g., James Obelkevich, review of *The Sixties: Cultural Revolution in Britain, France, Italy, and the United States, c1958–c1974* (1998) by Arthur Marwick, *Twent. Cent. Brit. Hist.*, 2000, *11* (3): 333–36.

8. The work of Dorothy Porter on social medicine and the organizational relationship with the social sciences is the main example: see Dorothy Porter, ed., *Social Medicine and Medical Sociology in the Twentieth Century* (Amsterdam: Rodopi, 1997).

9. Jane Lewis, *What Price Community Medicine? The Philosophy, Practice and Politics of Public Health since 1919* (Brighton: Harvester, 1986), pp. 1–12.

Fitzpatrick have discussed the subsequent history of public health. They have criticized the rise of a new "health tyranny" through health promotion, but they have focused primarily on later events and key issues like the government health-education campaigns on AIDS in the 1980s.[10]

I argue in this paper that both sets of historical debates need to incorporate consideration of the 1962 Royal College report and the rise of an ethos of public health not tied to health services, to MOsH, or to community physicians. The 1962 report was highly significant for the history of smoking policy, but its significance was also a wider one. *First, it signified a new willingness on the part of medicine to speak to the public, and to use the media to do so.* The media became central to public health. Doctors reoriented their role so that they spoke to the public, not just to the rest of the profession. The role of the media also became central to debates within public health: on the one hand, mass-media campaigns were increasingly important as a strategy and began to focus on the role of individual risks to health, to urge the reformation of behavior; on the other, the control and even prohibition of advertising deemed detrimental to health was to become an important public health strategy. The wartime and immediate postwar emphasis on responsibility and citizenship gave way to an emphasis on propaganda and persuasion using consumerist techniques. *Second, it marked the emergence of a "policy community" around public health, linking civil servants within government with medical experts outside.* This model of health policymaking was, with variations, to dominate the process of British health-policy formation into the twenty-first century. British government carried on a policy-balancing act in which the role of insider/outsider organizations and formal interconnections with scientific expertise were increasingly important. *Third, it emphasized the role of individual behavior, legitimated through population-based epidemiology, as the dominant focus of public health endeavor in postwar Britain.* The report gave public significance to a new type of public health and to different scientific ways of studying it. The new epidemiology of the 1950s and the new focus on the risk of chronic disease were translated into a wider public and policy agenda. *Fourth, it stimulated new attitudes on the part of government regarding its relation to the public on matters of health, and a heightened significance for research-based surveillance.* Medicine and consumerism were allied through a focus on the role of the individual in society, and through a new emphasis on

10. James Le Fanu, *The Rise and Fall of Modern Medicine* (London: Little Brown, 1999); Michael Fitzpatrick, "Take Two Aspirins and Thank Your Caring PM," *Times Higher Educ. Suppl.*, 19–26 December 2003, pp. 28–29. See also Fitzpatrick, *The Tyranny of Health: Doctors and the Regulation of Lifestyle* (London: Routledge, 2001).

individual persuasion. At the same time, research and the social survey began to outline a new view of "the public" and to establish a relationship between medicine and the social sciences, one that built on the alliances within social medicine but also turned them in a new consumerist direction. It was part of the rise of evidence-based medicine.

The report therefore signified a new style and outlook for public health that was emergent at around the same time as the organizational and professional changes, but was, in many respects, separate from them. The smoking activists were not MOsH or even the new community physicians: a new public "public health" was emerging, distinct from the profession and its service role. This was research- and "evidence-based," using the social sciences as technical tools. Such developments also invite reflection about the nature of the permissiveness of the 1960s and the roots of the "health tyranny" that the journalists have criticized. The health discussions of the 1960s were marked by contradictory tendencies: in one sense, by the very antithesis of permissiveness; in the other, by a new style of "coercive permissiveness" in health.

The Prehistory of Smoking and Lung Cancer

The early history of the smoking-and-lung-cancer connection is well known and has been recounted in a number of different works.[11] Concern was roused by the gradual increase in the incidence of cancer; by a change in the balance of the sexes, toward men; and by the increasingly important role of lung cancer. The greatest increase in lung cancer came in males over forty-five, where the incidence increased sixfold between 1930 and 1945. At first it was thought that these changes might be due to improved diagnosis and better recording and registration. Work carried out by Sir Ernest Kennaway in the 1930s and published in 1947, a detailed examination of postmortem certificates, helped eliminate occupational and environmental factors. Kennaway pointed to a connection with cigarette smoking, but his work, based on statistical correlations, carried little weight because of the perceived lack of legitimacy of this mode of explanation at the time. Laboratory studies tended to support the connection. Research had also been undertaken before the war in Nazi Germany, and by the American biometrician Raymond Pearl, for the insurance indus-

---

11. E.g., Joan Austoker, *A History of the Imperial Cancer Research Fund, 1902–1986* (Oxford: Oxford University Press, 1988), pp. 186–99; Charles Webster, "Tobacco Smoking Addiction: A Challenge to the National Health Service," *Brit. J. Addict.*, 1984, *79*: 8–16.

try.[12] The issue became more urgent after the war, and discussions between the Ministry of Health and the Medical Research Council (MRC) led to the council's convening an informal conference on cancer of the lung in February 1947. The MRC agreed to initiate a large-scale statistical study of the past smoking habits of those with cancer of the lung, and of two control groups. This was the origin of the work carried out in the Statistical Research Unit at the London School of Hygiene and Tropical Medicine (LSHTM) by Professor Austin Bradford Hill and Dr. Richard Doll. The results, published in the *British Medical Journal* in 1950, concluded that there was a "real association" between carcinoma of the lung and smoking, and that smoking was a factor, and an important one, in the production of lung cancer.[13] Work by Ernest L. Wynder and Evarts A. Graham in the United States had come to similar conclusions.[14] Later prospective studies carried out by Doll and Bradford Hill and by Edward Cuyler Hammond and Daniel Horn in the United States appeared to implicate cigarette smoking even further.[15]

Charles Webster has shown in detail how the issue fared over the next seven years.[16] A written parliamentary answer from Ian Macleod as Conservative minister of health in February 1954 accepted that there was a connection, but that it was not a simple one.[17] When the MRC issued its own report on smoking and lung cancer in June 1957, the Ministry of Health adopted the argument more fully. The parliamentary secretary to the Ministry of Health (MH) for the first time on 27 June 1957 expressed unambiguous support for the conclusions reached by Doll and Hill in

12. George Davey Smith, S. A. Strobele, and Matthias Egger, "Smoking and Health Promotion in Nazi Germany," *J. Epidemiol. & Commun. Health*, 1994, *48*: 220–23; Robert N. Proctor, *The Nazi War on Cancer* (Princeton: Princeton University Press, 1999), pp. 173–247.

13. Richard Doll and Austin Bradford Hill, "Smoking and Carcinoma of the Lung: Preliminary Report," *Brit. Med. J.*, 1950, *2*: 739–48.

14. Ernest L. Wynder and Evarts A. Graham, "Tobacco Smoking as a Possible Etiologic Factor in Bronchiogenic Carcinoma: A Study of Six Hundred and Eighty-four Proved Cases," *JAMA*, 1950, *143* (4): 329–36.

15. Richard Doll and Austin Bradford Hill, "The Mortality of Doctors in Relation to Their Smoking Habits: A Preliminary Report," *Brit. Med. J.*, 1954, *1*: 1541–55; Doll and Austin Bradford Hill, "Lung Cancer and Other Causes of Death in Relation to Smoking: A Second Report on the Mortality of British Doctors," ibid., 1956, *2*: 1071–81; Edward Cuyler Hammond and Daniel Horn, "The Relationship between Human Smoking Habits and Death Rates: A Follow- up Study of 187,766 Men," *JAMA*, 1954, *155* (15): 1316–27.

16. Webster, "Tobacco Smoking Addiction" (n. 11).

17. Written answer from Ian Macleod, Minister of Health, 12 February 1954, *Parliamentary Debates*, Commons, 5th ser., vol. 523 (1954), cols. 173–74.

1950. Webster locates this sequence of events in the machinations of the powerful and complex advisory machinery that stood between the MRC and the MH: the main advisory body was the Cancer and Radiotherapy Standing Advisory Committee, reporting to the Central Health Services Council, which in turn advised the Ministry of Health. Horace Joules of the Central Middlesex Hospital, a member of both bodies, was the only person within the advisory-committee machinery consistently to press the issue; Paolo Palladino has recently related his stance to a continuing Christian Socialist tradition.[18] The initial governmental response focused on a Ministry of Health circular encouraging local authorities to develop health-education campaigns on smoking. Further action under the Labour government of the 1960s saw the banning of cigarette advertisements on television in 1965, and attempts by the Labour minister of health, the GP Kenneth Robinson, to introduce legislation to ban cigarette coupon schemes and to limit other forms of advertising. Health warnings on cigarette packets appeared in 1971. This was the "end of the beginning" of the first phase of the policy response.

The Doll/ Hill research of the 1950s had impacted upon a fluid policy situation in that decade in which the governmental response was conditioned by a number of factors, not all of them directly smoking-related.[19] The economic importance of smoking to the exchequer was considerable, and the tobacco industry was a valued partner of government, building on formal controls that had operated during wartime. But also in play were changes in the nature and role of public health; the role of air pollution as a contentious political issue; the contested nature of the evidence; the central governmental politics of health education; and the general culture of smoking, with its electoral implications. The last of these was a crucial issue for politicians: did governments have the right to tell the public what to do about a culturally sanctioned, acceptable habit that might possibly lead to disease many years hence? and, what would this mean in terms of political popularity?

It was also a crucial issue for public health. The British social-medicine ideology of the 1930s and 1940s had stressed the need for a holistic vision of medicine, and key research papers had talked of occupation and of class as crucial dynamics. But, as Dorothy Porter's work has shown, the

18. Paolo Palladino, "Discourses of Smoking, Health, and the Just Society: Yesterday, Today, and the Return of the Same?" *Soc. Hist. Med.*, 2001, *14*: 313–35.

19. This is discussed in Virginia Berridge, "Denial and Delay? Analysing the Policy Response to the Smoking and Lung Cancer Connection in the 1950s and 60s," *Hist. J.*, 2006, *49*: 1185–209.

ethos of social medicine was changing in the 1950s, with a new emphasis on the role of individual psychology and of issues such as "stress."[20] Social medicine was reorienting itself to a focus on chronic-disease epidemiology, of which the smoking work formed part, and which laid stress on the role of the individual. Central to this reorientation was the classic text by the social-medicine pioneer Jerry Morris, *Uses of Epidemiology*, published in 1957.[21] Morris's paper on the impact of exercise on heart disease tellingly compared the rates of heart disease of sedentary bus drivers with those of active conductors, combining the occupation and class emphasis of 1940s social medicine with the emergent interest in individual behavior.[22] Increasingly, too, such interests were looking outside the confines of the closed medical world and reaching out to a new engagement with "the public," an activity that previous bans on medical advertising had prevented.[23] The involvement of Charles Fletcher (who was a pioneer of the new media- and public-focused developments) and of Morris in the 1962 Royal College committee was thus highly significant.

The Origins and Membership of the Royal College Committee

Nevertheless, the Royal College of Physicians (RCP) was not the most obvious body to produce a report on the link between smoking and lung cancer, and it had already turned down the opportunity once. In November 1956, Francis Avery Jones, a gastroenterologist from the Central Middlesex Hospital with whom Doll had originally worked, wrote to the president of the College, Lord Brain, urging that the College put out a statement on the effect of smoking on health, "with particular reference to the rising generation."[24] Brain—a shy, reserved man—took a month to reply, only to turn the proposal down. The reasons for his refusal were, in their dislike of giving public advice, typical of the profession's attitude at the time:

20. Dorothy Porter, "From Social Structure to Social Behaviour in Britain after the Second World War," in *Poor Health: Social Inequality Before and After the Black Report*, ed. Virginia Berridge and Stuart Blume (London: Cass, 2003), pp. 58–80.

21. Jerry Morris, *Uses of Epidemiology* (Edinburgh: Livingstone, 1957).

22. J. N. Morris, J. A. Heady, P. A. B. Raffle, C. G. Roberts, and J. W. Parks, "Coronary Heart Disease and Physical Activity of Work," *Lancet*, 1953, 2: 1053–57, 1111–20.

23. Kelly Loughlin, "Spectacle and Secrecy: Press Coverage of Conjoined Twins in 1950s Britain," *Med. Hist.*, 2005, 49: 197–212.

24. Francis Avery Jones to Lord Brain, quoted in Christopher Booth, "Smoking and the Gold Headed Cane," in *Balancing Act: Essays to Honour Stephen Lock*, ed. Christopher Booth (London: Keynes Press, 1991), pp. 49–55, on pp. 51–52.

The work of Richard Doll and Bradford Hill has received very wide publicity and must be known, I should imagine, to every doctor in the country, so it is difficult to see that the College could add anything to the knowledge of the existing facts. If we go beyond facts, to the question of the giving of advice to the public as to what action they should take in the light of the facts, I doubt very much whether that should be a function of the College.[25]

Subsequently, the College's attitude changed. In 1957 Robert Platt was elected president as successor to Brain. Platt had a modernizing agenda for the profession, which smoking fitted admirably. He was first approached on the subject of smoking by Charles Fletcher, first director of the MRC's pneumoconiosis research unit in Cardiff, who at the time of his approach was working as a respiratory physician in the department of medicine at Hammersmith Hospital. Fletcher had been invited to lunch by the deputy chief medical officer, George Godber, who was frustrated by the lack of activity within his Ministry, and the two had agreed to sound out Platt about taking on the smoking issue.[26] Godber was a member of the RCP's Council and a close friend of Platt. Avery Jones also heard what was afoot and wrote again in January 1959 to urge the Royal College to action. The first informal meeting was held on 16 February 1959, and in April the Comitia of the College agreed that a committee should be formed "to report on smoking and atmospheric pollution in relation to carcinoma of the lung and other illnesses"; the first formal meeting was held at the College on 15 July 1959 at 5 p.m.[27]

This sequence of events was illustrative of wider changes in postwar medicine. Smoking was a chance for the Royal College to position itself in relation to new agendas emerging in health. Medical interest had been in occupational health and in the environment and disease—symbolized by Fletcher's own previous occupational work on miners' lung disease and his interest in air pollution and chest disease—but these interests were giving place to a new focus on chronic diseases of the individual brought on by habits like smoking. The networks that operated in this instance were also significant for the future: Godber was a graduate of the London School of Hygiene and Tropical Medicine (LSHTM), the foremost public health school. His position as a medical civil servant in

25. Ibid.

26. Fletcher continued this "pressure from without" during the course of the committee. See his correspondence with Godber on what the Ministry was doing on lung cancer and on health education; e.g., Fletcher to Godber, 18 January 1960, NA MH 55/2226.

27. Committee to Report on Smoking and Atmospheric Pollution (hereafter RCP Committee), Minutes, vol. 1, 1959–63, n.p., Royal College of Physicians Archive, London, U.K.

the Ministry of Health, but working closely to a health agenda with medical and health interests outside, was illustrative of the emergence of the "policy community"—the term used by political scientists to analyze how policymaking interests work, with interests within government forming alliances with those outside. These alliances were to become important in the making of postwar health policy, particularly in relation to the medical profession.[28] British civil servants are neutral and nonpolitical figures who do not change when governments change; the role of the Chief Medical Officer in government was as a neutral adviser, and the Ministry of Health had a twin-track bureaucratic organization with both specialist medical and generalist civil servants.[29] The links between the former group of civil servants and outside medical interests were important in this instance and for other issues in postwar health policymaking. Platt's interests in medical modernization extended widely—he was a leading figure behind the subsequent Todd committee on medical education in 1968, and was also important in new moves around genetic disease in Manchester.[30] The creation of the College committee symbolized the changing role of medicine.

The membership of the committee was also symbolic. It was decided informally through the networks of British social medicine, with Fletcher and Platt in leading roles and Godber behind the scenes. Platt was in the chair, but Fletcher as its secretary was the moving spirit of its work. Fletcher was the son of Walter Morley Fletcher, former secretary of the MRC; he had "all the confidence of the Old Etonian" and impeccable connections in medical circles, but also a social conscience and a commitment to communicating with the public through the media.[31] In 1958 his series *Your Life in Their Hands*, showing surgical procedures on television, had caused huge controversy. The series had been part of developments in medical broadcasting. It had originated in a set of programs called *Thursday Clinic* transmitted in 1954 and 1956, consisting of outside broadcasts from St. Mary's hospital in Paddington. The work of NHS hospitals had been seen in earlier programs such as *Matters of Life and Death*

28. There is a wide literature on this which is summarized in Virginia Berridge, ed., *Making Health Policy: Networks in Research and Policy since 1945* (Amsterdam: Rodopi, 2005).

29. Virginia Berridge, "Doctors and the State: The Changing Role of Medical Expertise in Policy-making," *Contemp. Brit. Hist.*, 1997, *11* (4): 66–85.

30. Peter A. Coventry and John V. Pickstone, "From What and Why Did Genetics Emerge as a Medical Specialism in the 1970s in the UK? A Case History of Research, Policy and Services in the Manchester Region of the NHS," *Soc. Sci. & Med.*, 1999, *49*: 1227–38.

31. Comment made in interview with Roger Braban, June 1996, London School of Hygiene and Tropical Medicine, London.

(1951) and *Matters of Medicine* (1952), and medical procedures were also shown in *The Hurt Mind* (1957), which dealt with new developments in the treatment of mental illness and in which Fletcher was also involved.[32] Such programs, and the media controversy over cases of conjoined twins in the 1950s, had begun the reordering of relationships around medical confidentiality which had up until then been a constraining issue for public depictions of medicine.[33]

Fletcher was a leader of these developments—but other members of the committee were also closely involved in the new relationships between medicine and the media: Dr. Guy Scadding had appeared in *Matters of Medicine* explaining the complexities of the interactions between lung cancer, smoking, and air pollution. Jerry Morris, of the MRC-funded Social Medicine Unit, had given radio talks, including one in 1955 whose content foreshadowed the new developments in public health that the RCP committee came to symbolize:

> We are dealing with a different social situation. The nineteenth-century epidemics, bred in poverty and malnutrition, arose from the failures of the social system. . . . But coronary thrombosis . . . with its origins apparently in high living standards . . . seems to be arising from what we regard as successes of the social system. . . . It is becoming clear that in the modification of personal behaviour, of diet, smoking, physical exercise and the rest, which look like providing at any rate part of the answer, the responsibility of the individual for his own health will be far greater than formerly. It will not be possible to impose from without (as drains were built) the new norms of behaviour better serving the needs of middle and old age. They will only come about in a new kind of partnership between community and individual.[34]

Morris's advocacy of media and advertising initiatives on the committee was strong and a continuing strand in his long career; in 2000 at his ninetieth-birthday conference at LSHTM, the leading epidemiologist Michael Marmot remarked that "Jerry has always told me that I should watch more television rather than less."[35] Others on the committee, like

---

32. Fletcher's media work is discussed in Kelly Loughlin, "'Your Life in Their Hands': The Context of a Medical-Media Controversy," *Media Hist.*, 2000, 6 (2): 177–88.

33. Loughlin, "Spectacle and Secrecy" (n. 23).

34. Jerry Morris, "Twentieth Century Epidemic: Coronary Thrombosis" (transcript of BBC Third Programme talk, 1 December 1955), BBC written archives, Caversham, Reading. The printed version is "Coronary Thrombosis: A Modern Epidemic," *Listener*, 8 December 1955, pp. 995–96.

35. See Virginia Berridge and Suzanne Taylor, eds., *Epidemiology, Social Medicine and Public Health*, transcript of the witness seminar held on 21 July 2000 on the 90th birthday of Pro-

Avery Jones, the gastroenterologist who had originally suggested action to the RCP, symbolized the new medical interest in smoking and chronic disease, while the presence of Sir Aubrey Lewis of the Institute of Psychiatry indicated the role that psychological insights were to play in the new developments in public health. The committee subsequently added Dr. N. C. Oswald to its number; he was a smoker, and all the rest of the committee were by then nonsmokers. The committee also consulted experts including Richard Doll and Alexander Haddow of the Chester Beatty Institute, and Godber was also available, although not a member of the committee. In an interview, Morris remembered that they had tried to involve a Medical Officer of Health with an interest in smoking, but could not find one.[36] That comment was indicative of the gulf between academic and practice-based public health. The committee's membership emphasized the networks that were beginning to coalesce around the new risk-based public health. It also symbolized an alliance between Fletcher's prestigious medical connections and the clinicians and social-medicine people and epidemiologists, who had lower status within the profession.[37] (They had originally been located at the Central Middlesex Hospital in Willesden, a North London suburb; as a former local government hospital under the aegis of the London County Council, this had much lower status than the prestigious London teaching hospitals.)

The Work of the Committee

The work of the committee proceeded through nine meetings between 1959 and 1961, often with long gaps between them. Much was done outside the committee, with members preparing papers and gathering evidence. Early on it made two key decisions that emphasized the new directions in public health. First, it decided to speak directly to the public rather than to the profession. The minutes of the fourth meeting, on 17 March 1960, recorded that a discussion was opened by the president on how the report should be presented: "The usual College report had limited circulation among the medical profession"; therefore,

---

fessor Jerry Morris (London: Centre for History in Public Health, 2005), p. 18; available at **http://www.lshtm.ac.uk/history/jerrymorris.html** (last accessed 31 October 2006).

36. Interview with Jerry Morris, June 1995, London School of Hygiene and Tropical Medicine.

37. Older colleagues at LSHTM remember how it was customary for the epidemiologists to wear white coats to show that they were doctors, even though they did not see patients. Photographs of Morris from the 1970s show him with a white coat.

it was agreed that the Committee's report should have more publicity and a wider circulation than the usual College reports. It could not advise government on any course of action, but it could suggest lines of action.[38]

Second, it disposed of the air-pollution connection. Although the Comitia of the Royal College had wanted a report that combined discussion of both issues, the committee decided not to produce this:

It was agreed that the evidence would be of an entirely different quality and nature. It was pointed out that individuals could avoid the dangers of smoking but not those of pollution. It was also thought that a section on atmospheric pollution within the main report might detract from the main arguments on smoking and lung cancer.[39]

The committee did eventually produce a separate report on air pollution, but this was not published until the early 1970s and without much sense of urgency. The committee recognized that the issue of smoking and lung cancer was a much more clear-cut case where individual action could be stressed. On both counts, the committee was moving toward a concept of health that focused more clearly on individual responsibility and that could be expressed through appeals to the public rather than to the profession.

The areas of the committee's work were divided between members according to their own interests, so memoranda appeared through the meetings on diseases of the lung, on the chemistry and pharmacology of smoking, on smoking and the gastrointestinal tract. Interest in consumer issues, in advertising and the media, and in what the public thought and how it could be influenced formed significant threads in the discussions. Early on, Aubrey Lewis produced a paper on the psychological aspects of smoking that pointed out the lack of evidence that health education could discourage inveterate smokers; school-based prevention might be more effective, but there was little information on projects that had been undertaken.

Lack of information on these newer strategies and aspects of health interest was a theme throughout the work of the committee. Economic issues and consideration of the role of the media were to be of growing importance within the new ideology of public health—but in the late 1950s and early 1960s the profession of health economics was still in the future, and it was the social-medicine interests that took up the economic and media issues. It was the social-medicine pioneer Jerry Morris who was

38. RCP Committee, Minutes, 17 March 1960.
39. Ibid.

active throughout the life of the committee in investigating consumer expenditure and the role of tobacco advertising. His work showed the expanding importance of television advertising in the situation; the committee therefore pressed for an official survey of smoking habits in children and inquired into advertising controls on television.[40] Morris also brought the issue of coronary heart disease (CHD) into the committee's discussions, influenced by the early publications of the Framingham study that had investigated CHD in the United States.[41]

Fletcher drew together the final report, making it accessible to the lay public, but clearly other members of the committee played an important role; Morris's work was particularly significant for the public, media, and consumerist emphasis. It was agreed that the report should include a section on the use of advertising against smoking: "modern methods should be employed to combat modern methods."[42] Public health at this stage had close relationships with the British tobacco industry. Imperial Tobacco, the main industry organization, was seen by some public health interests and by government as a partner in a shared enterprise to reduce harm from smoking.[43] Geoffrey Todd, the Imperial Company's lead statistician, and others from the Tobacco Manufacturers Standing Committee provided information and statistics for the final report; the report was also shown informally to the Tobacco Manufacturers Standing Committee before publication.[44]

The report was finally published in March 1962. Its form, content, and presentation were significant. Surveying the history of smoking, the chemistry and pharmacology of tobacco smoke, and the latest scientific evidence about the relationship with cancer, gastrointestinal diseases, lung disease, and coronary heart disease, as well as the psychology of smoking, it laid out a possible seven-point agenda for governmental action. Five of the seven points were consumerist and media oriented: public education, restrictions on sale to children, restriction of tobacco advertising, tax increases (and perhaps differential taxation for less harmful pipes and cigars), and information on the tar and nicotine content of cigarettes. Only two points came from different traditions: the environmentalism

40. Ibid., 18 February 1960.
41. Ibid., 17 March 1960.
42. Ibid., 4 January 1961.
43. For the history of this relationship, see Virginia Berridge and Penny Starns, "The 'Invisible Industrialist' and Public Health: The Rise and Fall of 'Safer Smoking' in the 1970s," in *Medicine, the Market and the Mass Media*, ed. Virginia Berridge and Kelly Loughlin (London: Routledge, 2005), pp. 172–91.
44. RCP Committee, Minutes, 23 February 1961.

of restrictions on smoking in public places, and the "medical model" of antismoking clinics.[45] The agenda for government thus largely dropped action on the environment (air pollution) and gave full rein to the new appeal to the public, to economic and consumerist trends.

The 1962 Report and the Appeal to the Public

The manner of the report's presentation and publication symbolized this. The College hired a public relations consultant, Roger Braban, to manage the launch of the report, and held its first-ever press conference. Braban recalled:

> I came in as PR consultant to the RCP a few months before the smoking report—they had never used a professional launch . . . then they got a taste for it and used it for every report. . . . I spent a lot of time in finding the right team. . . . the President and Charles Fletcher, he was a popular figure with the media. . . . I timed it so that Ministers had the report before it was published—they feel they're party to something.[46]

Charles Fletcher later gave a flavor of that first press conference:

> On the day before publication a press conference was held at the College and it was crowded. Many questions were asked. When one reporter quoted that the annual risk of lung cancer in heavy smokers aged 55 was only one in 23, the President asked him if he would fly with an airline only one in 23 of whose planes crashed he agreed he would not. Next day there was fortunately no big news and the report got major headlines, Robert Platt on the BBC and I was interviewed on ITV.[47]

The report was also marked by a special program on *Panorama*, the flagship TV vehicle for current affairs, which went out on television on 12 March, just after the publication of the report. Fronted by the commentator Richard Dimbleby, the program interviewed scientists (mostly laboratory based) and members of the public about their response, and about giving up smoking. The centerpiece of the program was an interview by the presenter Robert Kee with John Partridge (chairman of the Tobacco Manufacturers Standing Committee) and Sir Robert Platt. The standoff between the two, with Platt robustly interrupting Partridge's defense of the industry, made good television:

45. Royal College of Physicians, *Smoking and Health* (London: Pitman, 1962).

46. Braban interview (n. 31).

47. Charles Fletcher, "The Story of the Reports on Smoking and Health of the Royal College of Physicians," in *Ashes to Ashes: The History of Smoking and Health*, ed. Stephen Lock, Lois Reynolds, and E. M. Tansey (Amsterdam: Rodopi, 1998), pp. 202–5, on p. 203.

KEE: Mr Partridge, would you agree that we must stop young people smoking?

PARTRIDGE: No I would not, and let me, just while I can, take up one point that Sir Robert made just now. The *Observer* had no right to make that remark in its editorial yesterday, Sir Robert, and nor, with respect, have you.

(INTERRUPTION) . . . about only a tobacco manufacturer could deny this.

KEE: Well that is the position we have here now isn't it?

PARTRIDGE: It is so, but the implication is some dishonest approach to this problem, and that is not well founded.

(INTERRUPTION) . . . May I just finish here . . . [48]

This was unusual television for the time, but it was a portent of the future "mediatization" of health issues and the premium it put on conflict and opposition.

The report was popular with the public. Originally the College had wanted only 5,000 copies printed, and when Fletcher insisted on double that number, it had required the committee to pay for any copies that were unsold. But the report sold out within a few days, and a second printing was needed. It had sold more than 33,000 copies in the United Kingdom by the autumn of 1963, and more than 50,000 in the United States.[49] It was followed the next year by Fletcher's "Penguin Special" volume, *Common Sense about Smoking*, which symbolically linked the medical evidence with a chapter on economic effects and others on social implications and how to stop. Here was a further attempt to appeal to the public, which brought together what was to become a common combination in public health: a review of the science coupled with a self-help guide to individual reformation.[50]

The Work of the Cabinet Committee on Smoking

What was the government's response? Governments of the period have often been criticized for inadequate responses, reliant on health education rather than more stringent measures of control. But the choice of health education as the main response, and the change in the nature of that education, was significant. Just as medicine in this period was reorienting toward a public advice role, so too can we see governments of both

48. There is a transcript of the program in the Ministry of Health papers; see Public Health Propaganda: Smoking and Lung Cancer, Publicity Policy, 1961–, NA MH 55/2204.

49. Fletcher, "Story of the Reports" (n. 47); RCP Committee, Minutes, 6 December 1961.

50. Charles Fletcher, *Common Sense about Smoking* (London: Penguin Books, 1963).

political persuasions, Labour and Conservative, moving toward a new view of their role in relation to the population and health matters, in line with the changed profile of disease. Governments began to assume a new duty to advise and warn about health risk, to persuade their citizens rather than to assume that a sense of public duty inherent in the population would lead them to make up their own minds. Politicians remained concerned about the electoral implications of such a stance—but their opposition to intervention in such matters was in decline by the end of the 1960s.

Governments began to seek to influence the health habits of those whom they governed. To do this, they also began actively to seek out information about them—about the beliefs and habits of normal populations, and about their health—through surveys and other research mechanisms, a development that paralleled the increased emphasis on populations within chronic-disease epidemiology. This was an important change that again built on the wartime social surveys and gave a new role to research and also to quantitative social science.[51] The social science disciplines assumed heightened technocratic significance in relation to these developments. The 1962 report was an important catalyst for the "evidence-based" tendency within the new public health.

Let us look at how these responses developed in the 1960s. The main vehicle for governmental response to the report was the cabinet committee on smoking, which reported to the main cabinet. Cabinet committees had been briefly formed in the 1950s at the time of the various parliamentary statements, and had been chaired by the home secretary of the day. R. A. Butler, as home secretary, chaired the first meeting of the latest committee; but Harold Macmillan, the prime minister, did not want Butler in this role and Lord Hailsham, lord president of the Council, took over. The ministerial committee was paralleled by one of officials, which did the detailed work.[52] The officials moved swiftly: the first meeting of their committee was on 23 March, two further meetings followed, and a draft report was ready to go to the lord president by the middle of April.[53] The report, preceded by a flurry of activity in the relevant departments, was relatively anodyne, placing its reliance on health education and on voluntary agreements for advertising. The officials came down against

51. For the earlier history of surveys, see Martin Bulmer, K. Bales, and K. K. Sklar, eds., *The Social Survey in Historical Perspective, 1880–1940* (Cambridge: Cambridge University Press, 1991).

52. P. W. Cary, the civil servant who chaired this committee, was reluctant to reveal its existence: see note from him to the other officials on the committee, 27 April 1962, NA CAB 21/4648.

53. Minutes of third meeting, 13 April 1962, NA CAB 130/185 GEN 763.

differential taxation (taxation graded according to the harm occasioned by the product—so that pipes and cigars, thought to be less harmful, would attract lower tax rates than those for cigarettes) and the taxation option in general: taxation, it was argued, would penalize the poor, raise the cost of living, and have a serious effect on producer economies in the empire such as Rhodesia. This view reflected the belief that more-restrictive action could not be sustained without major change in public attitudes to smoking. Research in Edinburgh and the government's own pilot survey of public attitudes to smoking through the Central Office of Information (COI) had confirmed that most people knew about the link between smoking and lung cancer, but their views on why smoking was harmful to health were different from those of the scientists: the public view of smoking stressed the environmental-nuisance aspects rather than the risk-based epidemiology.[54]

The politicians did not agree on the sales-to-children issue, nor on differential taxation. The Treasury fought strongly against the latter, and ultimately the committee could not agree. In the event, education and voluntarism were the keynotes of the response, and the committee decided not to make a statement. As Hailsham told Macmillan, a small publicity campaign would not be welcomed, and in any case interest had abated for the present. He proposed to set up the machinery and start the campaign, perhaps issuing a statement later on. A meeting with the manufacturers might also result in an agreement to apply the TV restrictions voluntarily to other advertising, so the government could then claim credit for that also.[55] At a subsequent meeting in the House of Lords with representatives of the Tobacco Advisory Committee (TAC), the main industry representative organization, the lord president said that the government accepted the scientific case as in the RCP report but was against compulsion and action that would lead to pressure for similar measures in respect to alcohol, and even to foods like chocolate; it was "not the government's purpose to induce any catastrophic change in smoking habits."[56] The meeting resulted in a move toward overall agreement on advertising restrictions based on the code applicable to television. On 14 November, Hailsham wrote to Sir Alexander Maxwell, chairman of the TAC and previously wartime Tobacco Controller, that he felt the informal

54. For discussion of this point, see Public Health Propaganda: Smoking and Lung Cancer, Publicity Policy, 1957–60, NA MH 55/2203.

55. Lord President to Prime Minister, 25 July 1962, NA CAB 21/4878.

56. Notes of a meeting with representatives of the TAC (Tobacco Advisory Committee), 31 July 1962, NA CAB 21/4878.

way this matter had been dealt with was suited to other issues as they arose. But he was clear that he was no stooge for industry interests; someone at Carreras had sent him a box of filter-tipped Piccadilly cigarettes: "This was indeed bearding the lion in his den, but it was as ineffectual as the devil's attempt on St. Anthony."[57]

The governmental response was thus muted and focused on the strategy of health education. The multiplicity of interests in government was a key factor. The Treasury view ultimately prevailed over the taxation issue, but not before the implications had been fully aired at the political level. The role of the industry was important, although its representatives were called in after the political decisions had been taken. Also behind these decisions was a desire to achieve a balance in policy, and the realization that without a huge change in the social positioning of smoking there was little point in initiating a major program of activity. Discussion of health-education strategies and organization was not the only way in which government considered the implications of the RCP report: the debates about differential taxation and other strategies also led to important developments both in smoking policy and in public health later on, in the 1970s.[58]

But health education was the main response. We can trace the beginnings of the important change in attitude from the 1950s. It was one that also ultimately saw the responsibility for health education move from the local arena to become a national concern. In the late 1950s, at the time of the MRC's statement on smoking and lung cancer, the response had been at the local level through the Medical Officer of Health. The message that came across in public education in the 1950s was equivocal. The idea of outlining specific courses of action was anathema to a society that associated "propaganda" with wartime central direction, and with earlier Nazi propaganda. Health education at this time placed its faith in the citizenship of its recipients. One can see the government departments edging toward this change in the discussion of smoking, prodded also by tensions in the organization and funding of health education. The civil servant Enid Russell Smith, always an incisive analyst of events, commented in 1962 that government could draw in future on two things: parents' concern for their children, and the changes taking place in the medical profession. Publicity would have the authority of the profession. So far, she

57. Lord Hailsham to Sir Alexander Maxwell of the Tobacco Advisory Committee, 14 November 1962, NA CAB 21/4878.

58. For discussion of how the differential taxation question evolved, see Berridge and Starns, "'Invisible Industrialist'" (n. 43).

commented, the state had not sought to protect individuals from doing harm to their own health if they were not harming the health of others; alcohol was an exception to the rule, and also drugs of addiction, but for both it was the social consequences rather than individual health that was paramount. The new line might be that the costs fell on the state, and so government should stop people from damaging their health—but, she commented presciently, once government took on this role, it would not stop at smoking.[59] Lung cancer, argued the secretary of state for Scotland, the minister of education, and the minister of health, in an appendix to a policy document prepared just before the 1962 report was published, was a largely preventable disease, but "the question for us is whether it is our duty as a Government to set about preventing it."[60]

This was the central issue. The period encompassing the end of the 1950s and the beginning of the 1960s was suffused with discussion within government about a reorientation of its role in relation to the health of the public. Although the costs of the newly established NHS were a matter of concern elsewhere in the policy machine, there was no connection between that issue and the potential expansion of the role of government in relation to behavior. Here government was actively resisting its potential new role. It was feared, for example, that more cancer education would lead to greater fear of cancer and hence a greater demand for services, not a reduction. The discussion of the rise in lung cancer was affected by those considerations. The NHS, in any case, was recognized already to be a national *sickness* service rather than a national *health* service, concentrating on disease rather than on positive health. It was not until the 1973 oil crisis that costs and the role of individual behavior began to be considered in tandem. The 1962 report—produced by an "outside" body, not by an official committee—brought to a head the issue of whether government should have a role in health behavior, and also highlighted the organizational tensions. It led ultimately, through the Cohen committee report of 1964, to the formation in 1968 of the Health Education Council, a new technocratic central agency responsible for persuasive media campaigns.[61]

59. Minute from Enid Russell Smith, 5 February 1962, NA MH 55/2204.

60. Smoking and Health: Memorandum by the Secretary of State for the Home Department, 2 March 1962, Annex A 26, February 1962, Memorandum by the Secretary of State for Scotland, the Minister of Education and the Minister of Health, NA CAB 129/108 C(62)43.

61. These developments are discussed in more depth in Virginia Berridge and Kelly Loughlin, "Smoking and the New Health Education in Britain, 1950s to 1970s," *Amer. J. Pub. Health*, 2005, *95*: 956–64.

The Control of Advertising

Advertising for health was part of the emergent media and consumerist focus of public health—but advertising was also an activity to be opposed when it was promoting harmful products. The same combination of economics and statistical evidence began to mark governmental activity against tobacco advertising, the other key plank of the government's response to the RCP report. This new consumer strand in policy was symbolized by another report, which arrived in the Ministry of Health just after the publication of the RCP's, from the Advertising Inquiry Council, a body formed in March 1959 in order to represent the interests of the consumer in advertising.[62] It was a study of expenditure and trends in sales advertising on tobacco, researched and written by an economist and a doctor—a significant combination for the future of public health. It looked at the rise in expenditure on tobacco advertising in the early 1960s: advertising costs had risen by 50 percent in one year, 1960, and the public's expenditure on tobacco was also rising. Women's smoking was on the increase, and the teenage market was growing. Filter cigarettes had taken off in popularity in the mid-1950s after their introduction in the late 1940s to save leaf and to save smokers' money after increases in tobacco duty; the report noted that their sales now accounted for 20 percent of the cigarette market. The whole nature of tobacco and cigarette promotion had changed in recent years. The Council's report, which was mentioned in Parliament, added to fears already raised about trends within the tobacco industry: a Monopolies Commission report had drawn attention to its high degree of business concentration, with two firms, Imperial and Gallaher, accounting for over 90 percent of the market. Philip Noel Baker, MP, chairman of the Advertising Inquiry Council, was pressing Macmillan for an advertising ban.[63] Fletcher and Morris were also involved.[64] Advertising was an important component of the response to the 1962 report, and the tobacco companies voluntarily offered the removal of all advertising on television before 9 p.m. But concerns later arose on their part about this voluntary concession. Partridge of Imperial

62. The report was widely circulated within government. See Tobacco Smoking and Health: Restrictions on Advertising, 1962–65, NA CAB 124/1672.

63. Philip Noel Baker, MP, to Harold Macmillan, 29 May 1962, NA CAB 21/4878, 1962–63.

64. Ministry of Health, Note of a meeting with the Advertising Inquiry Council to discuss cigarette advertising, July 1963, Smoking and Health 16/2/3 part 4.24, NA CAB 21/5083, 1963–64. Fletcher and Morris were present at the meeting along with Noel Baker and representatives from the Baptist Union, the Methodists, and others. The Advertising Inquiry Council also met with the TAC on 13 May 1963 and agreed to differ about advertising control.

told a Board of Trade official in June 1962 that Imperial and Gallahers had seen advantages in the concession: they had expected to be able to reduce advertising expenditure by 50 percent because of the television restriction—but Rothman Carreras had increased its advertising, and so the manufacturers were beginning to break ranks.[65] Negotiations about further restrictions dragged on into the 1964 changeover to a Labour government—which took a stronger line.

The Social Survey, Social Research, and the New Role of the Public

What was also beginning to change in the mid-1960s was the view of "the public" held by politicians and by officials: this was to be a crucial component of future public health initiatives. The commercial techniques of market research expanded in the postwar years and government also began to survey the nature of public opinion and attitudes through the social survey. This surveillance of the population was part of a more general expansion of research and evaluation that was epitomized by the smoking issue. In 1962 a report from the PR firm Armstrong Warden, presented to the Ministry of Health's advisory group on publicity, had pointed out the long-term nature of trying to change public attitudes to smoking. The first job was to convince people that smoking did constitute a danger, and the effects of that should be measured by public opinion research.[66] As with the change of attitude toward the content of public education, government was edging toward this form of surveillance. A pilot social survey had been carried out in 1960 for the Home Affairs committee by the Social Survey division of the Central Office of Information. This had confirmed the impression given by earlier surveys carried out in Edinburgh to evaluate a campaign led by the MOH there in the 1950s: most of the population was aware of the association between smoking and lung cancer; only one person in the 1960 survey was not, an old lady of eighty-seven who was a nonsmoker. But both the Edinburgh and the pilot surveys had shown that a smaller proportion of the survey population accepted that the association was proved, and a negligible number had given up smoking because of it.[67]

65. G. J. MacMahon of the Board of Trade to Fife Clark of the COI, 15 June 1962, NA CAB 21/4878, 1962–63.

66. "The Role of Publicity in the Smoking and Health Campaign," April 1962, Report for the COI by Armstrong Warden Ltd., NA MH 55/2237.

67. Ann Cartwright, Fred M. Martin and J. G. Thomson, "Health Hazards of Cigarette Smoking: Current Popular Beliefs," *Brit. J. Prevent. & Soc. Med.*, 1960, *14*: 160–66; Cart-

In the mid-1960s the surveillance of public attitudes went further. For the first time, survey research and evaluation accompanied a campaign almost from the start, and research into young people's attitudes to smoking was undertaken. There was also research into medical students' attitudes. The research was carried out by Drs. Aubrey McKennell and R. K. Thomas of the Social Survey division and by the social psychologist John Bynner. Bynner's work on adolescent smoking was based on the smoking questions in a wartime survey of adolescent sexual behavior by the Central Council for Health Education.[68] The results of the McKennell survey, started in 1963 and first reported to the officials' committee in 1964 when the American surgeon general's report was under consideration, emphasized the potential new role for government health education: "The ethics or appropriateness of using such an approach in Government publicity needs to be faced. The use of somewhat devious, emotional rather than straightforward means of persuasion is of course, for better or worse, a characteristic of much successful commercial advertising."[69]

Other survey research was carried out by social scientists and epidemiologists, and increasingly this focused on the young. The sociologist Margot Jefferys was involved in the 1950s and early 1960s in a study of Harlow New Town with other researchers from the London School of Hygiene; her study of the impact of health education on children's attitudes toward smoking was one of the first academic publications in the field.[70] The choice of smoking and of children also indicated the reorientation of this type of "community study," which had until then concentrated on the environment rather than individual issues. Jefferys, as a key figure in the Society for Social Medicine in this period, was part too of the transformation of social medicine into a new form of public health that the smoking work symbolized.[71] In the discussions of the ongoing research

wright, Martin and Thomson, "Distribution and Development of Smoking Habits," *Lancet*, 1959, 2: 725–27.

68. Louis Moss, *The Government Social Survey: A History* (London: HMSO, 1991), pp. 134–36.

69. Study by the Social Survey, report to Cabinet committee on smoking, February 1964, NA CAB 130/185 GEN 763.

70. Margot Jefferys and W. R. Westaway, "'Catch Them Before They Start!' A Report on an Attempt to Influence Children's Smoking Habits," *Health Educ. J.*, 1961, *19*: 3–17.

71. Margot Jefferys, "Social Medicine and Medical Sociology, 1950–70: The Testimony of a Partisan Participant," in Porter, *Social Medicine* (n. 8), pp. 120–36. Smoking among schoolchildren was also one of the early pieces of research carried out at St. Thomas's where one of the first health-services research units was set up by Walter Holland, a pioneer of such research in the United Kingdom: Interview with Walter Holland, 6 March 1997, London School of Hygiene and Tropical Medicine.

in the Central Office of Information and the Ministry of Health can be seen in embryo the emergent evaluative paradigm of "relevant research," a precursor of later evidence-based tendencies in health research.[72]

The Electoral Argument Diminishes

The publication of the American surgeon general's report in 1964 led to a further officials' report and to political interest. The American report extended associations between smoking and health risk to diseases other than lung cancer, but British officials did not feel that this warranted further action. On 30 June 1964 the cabinet committee approved the officials' suggestion of a modest extension of the government's health-education campaign. There was no support for a ban on TV advertising or on smoking in cinemas. Least opposition was attracted by packet warnings. Lord Hailsham wanted more action. On 6 April 1964, he wrote in response to his officials' lack of enthusiasm: "I consider that the American Report, the American action and the Social Survey *have* strengthened the case for action, and that it is *not* too early to say that our limited campaign is failing and that unless we can bare our teeth nothing that we do *will* be taken seriously."[73] He also inserted a significant change in the inequality argument deployed by officials: the words "it would bear more hardly on the poor than on the rich" were replaced by "it could be harder for a poor man than for a rich man to continue his existing level of smoking and while this element of discrimination might be said to be more to the poor man's benefit, it would be unlikely to go uncriticised."[74] But Hailsham's response in 1964 was unusual for the time. As he pointed out in the Commons adjournment debate on the surgeon general's report, he was a nonsmoker in a Parliament of smokers, a cabinet of smokers, and an electorate of smokers. His views did not at that stage represent either the cultural or the political norm.[75]

In 1961, Enoch Powell, the Conservative minister of health when the RCP report was published, had expressed his opposition to media

72. The connection with smoking and research is not noted in Jeanne Daly, *Evidence Based Medicine and the Search for a Science of Clinical Care* (Berkeley: University of California Press, 2005), in her discussion of the lineages of evidence-based medicine (pp. 128–53), although the connection between social medicine and the rise of health-services research in Britain is made.

73. Note from Lord Hailsham, 6 April 1964, NA CAB 21/5083.

74. Ibid.

75. Adjournment debate speech by Lord Hailsham, 12 February 1964, *Parliamentary Debates*, Commons, 5th ser., vol. 630, col. 522.

strategies.[76] In an interview conducted in 1975, Powell was more forthcoming about the roots of his opposition. Governments did not like to reorganize taxation, and then there was the question of harm, which, in the case of smoking, was fluid and vague. Legislating against a widespread and common form of behavior was very different from legislating against an uncommon and marginal form. Governments would be very foolish to act without overwhelming evidence—and here the 1962 report, in his view, did make a difference to the clarity of the issue.[77]

Kenneth Robinson, as Labour minister of health in the mid- to late 1960s, was more active against smoking, but his view of policy was also that it was constrained by public opinion, not by financial considerations. He also stressed that the main constraint on government had been that there was no public support for action against smoking. The answer, as he saw it, was to change the climate of opinion through health education, in particular with themes like smell and attractiveness that appealed to young people.[78] The Labour politician Richard Crossman's opposition to Robinson's proposed changes in smoking policy in the later 1960s was also prompted by electoral considerations.[79] But this argument began to change in the 1970s when Conservative politicians like Keith Joseph and Labour politicians like David Owen and Dennis Healey as chancellor of the exchequer saw dawning electoral advantage in antismoking measures.

Conclusion

The RCP report of 1962 was the forerunner of later College reports on smoking and a host of other health-related subjects, all of which were aimed at both government and the public. The "medical voice" developed important relationships with both government and the public in areas that would not previously have been considered the province of either. In the 1970s this insider/outsider relationship for medicine developed further into a host of expert committees with close relationships within government. The RCP report in 1962 was a significant stage in moves toward a new era in which the presentation of science to the public through the

76. Minute from Enoch Powell, 11 November 1961, NA MH 55/2227.

77. Interview with Enoch Powell, October 1975, William Norman Papers, ASH (Action on Smoking and Health) archive, SA/ASH R.27, box 79, Wellcome Library, London.

78. Interview with Kenneth Robinson, 18 January 1976, ibid., SA/ASH R.31 box 79.

79. R. Crossman, *The Diaries of a Cabinet Minister*, vol. 3, *Secretary of State for Social Services 1968–1970* (London: Hamish Hamilton and Jonathan Cape, 1977), entry for 19 July 1968, p. 147.

media, with the authority of scientists and the medical profession, became central. As consumerist trends in society consolidated, and medicine and public health both sought "modernization," the old tradition of "giving the facts" to citizens was transformed into warnings about health risk. The nature of public opinion and "the public" was exposed to research-based surveillance. The techniques of social as well as medical science were brought into play. These changes were recognizably rooted in some of the postwar transformations of social medicine, but they also incorporated new commercial techniques of persuasion and commercial ideas about research. The permissive-society analysts have argued for a diminished state role for some health-related issues—but the case of smoking, and the new ideas within public health, show the influence of the state as increasing, not diminishing. This influence was exerted through new relationships with the medical profession and with research, and through new agencies. Government and the medical profession began to share a belief in the power of the media and of advertising to alter public attitudes.[80] This is what I have called "coercive permissiveness": members of the public could modify their own habits and lifestyle to gain better health, but increasingly that modification was state ordained and supported. The case of smoking and the RCP report shows how such ideas and interests were beginning to shape a distinctive postwar British public health ideology, separate from the organizational base of the profession in health services and community medicine that has attracted most commentary. The report mediated between social medicine in flux and the new evidence-based medicine and public health.

❖

VIRGINIA BERRIDGE is Professor of History at the London School of Hygiene and Tropical Medicine, University of London, Keppel Street, London WC1E 7HT, U.K. (e-mail: virginia.berridge@lshtm.ac.uk). She is head of the Centre for History in Public Health. Her research interests include substance use and policy, HIV/AIDS, public health, and the relationship between evidence and policy. Her recent publications include *Making Health Policy: Networks in Research and Policy after 1945* (editor and author) and *Medicine, the Market and the Mass Media: Producing Health in the Twentieth Century*, both published in 2005. Her book on postwar public health will be published in 2007.

80. It is arguable that this belief in the power of the mass media may have been a distinctive "stage" in British public health, which is now undergoing significant change. See V. Berridge and K. Loughlin, *Records Relating to the Health Education Council, Health Education Authority, and Health Development Agency: Thematic Mapping Exercise, July/August 2006*, Report produced for NICE (National Institute for Clinical Excellence), September 2006.

As Depressing as It Was Predictable? Lung Cancer, Clinical Trials, and the Medical Research Council in Postwar Britain

CARSTEN TIMMERMANN

SUMMARY: In recent years lung cancer specialists have complained that due to stigma resulting from the association of the disease with smoking, theirs is a neglected field. This paper demonstrates that in the 1950s and 1960s, when the British Medical Research Council (MRC) started to organize clinical trials for various forms of cancer, this was not the case. Rather, the organizers of these trials saw lung cancer as a particularly promising object of research, for much was known about the disease. The cancer trials were part of a strategy to use the Randomized Controlled Trial (RCT) technology to cement the role of the MRC as the dominant body overseeing medical research in Britain. The organization of the trials, however, turned out to be very difficult, due to ethical problems and the dominance of one form of therapy, surgery. The trial results were deeply disappointing. I argue that these frustrating results contributed to the notion of hopelessness that has come to surround lung cancer, and to the shift of focus from cure to prevention that was triggered by epidemiologic studies identifying tobacco smoke as the main cause of the disease. The paper deals with an important episode in the history of clinical cancer research in postwar Britain, illustrating the ethical and practical problems faced by the organizers.

KEYWORDS: lung cancer, smoking, surgery, radiotherapy, chemotherapy, clinical trials, ethics, Britain, Medical Research Council

My thanks to my Manchester colleagues Emm Barnes, John Pickstone, Elizabeth Toon, and Helen Valier (now Houston); and to the participants in the Bethesda workshop on Cancer in the Twentieth Century, for many useful suggestions. The research for this paper was generously funded by a Wellcome Trust Programme Grant.

Introduction

It has been a common complaint in recent years among lung cancer specialists that theirs is a neglected field, and that the main reason for this is a stigma resulting from the association of the disease with smoking. Claudia Henschke and Peggy McCarthy, for example, in a recent book have argued that "in part because of pervasive negative feelings about smokers (and even ex-smokers), many lung cancer patients aren't offered the aggressive treatments routinely provided for those with other types of cancer."[1] In an informal conversation with this author, a leading British medical oncologist specializing in lung cancer therapy reported similar attitudes: medical researchers who wanted to undertake research on lung cancer, he suggested, always struggled for resources because finding cures and treatments for other cancers is seen as more important, for lung cancer is perceived as a self-inflicted disease. Whatever the truth of these arguments today, I argue here that such claims do not hold for Britain in the 1950s and 1960s. On the contrary, the British devoted considerable research attention to lung cancer therapy in these decades, and the failure to develop a successful treatment had more to do with technical difficulties than with any stigma associated with the disease.

Looking at a series of clinical studies of lung cancer funded by the British Medical Research Council (MRC) between the mid-1950s and the mid-1970s, I will argue that when planning for these trials started, the expectations in lung cancer treatment were not significantly different from those for other cancers. The lung cancer trials, as we will see, were part of an attempt to introduce the Randomized Controlled Trial (RCT) technology, which had been used successfully to evaluate the effectiveness of streptomycin in the treatment of tuberculosis, to clinical cancer research. While only a minority of lung cancer patients in the 1950s could expect to be cured, and there was little hope of long-term survival for the majority, there was also no general notion that lung cancer would remain incurable. Neither, as work by Charles Webster, Virginia Berridge, Paolo Palladino, and others indicates, was there much of a stigma attached to smoking in the 1940s and 1950s.[2] Lighting up in the wrong place or at

1. Claudia I. Henschke and Peggy McCarthy, *Lung Cancer: Myths, Facts, Choices—and Hope* (New York: Norton, 2002), p. 13.

2. Charles Webster, "Tobacco Smoking Addiction: A Challenge to the National Health Service," *Brit. J. Addict.*, 1984, *79*: 7–16; S. Lock, L. A. Reynolds, and E. M. Tansey, eds., *Ashes to Ashes: The History of Smoking and Health* (Amsterdam: Rodopi, 1998); Virginia Berridge, "Medicine and the Public: The 1962 Report of the Royal College of Physicians and the New Public Health," in this issue; Paolo Palladino, "Discourses of Smoking, Health, and the Just

the wrong time was viewed as an expression of bad manners, but smoking was seen as a legitimate pleasure (and at worst, as a minor vice). Concerns over the health of nonsmokers were rare. Risk and the long-term implications of the habit entered the debate from the mid-1950s, when the results of epidemiologic studies on smoking and health made it into the newspapers and started to inform a new agenda in public health and health education.[3] Only since the 1970s, and, as Berridge shows, partly in response to the debates over smoking and health, has this new agenda centered on risk factors and individual lifestyle choices come to dominate public health debates in Britain.[4]

In the absence of stigma, how do we explain the apparent neglect of lung cancer research that current-day authors point to? I will argue that an explanation can be found in the history of treatment trials, whose organization was made complicated by the fact that there was a well-established treatment, surgery. This, along with the new ideal of randomization, led to ethical problems for the organizers of the trials. Could researchers withhold the option of surgery from patients if there was only a slight chance that these patients might benefit from an operation? A trial that was not ethical was also not feasible, even if it might provide interesting results. Moreover, the main groups involved with the preparation of the trials at this stage, radiotherapists and surgeons, had different opinions as to what was good practice. While the organizers of the MRC cancer trials initially considered lung cancer as a particularly suitable target for therapeutic trials, these problems, as we will see, led to trials about which hardly anybody was enthusiastic. References to the link with smoking and the perception that individuals brought the cancer upon themselves provided the clinical researchers conducting these trials with a way of dealing with the disappointing outcomes by shifting the focus of attention from cure to prevention.

Society: Yesterday, Today, and the Return of the Same?" *Soc. Hist. Med.*, 2001, *14*: 313–35; Matthew Hilton, *Smoking in British Popular Culture 1800–2000* (Manchester: Manchester University Press, 2000); Allan M. Brandt, "The Cigarette, Risk, and American Culture," *Daedalus*, 1990, *119*: 155–76; John Burnham, *Bad Habits: Drinking, Smoking, Taking Drugs, Gambling, Sexual Misbehaviour, and Swearing in American History* (New York: New York University Press, 1993).

3. See Virginia Berridge and Kelly Loughlin, "Smoking and the New Health Education in Britain, 1950s–1970s," *Amer. J. Pub. Health*, 2005, *95*: 956–64.

4. Berridge, "Medicine and the Public" (n. 2).

MRC Trials and Lung Cancer Therapy, 1957–1973

Lung cancer therapy today certainly seems less innovative, with fewer headlines about advances than in other cancers. Hopes for new cures and research progress, which dominate debates around other forms of cancer, are often absent in discourses centering on lung cancer. However, this was not the case in the 1950s. On 31 January 1957, five months before the publication of its important "Statement on Tobacco Smoking and Cancer of the Lung," the Medical Research Council held a Conference on the Evaluation of Different Methods of Cancer Therapy.[5] The conference, under the chairmanship of the renowned professor of radiotherapy at Middlesex Hospital Medical School, Brian W. Windeyer, recommended that the Council "should consider undertaking an investigation into the treatment of certain tumours which appeared particularly suitable for short-term study."[6] They included in this group carcinoma of the bronchus, esophagus, and bladder; bone sarcoma; and medulloblastoma. Carcinoma of the bronchus was chosen "after considerable discussion" because of "the vast amount of material which was available and the existence of a good deal of confusion of thought about the best form of treatment."[7] It seems that a strong argument for the inclusion of lung cancer was that this was a malignant disease that was particularly well researched and understood and yet was also the focus of disagreement about the best treatment.

The notion that lung cancer was particularly well understood had its origins in the intense interest generated by the mysterious increase in the incidence of this once rare and obscure disease, which clinicians and pathologists observed to have occurred since the beginning of the twentieth century. Debates over whether this increase was real, and its possible causes, grew more intense toward the 1950s; the suspects, besides cigarette smoking, were the tarring of the roads, exposure at work, or car fumes and smog. These well-documented debates provided the background for the epidemiologic studies by Richard Doll and Austin Bradford Hill in Britain and by Evart Graham and Ernst Wynder in the United States, and for the reports by the MRC, the Royal College of Physicians (see the

---

5. Medical Research Council (hereafter MRC), "Medical Research Council's Statement on Tobacco Smoking and Cancer of the Lung," *Lancet,* 1957, *269*: 1345–47.

6. "Evaluation of Different Methods of Cancer Therapy," Recommendations of the Council's Steering Committee, National Archives (hereafter NA), FD 7/327.

7. Working Party for the Evaluation of Different Methods of Therapy in Carcinoma of the Bronchus (hereafter Working Party), Minutes, 24 June 1958, p. 1, NA FD7/327.

article by Virginia Berridge in this issue), and the U.S. Surgeon General on smoking and health.[8] While among the medical profession consensus formed fairly quickly regarding the dangers of smoking, wider debates over the meanings of smoking and the political consequences that were to be drawn from the results of these epidemiologic studies, as Berridge shows, lasted much longer. Contrary to current assumptions, however, the high profile that lung cancer gained through these debates stimulated therapeutic research.

The standard treatment for most lung cancers was (and still is) surgery. A typical lung cancer patient in the 1950s (usually a middle-aged man) would see his GP about chest problems: difficulties with breathing, or even blood in the sputum. The task of the GP was then to decide whether or not the patient was suffering from one of the "conventional" chest problems, such as TB or bronchitis. Usually, the patient would be referred to the local chest X-ray service.[9] If a shadow was visible in the X ray, and there were no TB bacilli in the sputum, cancer was a possibility. A sputum sample would be screened for malignant cells, and the patient would be referred to a chest surgeon for a bronchoscopy.[10] If the patient's general condition was good and there were no metastases, the surgeon would perform an exploratory thoracotomy, a pneumonectomy (resection of a whole lung), or, increasingly, a lobectomy (resection of

8. Richard Doll and Austin Bradford Hill, "Smoking and Carcinoma of the Lung," *Brit. Med. J.*, 1950, *2*: 739; Doll and Hill, "The Mortality of Doctors in Relation to Their Smoking Habits: A Preliminary Report," ibid., 1954, *1*: 1451; Ernst L. Wynder and Evart A. Graham, "Tobacco Smoking as Possible Etiologic Factor in Bronchiogenic Carcinoma," *JAMA*, 1950, *143*: 329; Royal College of Physicians, *Smoking and Health: A Report of the Royal College of Physicians on Smoking in Relation to Cancer of the Lung and other Diseases* (London: Pitman Medical Publishing, 1962); The Surgeon General's Advisory Committee on Smoking and Health, *Smoking and Health: Report of the Advisory Committee to the Surgeon General of the Public Health Service* (Washington, D.C.: U.S. Department of Health, Education, and Welfare, 1964). On the Surgeon General's Report, see also John C. Burnham, "American Physicians and Tobacco Use: Two Surgeons General, 1929 and 1964," *Bull. Hist. Med.*, 1989, *63*: 1–31.

9. Some lung cancers were also picked up by mass X-ray service in routine screenings. With TB declining, a long debate unfolded over the potential value of such screening services for lung cancer. The provisional verdict, in the early 1970s, was that the benefit was negligible compared to the cost: see "Survival in Lung Cancer" (editorial), *Lancet*, 1971, 298: 648–49. Henschke and McCarthy argue, however, that CT scanners make it necessary to reevaluate screening, since with these new technologies far smaller tumors can be made visible than with the old chest X ray: *Lung Cancer* (n. 1), pp. 43–61.

10. Brenda Gray, "Sputum Cytodiagnosis in Bronchial Carcinoma," *Lancet*, 1964, *284*: 549–52.

the affected lobes).[11] These were serious operations, which carried considerable risks, and patients frequently died from complications. A focus of innovation, therefore, apart from the operation as such, was diagnosis: the search for methods that allowed the distinction between operable and nonoperable cases. But what was to be done with the patients whose tumors were already too large for surgery at the time of diagnosis, or had metastasized or belonged to a cell type that was likely to do so? Should they simply be sent home to die? Or did new methods in radiotherapy or chemotherapy offer new means of intervention, for purposes of palliation or even cure?

The agenda set by the recommendations of the 1957 conference was heavily geared toward the evaluation of new approaches in radiotherapy, which was the form of therapy from which British cancer specialists most expected innovative impulses—in spite of disappointments with the treatment of lung cancer.[12] This was perhaps not surprising, given the strength of the field in Britain and the strong presence of radiotherapists on the committee. The MRC had played a central part in the rise of radiotherapy in the United Kingdom in the interwar years.[13] Radiotherapists were increasingly discontent with the key position of surgeons in the treatment of malignant disease, and with the notion that surgery was the default treatment for all patients who had any hope of survival, while radiotherapists had difficulties in recruiting trial subjects.

11. W. P. Cleland, "The Treatment of Carcinoma of the Lung: Surgical Treatment," in *Carcinoma of the Lung*, ed. John R. Bignall (Edinburgh: Livingstone, 1958), pp. 213–33; J. R. Belcher, "Lobectomy for Bronchial Carcinoma," *Lancet*, 1956, *267*: 349–53; R. Abbey Smith, "Development of lung surgery in the United Kingdom," *Thorax*, 1982, *37*: 161–68; Clifton F. Mountain, "The Evolution of the Surgical Treatment of Lung Cancer," *Chest Surg. Clin. North America*, 2000, *10*: 83–104.

12. "Radiotherapy and Bronchial Carcinoma" (editorial), *Lancet*, 1953, *262*: 1298–99; Gerald Blanshard, "The Palliation of Bronchial Carcinoma by Radiotherapy," ibid., 1955, *266*: 897–901; "Radiotherapy for Lung Cancer" (editorial), ibid., p. 963.

13. For the history of radiotherapy in Britain, see Caroline C. S. Murphy, "A History of Radiotherapy to 1950: Cancer and Radiotherapy in Britain 1850–1950" (Ph.D. diss., University of Manchester, 1986); David Cantor, "The Definition of Radiobiology: The Medical Research Council's Support for Research into the Biological Effects of Radiation in Britain, 1919–1939" (Ph.D. diss., University of Lancaster, 1987).

Randomized Trials

In June 1957 the Council appointed a Steering Committee, also chaired by Windeyer, to prepare the appropriate trials.[14] The Steering Committee then appointed five ad hoc working parties for the chosen forms of cancer, to assist with the task of "drawing up a co-ordinated scheme of investigation."[15] A sixth working party was to be appointed to work on leukemia. The composition of all these subcommittees followed the same pattern: each included a physician, a surgeon, a pathologist, a radiotherapist, and a statistician. With the proposals of the working parties in hand, the committee recommended that

> favourable consideration should be given, if possible, to the support of any suitable clinical trials in the field of cancer therapy which can be carried out without too elaborate an organisation and with reasonable promise of yielding useful information.[16]

The research program drawn up by the committee was, it seems, at least as much about the development of new methods of clinical research as about finding new cancer therapies. The committee was a vehicle for applying the new RCT approach to the evaluation of well-established and new therapeutic methods, especially in radiotherapy. The use of the new technology for establishing the effectiveness of streptomycin in the treatment of tuberculosis had provided the MRC with a much-publicized success.[17] The timing of the 1957 conference, with the results of a number of conventional trials already published or about to be published, as well as the subsequent discussions in the Working Party, suggests that the use of the RCT may even have had priority over the development of specific new therapeutic techniques. Extending the Council's activities to cancer research (the domain of the Imperial Cancer Research Fund and the British Empire Cancer Campaign) was part of an MRC strategy to establish the Council as the main body controlling clinical research in Britain.[18] The RCT technology, which built on some of the key strengths

---

14. See Table 2.

15. "Evaluation of Different Methods of Cancer Therapy" (n. 6), p. 1.

16. Ibid., p. 2.

17. Alan Yoshioka, "Streptomycin in Postwar Britain: A Cultural History of a Miracle Drug," in *Biographies of Remedies: Drugs, Medicines and Contraceptives in Dutch and Anglo-American Healing Cultures*, ed. M. Gijswijt-Hofstra, G. v. Heteren, and E. M. Tansey (Amsterdam: Rodopi, 2002), pp. 203–27.

18. On the history of the ICRF, see Joan Austoker, *A History of the Imperial Cancer Research Fund, 1902–1986* (Oxford: Oxford University Press, 1988).

of MRC-funded clinical research and came to embody its ethos, was a vehicle for this strategy.[19]

The members of the ad hoc Working Party (Table 1) appointed to assist the Steering Committee (Table 2) with the organization of the trials on carcinoma of the bronchus were Dr. John Guyett Scadding, Dr. L. G.

Table 1. Members of the Working Party on the
Treatment of Carcinoma of the Bronchus

John G. Scadding (Chairman)	Chest physician, Brompton Hospital; Dean and Director of Studies, Institute of Diseases of the Chest; Physician and Senior Lecturer in Medicine, Postgraduate Medical School, Hammersmith Hospital, London
Leslie G. Blair	Radiologist; Director of the X-Ray Department, Hospital for Sick Children, Great Ormond Street; Radiologist to the Brompton Hospital, the Harefield Sanatorium and Hospital, and St Vincent's Hospital. Published on the diagnosis and radiological treatment of chest injuries and chest diseases.
Alphonsus L. d'Abreu	Thoracic surgeon, United Birmingham Hospitals; Reader in Thoracic Surgery, University of Birmingham; Hunter Professor, Royal College of Surgeons, 1939 and 1946
Jethro Gough	Pathologist; Professor of Pathology and Bacteriology, Welsh National School of Medicine, Cardiff. Published on pneumoconiosis in coal miners.
Austin Bradford Hill	Epidemiologist and statistician; Professor of Medical Statistics at the London School of Hygiene and Tropical Medicine
Brian W. Windeyer	Radiotherapist; Director of the Meyerstein Institute of Radiotherapy, Middlesex Hospital, and the Radiotherapy Department, Mount Vernon Hospital; Professor of Therapeutic Radiology at the University of London; Dean of the Middlesex Hospital Medical School

19. On clinical research and the MRC, see also Christopher C. Booth, "From Art to Science: The Story of Clinical Research," in Booth, *A Physician Reflects: Herman Boerhaave and Other Essays* (London: Wellcome Trust Centre for the History of Medicine, 2003), pp. 79–101.

Table 2. Members of the MRC Steering Committee

Brian W. Windeyer (Chairman)	See Table 1
Joseph S. Mitchell	Radiotherapist; Honorary Director of the Radiotherapy Centre at Addenbrooks Hospital, Cambridge; Regius Professor of Physic at the University of Cambridge, 1957–1975
Robert B. Hunter	Clinician; Professor of Materia Medica and Lecturer in Clinical Medicine, University of St Andrews
Robert W. Scarff	Pathologist; Director of the Bland-Sutton Institute of Pathology, Middlesex Hospital, and Professor of Pathology at the University of London; Honorary Secretary of the British Empire Cancer Campaign
Austin Bradford Hill	See Table 1
Leslie J. Witts	Hematologist; Nuffield Professor of Clinical Medicine, Radcliffe Infirmary, Oxford

Blair, Mr. A. L. d'Abreu, Professor J. Gough, Professor Austin Bradford Hill, and Professor Windeyer. The chairman, Scadding, was consultant chest physician at the Brompton and Hammersmith Hospitals and professor at the Institute of Diseases of the Chest, the specialist medical school associated with the Brompton Hospital. He is hailed as one of the founding fathers of respiratory medicine in Britain, and was one of the founders and later president of the Thoracic Society and the first editor of the journal *Thorax*.[20] Along with Bradford Hill, who was consulted whenever the Council needed statistical expertise, he had been involved in the streptomycin trials.[21] The Working Party recommended that the Steering Committee undertake a randomized trial of different forms of radiotherapy in a small number of centers (they explicitly mentioned Edinburgh, Newcastle, Manchester, Liverpool, the Middlesex Hospital, and Hammersmith Hospital). Reconstituted for this purpose, under the same chairman, the Working Party was to prepare and oversee the trial.

20. John Crofton, "John Guyett Scadding" (obituary), *Brit. Med. J.*, 2000, *320*: 189.
21. Ibid. See also I. Chalmers and M. J. Clarke, "Guy Scadding and the Move from Alternation to Randomization," The James Lind Library, **http://www.jameslindlibrary .org/ trial_records/20th_Century/1940s/scadding/scadding_commentary.html** (accessed 3 August 2004).

In 1959, Scadding's colleague at the Brompton, the chest physician John Reginald Bignall, was appointed as secretary.[22]

Ethics and Feasibility

The discussions among both the Steering Committee and the Working Party centered predominantly on what kinds of studies were (a) technically and (b) ethically doable. However, as it turns out, the two realms, the technical and the ethical, were difficult to keep separate. Ethical concerns, for example, were frequently raised by the prospect of randomization—an issue that, as we have heard, was central to the committee's work. One of its members, Professor Robert W. Scarff, wondered "if strict randomisation was necessary since so many clinicians had a clear-cut impression of what was best for the patient and might feel random selection to be a little unethical."[23] Bradford Hill, seconded by Joseph S. Mitchell and Robert B. Hunter, argued that randomization was in fact necessary in order to detect marginal differences. To Hunter, this "raised in its train the question of feasibility again."[24]

How were such problems to be overcome and appropriate trials organized? And why did they choose to look at lung cancer therapy? At the Steering Committee meeting on 13 January 1958, Professor Mitchell proposed to look at a trial he was undertaking in Cambridge as a model, and his statement points to one of the reasons for including lung cancer in the recommendations. It had to be made sure, Mitchell suggested, that each patient received

> the best possible treatment appropriate to his particular case, and there should be the most careful clinical observation of each individual. Diagnosis, pathology and histology must be exact and unquestionable; a common type of tumour with a short natural history should preferably be studied to allow adequate numbers to be investigated in a reasonable time, a quantitative result without bias should be aimed at and criteria should be as objective as possible. His experience also showed that two forms of treatment, one new and one conventional, could be successfully compared and that randomisation was necessary for an accurate result.[25]

---

22. Working Party, Minutes, 23 June 1959, NA FD 7/327. Bignall was a central player in the field of clinical research on lung cancer in the 1950s. Interestingly, his obituary in the *BMJ* in 2001 mentions his work on tuberculosis but not that on lung cancer: John Bignall, "John Reginald Bignall" (obituary), *Brit. Med. J.*, 2001, *322*: 176.

23. Steering Committee for the Evaluation of Different Methods of Cancer Therapy, Minutes, 13 January 1958, p. 2, NA FD 7/327.

24. Ibid.

25. Ibid., p. 1.

Another member of the committee, Professor Hunter, was concerned that "there were many forms of cancer which could not be suitably used in such an investigation because the pattern of treatment was so well established and so widely accepted that any deviation would cause ethical difficulty, and that this left free for investigation only the fringe of cases of hopeless prognosis."[26] Windeyer disagreed, arguing that there were cancers, such as carcinoma of the bladder, for which several forms of therapy were successfully used, but where confusion existed over the relative merits of the different treatment regimens. The committee members viewed lung cancer as particularly suitable because its high incidence and short natural history (after diagnosis) promised large numbers of trial subjects in a reasonable time.

Contrary to current notions, the members of the committee did not view carcinoma of the bronchus as exceptionally hopeless, but as "a representative problem." They agreed that retrospective surveys could not supply the answers they were looking for. Long-term studies were too expensive (and this was where the short natural history comes in handy), but at least five years of follow-up were necessary. However, not only survival should be recorded: other parameters should also be taken into account, which might allow conclusions concerning quality of life—such as time spent out of hospital, time spent out of work, the degree of pain and disability, dyspnea, and hemoptysis. For lung cancer it was especially important, Mitchell suggested, "to evaluate the ordeal of treatment against possible benefit, and to try to decide if, in the late cases, X-ray treatment was worth while as opposed to simple palliation."[27] But this is where the problems started. At a meeting in 1959 the Working Party found it almost impossible to define criteria that distinguished palliation from prolongation of life, and defining criteria was an important stage in the organization of trials.[28] It became increasingly obvious, as we will see in the following section, that ethical difficulties were not merely matters of procedure: they were integral to the whole enterprise of organizing clinical trials of cancer therapies.

Finding a Suitable Question

Soon after the constitution of the ad hoc working parties in 1957 it became clear that it was not easy to find a suitable, well-contained question that

---

26. Ibid., p. 2.
27. Ibid., p. 3.
28. Working Party, Notes for Discussion, 10 June 1959, NA FD 7/327.

could be answered by way of an ethically acceptable clinical trial, within the remits set by the committee's recommendations (promising, reasonably easy to organize, using randomization, and leading to further research). While the motivation for the trials partly derived from the streptomycin success, American cancer research also served as a model. P. Armitage of Hammersmith Hospital was invited to report on experiences with cooperative, multicenter trials in the United States. He also told the committee about a trial in progress at the Hammersmith comparing surgery with radical radiotherapy in operable cases, but with a very limited intake of patients; an attempt to compare different methods of radiotherapy had failed for technical reasons.[29] Scadding suggested three problems that might fit the remits of the recommendations and were worth studying: (1) the efficacy of surgery as opposed to radiotherapy, "which was as yet an unsolved question"; (2) the efficacy of different kinds of radiotherapy; and (3) the use of chemotherapy alone or in combination with other forms of treatment. However, he did not believe that there was satisfactory evidence for the beneficial effects of chemotherapy, and therefore he did not think that an evaluation of its use was a suitable subject for an MRC trial. There were also, he argued, considerable ethical objections to a comparison of surgery and radiotherapy, for about a quarter of the patients undergoing surgery survived for five years or longer. For these and other reasons, Scadding was skeptical about the Hammersmith trial.[30] The Working Party concluded that, while desirable, "a large-scale controlled investigation of the relative merits of surgery as opposed to radiotherapy did not appear feasible at the present time."[31] It was clear that the main factor that made such a study appear unfeasible was the expectation that it would be difficult to obtain the necessary cooperation of surgeons.

The discussions in the committee seemed to go in circles, and progress was frustratingly slow. Since so far only a minority of "some ten percent" of patients was considered for therapy at all, Windeyer asked, would it not be possible to study the remaining 90 percent, maybe by comparing different

29. Working Party, Minutes, 24 June 1958, p. 2, NA FD 7/327. See also R. Morrison, T. J. Deeley, and W. P. Cleland, "The Treatment of Carcinoma of the Bronchus: A Clinical Trial to Compare Surgery and Supervoltage Radiotherapy," *Lancet*, 1963, *281*: 683–84.

30. Working Party, Minutes, 24 June 1958, pp. 1–2, NA FD 7/327. Scadding argued that it had not been certain if the groups had been strictly comparable in terms of operability. Also, often the histological diagnosis was available only after thoracotomy, and in such cases, although potentially responding well to radiotherapy, patients could not be included in a randomly allocated series.

31. Ibid., p. 4.

forms of radiotherapy?[32] Representing the surgeons, who were more interested in improving diagnosis, d'Abreu argued that what was really needed was information about the relative prognosis in different kinds of cancer of the bronchus, and also an answer to the question whether the prolongation of life by a few months by means of radiotherapy was worth it in terms of the quality of the life so gained. Also, did the linear accelerator improve quality of life more than conventional radiotherapy? Finally they came to a conclusion that nobody was really enthusiastic about, "that a comparative trial of different methods of radiotherapy might be considered in patients not primarily suitable for surgical treatment but regarded suitable for an attempt at cure by radiotherapy."[33] The inclusion of chemotherapy was "not thought to be practicable at the present stage of knowledge in this field."[34] The details of the trial, however (and this was an indicator of the increasing frustration), were to be determined by a working party of different constitution.

The Working Party continued to pursue the idea of a trial comparing the effects of super- and orthovoltage irradiation. Despite a distinct lack of enthusiasm on his part, Bignall volunteered to draft a provisional protocol for the trial. It was decided to approach Philip D'Arcy Hart of the MRC's Tuberculosis Research Unit about coordinating the work in collaboration with the Statistical Unit, due to these units' previous experience with controlled trials.[35] It appears as if the Working Party hoped that they were going to be able to repeat their streptomycin success. D'Arcy Hart, initially reluctant because of staff shortages in his unit, accepted the offer and appointed a new member of staff, Dr. Joan Heffernan.[36] Letters were written to the centers that the Working Party considered as likely participants in the study, and a joint meeting with radiotherapists was organized.

It was important for the Working Party to get a sufficient number of radiotherapists on board, so it made sense to involve them in the preparation. A meeting with twenty-nine consultant radiotherapists took place on 21 January 1961 in the Council Room of the Royal College of Surgeons in London.[37] The chairman told those present that "considerable difficulty

32. Ibid., p. 3.

33. Ibid., p. 4.

34. Ibid.

35. Working Party, Memorandum, 8 October 1959, NA FD 7/327.

36. D'Arcy Hart to Gorrill, 15 March 1960, NA FD 23/1163.

37. Working Party, Minutes of a Special Meeting with Consultant Radiotherapists, 21 January 1961, NA FD 7/327.

had been encountered in making plans which would not only be ethically acceptable and feasible but which, at the same time, could produce information of value."[38] In preliminary consultations, the draft protocol had found little support; the purpose of this meeting, therefore, was "to find out whether the radiotherapists concerned were in agreement about the importance of the principle of controlled clinical trials and whether further agreement could be reached upon a subject worth trying and upon the methods involved."[39] Windeyer added that the MRC committee that appointed the various working parties "had felt that there was not enough controlled work at present and that not all of the claims which were being made for various forms of treatment could stand up to rigorous examination."[40] Would the radiotherapists provide the Working Party with clearer directions?

They did not. The radiotherapists, too, were unenthusiastic about the protocol. Most thought that, clearly, supervoltage was to be preferred to orthovoltage therapy.[41] Dr. Tudway from Bristol spoke for many when he remarked that "it was difficult for those with a choice of treatments to believe that it was not better to use supervoltage if this was available."[42] Some of the radiotherapists doubted whether a trial in carcinoma of the bronchus made much sense in the first place. Ralston Paterson from Manchester conceded that "some difficulties were implicit in random selection, but he hoped that radiotherapists would encourage the Medical Research Council to continue to organize a trial"; however, he suggested that "lung cancer was one of the more difficult fields for investigation as overall mortality is high and it is difficult to assess differences in response."[43] Others reinforced the questions that members of the Working Party had already raised about withholding treatment from patients who might benefit from it. Many suggested, instead, that a trial should be designed to "compare the progress and survival rate of patients with presumed undifferentiated carcinomas of the lung following surgical treatment, with that following radiotherapy."[44] The Working Party followed their suggestions, and in the next section we will look at the results.

38. Ibid., p. 1.
39. Ibid., p. 2.
40. Ibid.
41. Ibid.; Working Party, Draft Memorandum (not dated), NA FD 7/327.
42. Working Party, Minutes of a Special Meeting (n. 37), p. 3.
43. Ibid.
44. Working Party, Draft Memorandum (n. 41), p. 1.

Trial I: Radiotherapy versus Surgery, 1961–1973

Four years after the decision to organize lung cancer treatment trials, the at times frustratingly slow negotiations over the details of these trials appeared finally to draw to a conclusion. Another meeting was scheduled with both consultant surgeons and radiotherapists on 25 July 1961.[45] Scadding introduced the agenda by stating that "there appeared to be a clinical problem as to the right advice to give a patient with a histological report of an undifferentiated carcinoma of the bronchus—whether to advise surgery or radical radiotherapy."[46] Defining the problem in this way helped to overcome ethical problems: "For those who honestly felt they did not know which treatment to advise there were no ethical difficulties. If there were enough people with this doubt in their minds, the trial could be conducted."[47] As mentioned above, a comparison of surgery and radiotherapy was already the subject of a smaller trial at Hammersmith Hospital, but it had been difficult to find enough patients in the more than six years that the trial was running.[48] Dr. Gwen Hilton at University College Hospital had also reported results with radiotherapy in a small number of cases that were "apparently as good as surgery."[49] The discussion with the surgeons, moreover, indicated that there was indeed disagreement: while some saw it as proven that resection, where possible, was always superior to other forms of treatment, others argued that for this kind of tumor it was time to move away from surgical treatment whose results were uniformly poor, and to turn to radiotherapy or chemotherapy. In most places, according to one radiotherapist (Dr. Fleming, St. Thomas's), only "surgical rejects" were treated with radiotherapy.[50]

However, while the agenda was set, there were still difficulties. A central problem was the eligibility of patients for the study. After the consultation with the radiotherapists, the Working Party had returned to an option for a trial design that its members had dismissed at an earlier stage of

45. Working Party, Minutes of a Special Meeting with Consultant Surgeons and Radiotherapists, 25 July 1961, NA FD 7/327.

46. Ibid., p. 1.

47. Ibid., pp. 1–2.

48. See Working Party, Minutes of a Special Meeting (n. 37); Morrison, Deeley, and Cleland, "Treatment of Carcinoma of the Bronchus" (n. 29).

49. Working Party, Minutes of a Special Meeting (n. 37), p. 5. See also Gwen Hilton, "Radiotherapy and Bronchial Carcinoma" (letter), *Lancet*, 1954, *263*: 47; Joseph Smart and Gwen Hilton, "Radiotherapy of the Lung: Results in a Selected Group of Cases," ibid., 1956, *267*: 880–81.

50. Working Party, Minutes of a Special Meeting with Consultant Surgeons (n. 45), p. 4.

the discussion, but that they now gave a specific focus on what at this stage they described as either anaplastic or undifferentiated carcinoma of the lung.[51] Restricting eligibility on grounds of cell type made a study feasible that originally was unacceptable on ethical grounds to some members of the Working Party. But tumor grading was a difficult business. One of the surgeons present at the meeting with the Working Party (Mr. Nohl, Harefield) pointed out that in his experience nearly one-fifth (18 percent) of histological reports were mistaken.[52] Grading schemes had changed significantly since the first attempts to classify tumor cells in the nineteenth century, with new techniques and pathological material becoming available. Later, new forms of therapy encouraged further distinctions between cell types: some tumors proved to be more susceptible to certain treatments, which made distinctions meaningful that had not carried any meaning before.[53] In the early 1960s, some "undifferentiated" or "anaplastic" bronchial tumors were reclassified as carcinomas of small-cell or oat-cell type.[54] This reclassification exercise was partly driven by experiences with chemotherapy (small-cell carcinomas are very responsive to chemotherapy) and partly by attempts to establish an internationally consistent terminology. During discussions, the different terms were used interchangeably. By the time the first results were published in 1966, the trial was described as "Comparative Trial of Surgery and Radiotherapy for the Primary Treatment of Small-Celled or Oat-Celled Carcinoma of the Bronchus."[55]

The results of the trial were not encouraging: after two years, only 3 of the original 71 surgical patients and 10 of the 73 radiotherapy patients were still alive. According to the report in the *Lancet,*

> the number of survivors at 24 months is so small that further statistically significant differences between the series in this respect cannot now arise. Despite the

51. Another option considered (and later apparently dropped) was a trial in the fractionization of doses: see Working Party, Minutes of a Special Meeting (n. 37) and Draft Memorandum (n. 41).

52. Working Party, Minutes of a Special Meeting with Consultant Surgeons (n. 45), p. 3.

53. John G. Gruhn, "A History of the Histopathology of Lung Cancer," in *Lung Cancer: The Evolution of Concepts,* vol. 1, ed. John G. Gruhn and Steven T. Rosen (New York: Field & Wood, 1989), pp. 25–63.

54. W. Watson and J. Berg, "Oat Cell Lung Cancer," *Cancer,* 1962, *15*: 759–68.

55. J. G. Scadding et al. (MRC Working-Party on the Evaluation of Different Methods of Therapy in Carcinoma of the Bronchus), "Comparative Trial of Surgery and Radiotherapy for the Primary Treatment of Small-Celled or Oat-Celled Carcinoma of the Bronchus: First Report to the Medical Research Council by the Working-Party on the Evaluation of Different Methods of Therapy in Carcinoma of the Bronchus," *Lancet,* 1966, *288*: 979–86.

slightly higher proportion of short-term and long-term survivors in the radical radiotherapy series both policies have produced very poor results in this highly malignant form of carcinoma, confirming the findings in other series.[56]

The working party suggested that radiotherapy might be the slightly better choice, since postoperative complications would be avoided.

However, because the results of the treatment are so poor whether by surgery or radical radiotherapy there is an urgent need for further research to improve the treatment of this condition. There is also an urgent need to apply the knowledge already available, in particular that of the role of cigarette smoking . . . to the *prevention* of the disease.[57]

We can see how in the light of widening acceptance of the tobacco hypothesis the focus is shifting toward prevention, in line with what Berridge observes for policy formation. A note in the administrative file dealing with the study states: "It seems to me that there is nothing at all controversial about this report, which is a straightforward account of a difficult but well organized clinical trial, the outcome of which has been as depressing as it was predictable."[58] Nevertheless, follow-up for the thirteen survivors continued as planned. After five years, only one surgery patient and three in the radiotherapy group were alive, and after ten years the last surgery patient had died (this patient, while originally assigned to the surgery group, had become too breathless to withstand an operation and received palliative radiotherapy instead—and he was not the only member of this group who turned out to be inoperable when surgery was scheduled). The three survivors in the radiotherapy group were still alive and well after ten years.[59]

One official goal of this and other clinical trials was to provide evidence that would lead to closure in a controversy. The debate unfolding on the letter pages of the *Lancet* after the publication of the first report indicates that this was not achieved. The study was criticized by leading specialists such as Roger Abbey Smith of the Thoracic Unit at the King Edward VII

56. Ibid., p. 984.
57. Ibid., p. 985 (emphasis in original).
58. Note by J. R. H. [Herrald?], 22 August 1966, NA FD 7/1151.
59. A. B. Miller, Wallace Fox, and Ruth Tall, "Five-Year Follow-up of the Medical Research Council Comparative Trial of Surgery and Radiotherapy for the Primary Treatment of Small-Celled or Oat-Celled Carcinoma of the Bronchus. A Report to the Medical Research Council Working Party on the Evaluation of Different Methods of Therapy in Carcinoma of the Bronchus," *Lancet*, 1969, *294*: 501–5; Wallace Fox and J. G. Scadding, "Medical Research Council Comparative Trial of Surgery and Radiotherapy for Primary Treatment of Small-Celled or Oat-Celled Carcinoma of Bronchus: Ten-Year Follow-up," ibid., 1973, *302*: 63–65.

Memorial Chest Hospital in Warwickshire, who argued that the reason why the results for surgery were so bad was that only patients with particularly unsuitable, centrally located oat-cell tumors were included in the study. Nine of the 71 patients in the series were not operated on because their condition deteriorated too rapidly, and of 58 patients where exploratory surgery was performed, 24 were found to be inoperable. In all patients whose tumors were resected, this was done by pneumonectomy, a type of operation that posed greater risks to the patients than the less radical lobectomy. Abbey Smith argued that the results for surgery would have looked much better had peripheral tumors also been included, and the Working Group could therefore claim validity of these results only for centrally located oat-cell carcinomas.[60] John Rashleigh Belcher, another leading specialist, based at the Middlesex Hospital, doubted if the conclusion that radiotherapy was superior to surgery in this situation was valid, for the numbers of patients were small and only the patients who were really operated on should have been included in the statistics for the surgery group.[61] This was seconded by Kent Harrison (St. Thomas's), who argued that there was a risk that uncritical readers might now accept that surgery had no place in the treatment of small-cell carcinoma, which was clearly not the case. He believed that any apparently operable carcinoma of the lung should be operated on, no matter what the cell type, and for this reason he had not participated in the trial.[62] Surgeons still criticized the trial in the 1980s for the image of hopelessness they thought it had created around lung cancer surgery, especially for oat-cell carcinoma.[63]

Scadding defended the study that his Working Party had organized, arguing that, even taking these criticisms into account, the results were not significantly different and the outlook remained bleak:

> The facts should be publicised: the incidence of a disease which has assumed epidemic proportions, which has a high mortality, and for which no current method of treatment can be regarded as satisfactory, would be reduced to a small fraction of its present level if men and women as responsible individuals chose to give up, or never to take up, cigarette smoking.[64]

60. R. Abbey Smith, "Treatment of Bronchial Carcinoma" (letter), *Lancet*, 1966, *288*: 1134–35.

61. J. R. Belcher, "Treatment of Bronchial Carcinoma" (letter), ibid., pp. 1190–91.

62. Kent Harrison, "Treatment of Bronchial Carcinoma" (letter), ibid., p. 1254.

63. John A. Meyer, "Surgical Resection as an Adjunct to Chemotherapy for Small Cell Carcinoma of the Lung," in *Bronchial Carcinoma: An Integrated Approach to Diagnosis and Management*, ed. Michael Bates (Berlin: Springer, 1984), pp. 177–95.

64. J. G. Scadding, "Treatment of Bronchial Carcinoma" (letter), *Lancet*, 1967, *289*: 157.

It seems that the frustrating outcomes of a trial about which nobody was very enthusiastic in the first place reinforced an ongoing shift of focus from therapy to the prevention of lung cancer. However, by presenting experiences with the treatment of small-cell carcinoma, an especially malignant type of cancer, as representative of lung cancer more generally, it may be argued that Scadding made the outlook for lung cancer patients seem even bleaker than it may have been anyway.

Trial II: Adjuvant Chemotherapy, 1964–1976

The second trial overseen by the Working Party was a study of chemotherapy as an adjuvant to surgery. The trial started in 1964, after having been discussed at a Working Party meeting in 1963. Like the first trial, this second one was also coordinated by the MRC Tuberculosis Research Unit. In charge of both trials at the Unit was Anthony Bernard Miller, replacing Joan Heffernan.[65]

The preparation of the chemotherapy trial, it seems, was much smoother than that of the first trial: there were no extensive debates in the Working Party, and no big meetings with consultants. One explanation for this lack of controversy may be that chemotherapy was tested only as a secondary therapy, an adjuvant to surgery, to prevent the growth of secondary tumors. It may also be due to the fact that in chemotherapy (unlike radiotherapy) there were few entrenched positions. It was perceived as something new, an approach that promised new channels for intervention (and also something that the British were not particularly good at and still had to learn a lot more about).[66]

Patients were randomly assigned, in a double-blind set-up, to groups that were prescribed either a placebo or one of two chemotherapeutic agents, busulphan or cyclophosphamide.[67] The drugs were prepared as tablets, to be taken at home when the patients were discharged after

65. NA FD 7/327; NA FD 23/1163.

66. For critical remarks on studies undertaken with chemotherapy in lung cancer from France, the United States, and Denmark, see L. Israel, "Chemotherapy in Inoperable Bronchial Carcinoma" (letter), *Lancet*, 1971, *297*: 971–72; Franco M. Muggia, Heine H. Hansen, and Per Dombernowsky, "Treatment of Small-Cell Carcinoma of Bronchus" (letter), ibid., 1975, *305*: 692.

67. Medical Research Council Working Party, "Study of Cytotoxic Chemotherapy as an Adjuvant to Surgery in Carcinoma of the Bronchus," *Brit. Med. J.*, 1971, *2*: 421–28; H. Stott, R. J. Stephens, W. Fox, and D. C. Roy, "5-Year Follow-up of Cytotoxic Chemotherapy as an Adjuvant to Surgery in Carcinoma of the Bronchus," *Brit. J. Cancer*, 1976, *34*: 167–73.

their operations. Finding participants does not seem to have been too difficult: Miller's satisfied letters to the collaborators report on steady progress with patient intake. By 10 March 1965, fourteen surgeons and thirty-four chest physicians had declared that they were taking part.[68] By 26 July 1965, 122 patients had been admitted to the study.[69] According to Miller, the study was "running very smoothly from an organizational point of view and [would] clearly yield answers to the questions originally posed in the protocol."[70] There were, however, some unexpected problems with the toxicity of the drugs, and the dosage had to be reduced in December 1965. By February 1968, there were 749 patients in the study, and the Working Party decided that the intake could be stopped.[71] The final intake was 753 patients in twenty-three centers throughout the U.K. These were centers where chest physicians and surgeons had agreed to cooperate, and where patients could be transferred to the care of the chest physician after discharge from hospital.

The only other difficulty the organizers encountered, besides the unexpectedly high incidence of hazardous toxicity with busulphan in the early stages of the study, was one that is very common to treatment trials: the problem of ensuring that patients took the right number of tablets, not more and not fewer than they had been prescribed. The organizers suggested that patients should occasionally receive home visits by health visitors, who on these occasions could count the patient's remaining tablets.[72]

While the Working Group had shown that it was able to organize a clinical study in lung cancer that conformed to the new standards of a cooperative, double-blind, randomized controlled trial, the results did not fulfil its expectations: "The therapeutic results at two years are disappointing, for there is no evidence that either of the two cytotoxic drugs in the dosage used improved survival."[73] After five years, 27 percent of the patients who received cyclophosphamide were still alive, 28 percent of those on busulphan, and 34 percent in the placebo group.[74]

68. A. B. Miller to collaborators, 10 March 1965, NA FD 23/1163.

69. Miller to collaborators, 26 July 1965, ibid.

70. Miller to collaborators, 17 January 1966, ibid.

71. Miller to collaborators, 9 February 1968, ibid.

72. Miller to collaborators, 17 June 1966, ibid.

73. Medical Research Council Working Party, "Study of Cytotoxic Chemotherapy" (n. 67), p. 427.

74. Stott et al., "5-Year Follow-up" (n. 67).

Conclusion

Let us disregard the disappointing results of these trials for a moment. Judging from the attention that lung cancer received from the Medical Research Council in the 1950s and 1960s, it appears that this was not a particularly neglected form of malignant disease. Indeed, the remarkable increase in incidence also triggered interest among researchers, with a view to not only lung cancer etiology, leading to the work that linked this disease firmly with cigarette smoking, but also its treatment.[75] Explicitly because they considered it a well-researched form of cancer on which much was known, the members of the MRC Steering Committee in 1957 wanted to see studies on lung cancer included in the program of randomized controlled trials that they were preparing.

Nor did this interest disappear quickly. In 1979, still, about 10% of cancer treatment studies then under way in Britain were dealing with lung cancer, 21 studies out of 211 for which questionnaires were returned.[76] This compared to 49 trials concerned with breast cancer, 30 with lymphomas, and 25 with leukemia. However, the absolute figures may be slightly misleading: with an estimated total incidence of nearly 32,000 lung cancer cases per year, this meant that only 2% of the patients were entered into trials, compared to 8% of breast cancer patients, 9% of those diagnosed with melanoma, 17% of those suffering from Hodgkin's lymphoma, and an impressive 27% of lymphoblastic lymphoma patients.[77]

What makes the treatment of one form of malignant disease a more interesting and rewarding subject for research than another? As Ilana Löwy, Jean Paul Gaudillière, and others have shown, for blood and lymph cancers it was partly the convergence of interest between cell biologists and cancer researchers.[78] Moreover, while the results of most studies on

---

75. This included research on curative and palliative treatments. See, e.g., George A. Mason, "Cancer of the Lung: Review of a Thousand Cases," *Lancet*, 1949, *254*: 587–91; "Radiotherapy and Bronchial Carcinoma" (n. 12); David A. Karnofsky, Walter H. Abelmann, Lloyd F. Craver, and Joseph H. Burchenal, "The Use of Nitrogen Mustards in the Palliative Treatment of Carcinoma. With Particular Reference to Bronchogenic Carcinoma," *Cancer*, 1948, *1*: 634–56.

76. Helen C. Tate, Janet B. Rawlinson, and Laurence Freedman, "Randomised Comparative Studies in the Treatment of Cancer in the United Kingdom: Room for Improvement?" *Lancet*, 1979, *314*: 623–25. The authors ascertained that a further twenty studies were in progress, although the questionnaires were not returned.

77. Ibid.

78. Jean-Paul Gaudillière, *Inventer la biomédecine: La France, l'Amérique et la production des savoirs du vivant (1945–1965)* (Paris: La Découverte, 2002); Ilana Löwy, *Between Bench and Bedside* (Cambridge: Harvard University Press, 1997).

treatments for lung cancer were disappointing, in childhood leukemia (and this is the other extreme) it was increasingly discussed in the 1960s and 1970s whether it was not appropriate, after the highly visible, successful trials with new regimes of multidrug chemotherapy, to talk about cure rather than temporary remission.[79] Increasingly this approach to cancer therapy was seen as a model that clinical researchers sought to apply to other forms of malignant disease.[80] In lung cancer, in contrast, the only therapy that could really be expected to bring any prospect of longer-term survival was (and still is) surgery, following increasingly routinized pathways that separated operable from nonoperable patients.

Bronchial carcinoma turned out to be a particularly "recalcitrant" form of malignant disease. By the time Wallace Fox and Scadding published the ten-year follow-up results of the MRC trial of surgery and radiotherapy, carcinoma of the bronchi was by far the commonest malignant tumor in Britain and most other developed countries, and was still increasing in frequency. Its mortality, moreover, was little affected by treatment. A *Lancet* editorial in 1975 suggested that the outlook for sufferers was dire: the proportion of all patients "diagnosed and treated with the best means available" who could expect to survive for five or more years was estimated to be one in twenty in the late 1950s, and this had not changed significantly in the meantime.[81] Technically satisfactory resection was possible in about a quarter of cases and accounted for most of the long-term survivors, most of whom had squamous-cell carcinomas. Radiotherapy occasionally led to long-term survival, especially with oat-cell (or small-cell) carcinomas, and it was useful as a palliative treatment. Attempts to use cytotoxic chemotherapy had so far proved disappointing, especially with a view to the considerable impact this form of treatment could have on quality of life. Screening, too, did not seem to deliver any significant benefits.

In the light of these results, the authors of the editorial concluded that "the overwhelming importance of a preventive approach to this disease must always be emphasised. It would be a cruel deception to allow smokers to think that any improvement in treatment, or any procedure to which they might submit themselves to attain early diagnosis, is likely to diminish appreciably their risk of dying of lung cancer."[82] If there is

---

79. "Radical Treatment of Acute Leukaemia in Childhood" (editorial), *Lancet*, 1972, *300*: 910–11. See also Gretchen M. Krueger, "'A Cure Is Near': Children, Families, and Cancer in America, 1945–1980" (Ph.D. diss., Yale University, 2003).

80. See, e.g., G. A. Edelstyn and K. D. MacRae, "Treatment of Breast Cancer" (letter), *Lancet*, 1972, *300*: 1307.

81. "The Treatment of Bronchial Carcinoma" (editorial), *Lancet*, 1975, *305*: 375–76.

82. Ibid., p. 376.

really, as Henschke and McCarthy argue, a lack of interest in research on lung cancer today, the remarkable recalcitrance of this group of malignant diseases is at least partly to blame. The stigma that these authors project back into the past may be a result rather than a cause. In the crucial period up to the mid-1970s, the application of the innovative techniques that made other cancers interesting to researchers, funding bodies, and companies, in clinical trials that were feasible and ethically acceptable (criteria that were difficult enough to fulfil, as we have seen), simply did not seem to make much of a difference for lung cancer patients. It appears that it was partly frustration that has made lung cancer less visible than other cancers.

The apparent neglect of bronchial carcinoma in clinical research was not caused by stigma, as I have shown. Rather, the notion of hopelessness in lung cancer therapy and the stigma of the self-inflicted disease emerged around the same time. The tide may be turning, though. Books like that by Henschke and McCarthy, charities dedicated specifically to lung cancer (like the Roy Castle Foundation in Britain), and the mere fact that medical oncologists are specializing in lung cancer research may all be indicators of change. In a climate where smoking is increasingly medicalized and viewed as an addiction rather than a matter of choice, depicting lung cancer as a neglected field may be a good strategy for generating attention and increasing its visibility.

———————————————— ❖ ————————————————

CARSTEN TIMMERMANN is a Wellcome Research Fellow at the Centre for the History of Science, Technology and Medicine, University of Manchester, Simon Building, Brunswick Street, Manchester M13 9PL, U.K. (e-mail: carsten .timmermann@manchester.ac.uk). He has published on constitutional therapy and German medicine in the interwar period and on medical research in postwar Germany and Britain, especially on high blood pressure and cardiovascular disease. He has edited a book (with Julie Anderson) entitled *Devices and Designs: Medical Technologies in Historical Perspective* (2006) and is currently working on a history of lung cancer.

Index

Lightning Source UK Ltd.
Milton Keynes UK
UKHW01f2215210918
329308UK00001B/72/P